THE ADOLESCENT IN FAMILY THERAPY

THE GUILFORD FAMILY THERAPY SERIES

Michael P. Nichols, Series Editor

Recent Volumes

The Adolescent in Family Therapy

*Breaking the Cycle
of Conflict and Control*

JOSEPH A. MICUCCI

THE GUILFORD PRESS
New York   London

© 1998 The Guilford Press
A Division of Guilford Publications, Inc.
72 Spring Street, New York, NY 10012
www.guilford.com

Printed in the United States of America

This book is printed on acid-free paper.

Last digit is print number: 9 8 7 6 5 4

Library of Congress Cataloging-in-Publication Data

Micucci, Joseph A.
    The adolescent in family therapy : breaking the cycle of conflict
and control / Joseph A. Micucci.
       p.   cm. ---- (The Guilford family therapy series)
    Includes bibliographical references and index.
    ISBN 1-57230-389-1 (hc.)   ISBN 1-57230-588-6 (pbk.)
    1. Adolescent psychotherapy.   2. Family psychotherapy.   3. Family—
Psychological aspects.   4. Parent and teenager.   I. Title.
II. Series.
RJ503.M495   1998
616.89′156′0835—dc21   98-37859
                                       CIP

About the Author

Dr. Joseph Micucci received his A.B. in Psychology from Cornell University and his PhD in Clinical Psychology from the University of Minnesota. He has been on the staff of North Memorial Medical Center in Minneapolis, Minnesota and the Robert Wood Johnson, Jr., LIFE-style Institute in Edison, New Jersey. In 1984, Dr. Micucci joined the staff of the Philadelphia Child Guidance Center where he served as Director of the Adolescent Unit from 1987 to 1993 and as Chief Psychologist from 1991 to 1993. Currently, he is Associate Professor of Psychology at Chestnut Hill College in Philadelphia where he teaches graduate level courses in family therapy and psychological assessment. He is a member of the American Psychological Association, the American Family Therapy Academy (AFTA), and is an Approved Supervisor of the American Association for Marital and Family Therapy (AAMFT). Dr. Micucci also has a private practice in Bala Cynwyd, Pennsylvania and Rosemont, Pennsylvania.

Acknowledgments

The ideas in this book germinated during the late 1980s and early 1990s when I worked on the Child and Family Inpatient Service of the Philadelphia Child Guidance Clinic (PCGC). Though the Golden Age of PCGC under Salvador Minuchin had passed, I think it's fair to say that the late 1980s and early 1990s were a Silver Age for PCGC. We had the opportunity to work with extremely difficult (some might say impossible) cases in an environment that nourished teamwork and collaboration. We were given free rein to develop our creativity by the director of the inpatient service, Connell O'Brien, and the medical director, Michael Silver.

I owe my greatest intellectual debt to my colleagues at PCGC, especially Mike Silver and John Brendler. It was they who helped me prepare my first presentations at professional conferences, and without whose help those presentations would never had happened. Mike generously gave hours of his time, talking about cases and ideas. John encouraged me to begin writing, and it is with his editorial and moral support that I struggled over the early drafts of the unpublished papers that were eventually to become Chapter 2 of this book. In addition to teaching me practically everything I know about therapy, John and Mike stoked my confidence to move behind the one-way mirror and take on the role of supervisor.

My development as a therapist and supervisor took place at PCGC in a crucible formed by relationships with a talented staff like no other I have encountered before or since. I thank especially the members of the treatment team for the Adolescent Inpatient Unit that I directed from 1987 to 1993, particularly Molly Hindman, Guy Diamond, Peggy Spiegel, and Carolyn Robbins. I also owe much to my other teacher–

colleagues at PCGC: John Sargent, Anne Itzkowitz, Sam Scott, Iolie Walbridge, and Marion Lindblad-Goldberg.

Many of the ideas in Chapter 10 were refined while I was consulting supervisor at Southern Homes Services in Philadelphia. I thank the staff and students there for the opportunity to learn from them.

I am grateful to Dean Caroline Golab and Sister President Carol Jean Vale of Chestnut Hill College for granting me release time to work on the manuscript. Sister Mary Anne Celenza, Dean of the Graduate Division at Chestnut Hill College, has been a source of inspiration and has helped me keep my sense of humor.

Series Editor Michael Nichols read early drafts of the manuscript and offered detailed suggestions that not only improved what I had written but also gave me the opportunity to learn about writing from one of the best in our field. Molly Hindman and Steve Simms, good friends and colleagues, gave hours of their time to reading and commenting on early drafts of the manuscript. Kitty Moore, my editor at The Guilford Press, patiently answered my questions and kept me on track.

My mother, sister, and her family have been unwavering in their support and faith in me.

The companionship, devotion, and patience of Jim Davis sustained me through this process. It's not an exaggeration to say that this book would not have been written without him.

Contents

THE ADOLESCENT IN FAMILY THERAPY

CHAPTER 1

INTRODUCTION

Tina, age 16, *has lost over 20 pounds in the past 6 months because she won't eat. Her divorced parents, Bill and Rose, are at war with one another regarding how to save Tina.*

Jenny, age 16, *ingested a handful of acetaminophen tablets minutes after what both she and her mother described as a pleasant conversation over dinner.*

Keith, age 15, *is running wild, staying out all night and using drugs, and there is little that his beleaguered parents feel they can do about it.*

Jamal, age 13, *has been hospitalized twice in the past 4 months and is now on the verge of his third hospitalization because he has been hearing voices and acting in strange ways.*

Todd, age 13, *was in danger of failing three courses, and his parents are bewildered because Todd had assured them that he was doing well at school.*

———◆◆◆———

This book is about adolescents like Tina, Jenny, Keith, Jamal, and Todd. Along the way, we will meet other young people like them: Bart, whose intractable abdominal pain allowed him to say "no" to his overbearing father; Tyrone, on the verge of leaving for college, who can't seem to follow his mother's simple rules about curfew; Tammy, whose sexual promiscuity terrified her parents. If you are a therapist who works with adolescents, the stories I tell will have a familiar ring. If you are a therapist who is looking for a compass to orient you through the often frustrating journey of working with teenagers and their families, I hope to provide one in this book.

Although my focus in this book is on adolescents, many of the principles I present can be applied to work with individuals of all ages. I hope to highlight what I have found to be some unique features of work with adolescents, dispel some of the myths, and stimulate your interest in working with a group that many therapists find impossible to engage.

I see myself oriented more toward theory than technique: I place far more importance on how a therapist thinks than on how many clever techniques he or she can pull from her kit. Techniques are like tools: the more you have, the more options for getting a job done—but you have to know what you are building first. Familiarity with a variety of techniques can give a therapist security in versatility, but techniques without a theory are like a body without a soul.

Yet many therapists find theories too abstract and therefore not particularly relevant to what they are trying to accomplish in their work with families. Seeing the merits in a number of different schools of therapy, many therapists consider themselves "eclectic," which usually means that they have refrained from committing themselves to a particular model. Unfortunately, eclecticism can breed hopeless confusion, leaving the practitioner a "jack of all trades, master of none," with no guidance on how to weave together ideas from a variety of theories into a coherent whole.

I hope to address this dilemma in this book by striking a balance between theory and technique. What I offer are pragmatic solutions for common clinical problems. I have tried to spell out my rationale for my suggestions, and illustrate their use in clinical case examples.[1] Sometimes, I recommend a step-by-step approach. I trust that readers will realize that steps and phases are rarely discrete or invariably sequential in all cases, and so will exercise sound clinical judgment in applying these ideas.

MY ORIENTATION

My orientation is grounded in the model of structural family therapy as explicated by Salvador Minuchin in a number of well-known writings (Minuchin, 1974, 1984; Minuchin & Fishman, 1981; Minuchin, Lee, & Simon, 1996; Minuchin & Nichols, 1993; Minuchin, Rosman, & Baker, 1978), but I try to avoid being doctrinaire, freely augmenting this basic model with ideas and methods from other schools of family and individual therapy.

By no means am I proposing a new model for family therapy. Nor am I simply recommending "technical eclecticism," or, to put it more crudely, a "shotgun approach" to therapy. Rather, by starting with some of the basic principles of structural family therapy, I expand on these principles and supplement them with compatible ideas from other models.

For example, as I will describe in the next chapter, a basic idea in my approach is "the symptomatic cycle," a concept that has been associated with schools of family therapy labeled "strategic" or "systemic." Yet, through the lens of the cycle, one can readily see the patterns of dysfunctional family structure Minuchin describes: weak boundaries, inconsistent hierarchy, detouring, triangulation. Looking from a slightly different angle, one can see how each family member's uniquely selective view of reality complements and reinforces one another's in an "ecology of ideas" (Bogdan, 1984), a web of "interlocking narratives" or "reciprocal double binds" (Elkaim, 1997). From yet a different angle, we may see individuals who are poorly differentiated from each other (Kerr & Bowen, 1988), or who are responding out of a legacy of "destructive entitlement" (Boszormenyi-Nagy & Spark, 1973). What is important is not the language used to describe a family's predicament, but rather the hypotheses about why the family is stuck and what can be done to help it move forward.

THE IMPORTANCE OF RELATIONSHIPS

In my view, the most powerful resource for helping a person change is the relationships in which he or she participates. It's about as close as we get to an axiom in therapy that the quality of the therapeutic relationship is a key determinant of the success or failure of therapy. Certainly I agree that our relationships with clients are critically important. But I'm talking here not only about the therapeutic relationship, but also about the healing potential of the natural relationships in a person's life.

As I discuss in the next chapter, family members who come to therapy are often experiencing profound isolation and disconnection in their relationships with one another. Perhaps they have become so focused on solving the problem that brought them to therapy that they have lost sight of other aspects of their relationships. Perhaps they have followed a policy of conflict avoidance for so long that they have concealed parts of themselves from one another, only to realize one day that they no longer feel connected to one another.

The relationships in these families are no longer sustaining. The family members see each other as obstacles rather than resources. They have settled into patterns of interaction that inhibit growth. Sometimes relationships outside the family can compensate for unfulfilling family relationships. But in many cases, all relationships are poisoned to some degree by the absence of a "secure base" in the family (Bowlby, 1988).

One of the features that distinguishes individual therapy from family therapy is the relative emphasis placed on the relationship with the therapist versus the relationships with people in one's life. Individual therapists see the therapeutic relationship as the crucible for change. Family therapists see beyond the dysfunctional[2] patterns in the family to the potential healing power of family relationships. Thus, a family therapist strives to help family members change their relationships with one another, from relationships that inhibit growth to relationships that promote growth.

A major thrust of my therapeutic work is to use my relationships with family members to help them change their relationships with each other. The therapeutic relationship is crucial: It is in the context of a relationship with the therapist that family members experience parts of themselves that had been suppressed in family interactions. But I believe the therapeutic relationship is a means to an end, not an end in itself.

In my view, the purpose of therapy is to enable individuals to experience sustaining and growth-enhancing relationships with the real people in their lives. In the case of troubled adolescents who are still living with their families of origin, my goal is to help the family members become better resources to the youngsters and to one another. If an adolescent is not living with her family, and instead resides in a group home or residential facility, my goal is to help her make better use of the available relationships in her life. If an individual client is disconnected and isolated from other people, I cultivate a relationship with the client that will inspire him or her to seek out sustaining relationships with others.

I consider therapy successful when the family members (or individual clients) have discovered ways to get what they need from their relationships with people in their lives, so that their relationship with me is no longer necessary to sustain them. Like a chemical catalyst that facilitates a reaction between two other substances, the therapeutic relationship catalyzes the transformation of relationships in the lives of clients. But the real healing takes place not in the therapeutic relationship but in the client's relationships with significant others.

THE ARCH

Thus, I suggest that therapists pay particular attention to cultivating relationships with each member of the family and to use these relationships as springboards for facilitating change. Minuchin (1974) has called this process *joining*. But joining is not simply a technique. It requires an experiential change on the part of the therapist and is achieved by making a conscious and deliberate effort to engage each family member in a relationship. To join effectively, a therapist must listen carefully to each family member, try to see the problem from each family member's unique point of view, and find something about the person that he or she likes. Then the relationship is maintained just like any other relationship that is important to the therapist by communicating what I like to call the ARCH of therapy: Acceptance, Respect, Curiosity, and Honesty.

The therapist makes a commitment to the relationship, and by holding the relationship in high esteem he conveys to the other person the expectation that they also will hold the relationship with the therapist in high esteem. This is particularly important with adolescents, who often feel as if adults don't accept them, don't respect them, don't care what they think, and aren't honest with them.

This brings me to another point, and one that has been a major goal of mine in writing this book. In my opinion, most writings on therapy with adolescents present a contradictory picture. On the one hand, the major thrust is to support the process of individuation, to serve as midwife to the separation of the adolescent from the family. On the other hand, many approaches to family therapy with adolescents emphasize the importance of helping the parents "put their foot down" with the youngster. Much less emphasis is given to the relationship between the parent and the adolescent, and, in particular, the adolescent's ongoing need for nurturance from the parents.

Susan Mackey (1996) is one of the few authors who has addressed the importance of strengthening the quality of the relationship between parents and the adolescent as an essential component of treatment:

> I believe that a secure attachment to parents may lessen the influence of peers and consequently increase the likelihood that the adolescent will respond to parental limits. Similarly, I believe that secure attachment allows the parents to feel safer about the normal acting-out behavior which is characteristic of adolescents and thus less prone to overreactions. Because they feel that their children are attached, they have greater trust that the children will contact them when they find themselves in situations they cannot handle. Therefore, it may be a mistake to guide parents who may already be feeling insecure in their attachment to the adolescent to "back off" without first addressing the relationship issues to increase security within the attachment. (pp. 497–498)

Feminist scholarship has noted that the equation of maturity and separation does not apply to women, who strive to maintain continuity in relationships even as they develop a clearer conception of a personal identity (Gilligan, Lyons, & Hanmer, 1990; Jordan, Kaplan, Miller, Stiver, & Surrey, 1991; Josselson, 1987). Recently, the emphasis on independence and invulnerability has been cited as contributing to difficulties in the psychological development of boys as well (Bergman, 1995; Pollack, 1995). Olga Silverstein and Beth Rashbaum (1994) have pointed out that parents, especially mothers, are encouraged to pull away from their teenage sons to avoid stifling their masculinity. They write:

> Often, of course, in the teenage years just as in the earlier phases of our sons' lives, we don't recognize that it is we who are doing the withdrawing. There's a reciprocity to this dance of withdrawal that has been going on for so long, and there's our firmly held and culturally mandated belief that it is the inexorable destiny of the adolescent male to move away from his parents. If for some reason he doesn't—if he's not ready yet to make that move, or if he is comfortable and happy enough within his family circle not to see the necessity of making it—we become very alarmed. And then we are likely to force the issue, with results ranging from disappointing to disturbing to disastrous. (pp. 123–124)

In later chapters, I discuss how our culture's expectations for the proper raising of boys and girls can get translated into family interactional patterns that can contribute to the emergence of symptoms. Here, what I want to emphasize is the importance of supportive and sustaining relationships in the adolescent's life, particularly with parents.

In order to be appropriately nurturing—neither smothering nor overestimating the adolescent—the parents must be able to *empathize* with the adolescent. To borrow a term from Winnicott (1965), the "good-enough" parents for an adolescent will be attuned to the adolescent's needs and respond accordingly. It is for this reason that "how to" books on parenting adolescents can offer no more than general guidelines. Like a good therapeutic relationship, the essence of good parenting is a connection, one grounded in empathy and resting on the ARCH—Acceptance, Respect, Curiosity, and Honesty.

STAYING THE COURSE

One of my goals in family therapy is to discover what is preventing the family members from experiencing more sustaining relationships with one another. One way to describe what we see in troubled families is patterns of over- and underreactivity. Sometimes, family members respond to one another in an impulsive way, with little evidence that they have given much forethought to their actions. At other times, family members are so isolated from one another that nothing short of an earthquake will get a response.

Unfortunately, many therapists fall into a similar dichotomy in their work with families. They may be so discouraged by the family's apparent "resistance" to change that they lurch from one approach to another without really giving any approach a chance to succeed (or fail)—this is one of the greatest drawbacks of "eclecticism." Other therapists are so wedded to a particular point of view that they are blinded by it and insensitive to the feedback from the family.

I believe that a therapist must take a position with a family, one based on a thoughtful consideration of the factors contributing to the problem at hand, and hold firm to this position while the family struggles through the grueling process of change. The therapist should fix on this hypothesis (or frame or formulation) and attack it from every possible angle, but abandon it (more accurately, refine it) only after careful consideration.

At the risk of sounding glib, allow me to propose a rule of thumb: Once a therapist has set a course (e.g., asking a father and son to have a conversation about the son's grades), the therapist should persist in this course *at least* through the remainder of the session. Before adopting a new course (no sooner than the next session, remember), the therapist should be able to articulate why the course she had set failed with the family, and from this understanding refine her hypothesis about what needs to change. If the therapist is unable to articulate this rationale (using the assistance of a supervisor or colleague, if necessary), then she should stay with the original course until it succeeds or she has gathered enough information to revise her hypothesis.

The following are a few other suggestions about deciding how and when to intervene with families.

Look before You Leap

In some approaches to therapy, assessment (or diagnosis) precedes intervention (treatment). In family therapy, the distinction between assessment and intervention is seen as an artificial one: A therapist assesses a family by carefully tracking how the family responds to his attempts to alter or modify their usual ways of relating to one another. As articulated by "second-order" cybernetics, the therapist is always part of whatever he observes, and it is an illusion for the therapist to consider himself an outside or objective observer of the family system (Atkinson & Heath, 1990).

Without quibbling about what does and does not constitute an intervention, I wish to make the point that a well-conceived intervention evolves from a hypothesis about the family, and in order for such a hypothesis to be formulated, the therapist must have had some opportunity to observe the family and assess their ways of interacting with one another. A therapist will be much more secure in persisting with an intervention (as I have advised) if the intervention has evolved from a carefully articulated rationale based on his experiences with the family.

Certainly, a therapist can learn about a family by "testing the waters," floating a few interventions past them and then carefully reading the feedback. However, the therapist who relies too much on this strategy will easily fall into the trap of trial-and-error, "shotgun" therapy. At best, this is sloppy work. At worst, it confuses and frustrates family members and may lead to their dropping out of treatment. Thus, I am recommending that therapists derive a hypothesis about the family before selecting a goal for intervention. One way of doing so is to utilize the idea of the symptomatic cycle, introduced in the next chapter.

Start Simple

Though families and the people that make them up are complicated, therapists who refrain from taking a position because they are daunted by the family's apparent complexity run the risk of succumbing to paralysis. Let's take an example.

You are consulted by two parents about their adolescent son who is staying out past curfew, refusing to help out around the house, neglecting his schoolwork, and arguing with his parents. You observe the family for a while and notice that the mother dominates the session, the boy interrupts to defend himself, and the father participates only when you directly address him. You might hypothesize that the father and son are in a covert coalition against the mother, or that the boy is "acting out" in order to engage his father, or that the boy and his mother are overinvolved, while father is peripheral.

One way to proceed is to wait until you gather more information so that you can select among these hypotheses. Another option is to recognize that each of these hypotheses is consistent with another hypothesis: that mother and father are not working together as a parenting team. Being a good family therapist, you recognize that simply asking the parents if they work well together will not elicit the information you need to evaluate this hypothesis. You need to see what they do when you ask them to enact a process of making a parenting decision. So you ask mother and father to talk together about what to do the next time the boy comes home late.

Everything seems fine up to this point, but now things might get more complicated. Let's say that the parents begin the conversation you requested, but soon the boy interrupts. You expected this, so you are ready. You block his intrusion and request that the parents continue talking with one another.

They proceed, but within a few minutes, the mother is shouting at the father for "never having been there" to help in the past, declaring that the marriage is a sham, and threatening to leave if he doesn't shape up. In response, the father feebly defends himself and then just shuts down. Eventually, the mother turns to you, announces that she is "tired of trying to make this marriage work" and launches into a history of the relationship that includes the fact that the father drank heavily until 5 years ago and the family has been on the verge of financial ruin several times.

Observing what has just happened and hearing the mother's accusations, many therapists might be tempted to conclude that the "real problem" in the family has now surfaced: The boy is acting out in order to distract his parents from the marital problems that threaten to tear the family apart. You present this hypothesis to the family and suggest a contract that involves working on the marriage, perhaps even offering to meet individually with the adolescent from time to time to provide "support." You interpret their silent nods as assent to this contract and proceed.

Six sessions later, you wonder why nothing has changed. The marriage seems no better and no worse than before, the boy is continuing to break the rules, and the mother is muttering about not coming any more because "it's not helping." What went wrong?

Well, one thing that might have gone wrong is that the therapist too quickly abandoned his first hypothesis (that the parents were not working as a team) in favor of another, apparently more complex hypothesis (that the boy was acting out in order to regulate the degree of tension between the parents). What the therapist apparently failed to notice, however, is what happened in the first session when he asked the parents to collaborate. While they initially complied, they did not complete the task. Instead, somewhere along the line, the conversation shifted from "what to do about the boy" to "what is wrong with this marriage." Though the latter might at first blush appear to be a "deeper" issue for this family, the next 6 weeks leads us to doubt it. In fact, the parents could go on for weeks, ostensibly talking about marital issues, but they could hardly spend 5 minutes talking about parenting.

Perhaps the therapist might have noticed this early on, and

redirected the parents to the task at hand, with a comment like, "I'm sure there are many hurt feelings between you, and we can get into that later if you wish, but right now what I want you to do is to talk with each other about what to do the next time your son comes home late." The therapist might still entertain the hypothesis that the boy's acting out is a way of maintaining the family "homeostasis," but does not abandon his initial position in favor of this new hypothesis, at least not until it is absolutely clear that no progress will be made on parenting until some of the marital issues are addressed. Even so, before venturing into the new area of marital work, the therapist should have a clearer hypothesis about how the marital issues prevent parental collaboration, so that he can return to work on parenting as soon as possible.

Keep a Focus

One of the reasons I emphasize the importance of a therapeutic contract in the next chapter is that the contract will help prevent the pitfall just described.

In this case, the family had come to therapy because the son was not behaving. They did not come to address marital problems. Thus, the contract needs to include a statement of the problem (the son is misbehaving), a hypothesis about why this problem is present (because the two of you don't work as a team), and a plan for solving the problem (so we will work on helping the two of you work as a team while also taking into account that your son is growing up and should have some voice in making the rules). If the couple had come for help with the marital problems, then the focus of the contract should be on the couple's relationship, and any parenting issues, if they arise, should be linked back to the problem you and the family have contracted to solve.

In addition to having an overall focus for therapy, it is important for the therapist to have a focus for every meeting with the family. This is not to say that the therapist refuses to listen to what the family members bring up at the beginning of the session, but rather that the therapist should be working at a different level, namely, one that addresses basic relational patterns (*process*) rather than specific issues or conflicts (*content*).

The therapist can work at the level of process through any piece of content the family presents, but the goal should always be to help the family develop *more effective ways of resolving conflicts* rather than arriving at a resolution of a specific issue. Thus, in this example, if the parents are struggling around the issue of whether to allow the boy to come in at 10:30 or 11:00 P.M., the most important issue is not the specific hour of the curfew but rather helping the family find better ways of disentangling themselves when they reach such impasses.

Capitalize on Strengths

Effective interventions should encourage people to draw upon their strengths and to utilize these strengths in creative ways. Most of the time, families come to therapy preoccupied with problems and pathology. Therapists often comply by asking questions that are designed to elicit more information about the problem, and in so doing emphasize what is wrong with the family.

It is, of course, important for the therapist to get a clear picture of how the family is stuck, and how the family's previous attempts to solve the problem have failed. But in doing so, the therapist must not lose sight of the family's strengths and resources, because it is from these that new patterns and new solutions can be generated. One of the main tasks of the therapist is to introduce people to aspects of themselves that they did not realize they had, to stop underestimating themselves and to rediscover what has often long been hidden.[3] This attitude is perhaps no better expressed than in Minuchin's famous axiom, "You are richer than you know" (Minuchin & Nichols, 1993, p. 47).

Restrain Yourself

This point is closely related to the earlier one. Often, therapists will too quickly intrude on family interactions in order to help the family members find more productive ways of resolving their conflicts. Certainly, a therapist must be prepared to intercede in unproductively escalating arguments or chaotic discussions, but the therapist should be judicious in doing so. Therapists should take the stance of facilitator rather than director.

Therapists should spend more time watching families and less time telling them what to do. When a therapist repeatedly interrupts family transactions, the implicit message is that the family lacks the resources to handle problems on their own. This message can foster dependence on the therapist and abdication of responsibility for change by the family members. The therapist should intervene just enough to initiate or prolong a productive exchange among family members, gently blocking intrusions, redirecting them to the topic at hand, or simply encouraging them to continue beyond the point they usually stop. Here's an example taken from a case I have discussed elsewhere (Micucci, 1995).

Rob, age 15, had been hospitalized after brandishing a knife during a heated argument with his father. He was threatening to leave the hospital against the advice of the treatment team, so a family session was scheduled, to be attended by Rob's parents, Gail and Len, and Rob's 12-year-old sister, Monica. The therapist asked Gail and Len to discuss how they would like to handle Rob's demand to leave the hospital.

> As Gail and Len began to discuss their disagreement and conflict mounted, the therapist noticed that they attempted to involve a third party to stabilize the emerging conflict between them. First, they avoided their conflict by attacking Rob, telling him how miserable he was making them and how stubborn he was to reject the "help" the hospital was offering him. The therapist intervened to stop this sequence and redirected Len and Gail to each other. As the conflict between them again mounted, Monica offered a suggestion and both parents immediately turned to her. The therapist again intervened to block the triangulation. Len and Gail then turned on the therapist, attacking his competence and demanding that he tell them what to do. The therapist nondefensively acknowledged Len's and Gail's frustration, but pointed out that he had confidence in their competence to arrive at a solution together, and that his taking responsibility for this decision would be disrespectful of their role as Rob's parents. Eventually, after struggling together for several minutes, Gail and Len agreed that it was not appropriate to pay Rob to stay in the hospital; they needed to find another solution. The therapist promptly complimented the parents on reaching agreement, and then supported them in telling Rob in a calm but firm tone of their decision: "We will not allow you to return home today. We're sorry if we've failed you as parents, and we'd like to work things out so that you can come home, but we'll have to talk about the conditions under which you may come home. If you insist on leaving the hospital now, you will have to go to placement or to a shelter or to a foster home—but you can't come home with us." Though Rob protested and verbally threatened violence, he withdrew his request for discharge. (Micucci, 1995, p. 158)

Remember How Change Happens

As Michael Nichols (1987) has pointed out, family therapy has blurred the distinction between family change and individual change. It's individuals who change, Nichols argues, not families:

> Most discussions of change in family therapy are muddled by confusion over who changes. Therapists don't change, systems don't change; people change. To be more exact, therapists initiate change, systems

undergo change, but individual persons must make changes. One consequence of ignoring the individual is the shifting of responsibility for change to the therapist. This is unfortunate because change ultimately works through individuals within the system. We may think about families—structured with boundaries and triangles—and we may convene families. Yet in a real sense there are no families. The family is an abstraction. Regardless of how many people are in the treatment room, the only person who can change is the individual. (p. 38)

Actually, I do believe that therapists change during the course of therapy (at the very least, they become better therapists!) and that the distinction between "undergoing change" and "changing" depends on your frame of reference. However, I think that Nichols is making an important point that strikes at the very heart of doing therapy: Patterns can change only when one or more of the people who participate in the pattern changes something they are doing.

The concept of the symptomatic cycle (discussed in the next chapter) is based on the idea that families get stuck in repetitive patterns that keep the symptom going. Families get stuck in these patterns because the individual family members get stuck. A father responds the way he does because his wife responds the way she does and his son responds the way he does, and over and over. The pattern changes when at least one person changes and sustains the change long enough for the symptomatic pattern to be dislodged and new patterns of interaction take its place.

It is my belief that one's significant relationships are the crucible in which change occurs. Surely, a person could go off by himself, think over a situation, and then resolve to change, and no therapist is involved at all. But the change this person makes must be noticed by someone else in order for the change to be meaningful or sustained. Therapists can help to facilitate this process. As explained in the next chapter, a therapist can connect with a part of the person that is not usually present in his relationship with others, and then help the person use this part of himself more creatively. Or, a therapist might help other family members notice that a small change has occurred in the behavior of someone else, thus making the change more obvious and amplifying its potential impact on the other members of the family.

Move People

The most profound change (the kind we are hoping to initiate in therapy) involves a shift in the way a person *experiences* herself or others. Experience includes what we think, how we feel, what we do. One of my misgivings about the narrative methods of doing therapy is that they are too cognitive. In delving into the intricacies of a person's language, these practitioners are indeed trying to help create an experiential change, but seem to be doing so in a way that puts too much emphasis on thinking. One of the major benefits of a technique such as enactment—when family members are asked to engage with one another in the presence of the therapist—is that it can facilitate a very different experience in the moment, which then can be amplified by weaving a new "story" or "narrative" around this experience.

Movement in therapy occurs when someone is moved by something that someone else does or says. Family members move away from their usual ways of relating to one another when someone in the family is moved (on an emotional level) by something that someone else (often, but not always, the therapist) has said or done.

THE PLAN OF THIS BOOK

In the next chapter, I outline key principles for treating adolescents and their families. In Chapter 3, I present a brief overview of current knowledge about "normal" adolescence. I believe that familiarity with the literature on adolescent development is essential for any therapist who is working with this population. Therapists must be familiar with what is typical or atypical in adolescence in order to assess the severity of a presenting problem and to provide proper guidance to parents.

In the following six chapters, I apply the principles of treatment described in Chapter 2 to problems that families with adolescents commonly present to therapists: eating disorders, depression and suicide, aggressive and defiant behavior, psychosis, school-related problems, and the so-called "problems of leaving home." In Chapter 10, I discuss common pitfalls encountered in work with multiproblem, low-income families and suggest ways to avoid these pitfalls. Along the way, I present case examples, some detailed and some brief, that highlight the challenges and delights of working with adolescents and their families.

NOTES

1. Most of the examples discussed in this book are based on actual clinical cases, with identifying information suitably disguised to safeguard confidentiality.
2. The term "dysfunctional" has gotten bad press lately, because it has been

used inappropriately as referring to families (as in "dysfunctional families") rather than to patterns of behavior. I use the term to mean that a behavior pattern is harmful, unproductive, or inefficient. Whole families are rarely, if ever, dysfunctional, though the family members may frequently engage in dysfunctional patterns of interaction.

3. Some approaches to therapy, notably Steve de Shazer's (1985) "solution-focused therapy," concentrate almost entirely on searching for and encouraging strengths and even discourage lengthy discussions about the problem. I focus directly on problems and conflicts but utilize existing strengths to help family members resolve them.

CHAPTER 2

THE PROCESS OF THERAPY: PRINCIPLES AND PITFALLS

In this chapter, I present key principles for conducting treatment with troubled adolescents and their families. In the chapters that follow, these principles are applied to specific presenting problems, such as eating disorders, depression, and defiant behaviors.

Although I frequently refer to the "stages" or "phases" of therapy, I do not intend to imply that the therapist progresses from one stage to the next in a lockstep fashion. Rather, I am talking about general episodes in treatment, the beginning and end of which often will overlap. While all the principles I discuss are operative throughout therapy, certain of these principles come to the forefront at different points of the the therapy process.

My framework is built on the core assumption that the interpersonal context of the adolescent, in particular the family, plays a crucial role in the development and maintenance of symptoms.[1] While other contexts, notably the peer group and the school, become increasingly important during adolescence, the influences of these other contexts are mediated by the quality of the adolescent's relationship with the family.

A number of reports in the research literature support this claim. A tumultuous family environment affects an adolescent's mood and behavior both in and out of the home (see Larson & Richards, 1994). A good family environment is related to more positive peer relationships (Savin-Williams & Berndt, 1990) and better school performance

(Entwisle, 1990). Adolescents who have good relationships with both parents and peers are less likely to become depressed than youngsters who are more oriented toward peers than parents (Kandel & Davies, 1982), and problems at home are more important than problems with peers in determining whether an adolescent gets depressed (Asseltine, Gore, & Colton, 1994). Kids are less likely to get involved with troublesome peers if they maintain a strong attachment to their parents (Brown, Mounts, Lamborn, & Steinberg, 1993; Gottfredson & Hirschi, 1994; Steinberg & Silverberg, 1986). Among disadvantaged youth, family social support can buffer the negative impact of the ghetto environment and the influence of deviant peers (Frauenglass, Routh, Pantin, & Mason, 1997).

While the approach discussed in this chapter concentrates on work with the family, it is understood that physiological factors contribute to the emergence of some severe symptoms such as psychosis and major depression. It is not my intention to deny the importance of these factors, but rather to focus on one aspect of the treatment of severe symptoms in adolescence: the family and social context. Interrupting symptomatic patterns and introducing the family members to new ways of relating to one another may enhance the effectiveness of biological treatments, and in some cases may even obviate the need for these treatments.

FOUR BASIC CONCEPTS

The Symptomatic Cycle

My central thesis is that symptoms in families evolve in a context of interpersonal isolation, characterized by conditional acceptance and efforts to control one another. As family members struggle to eliminate or control the symptoms, their preoccupation with the symptoms leads them to neglect other important aspects of their relationships with each other. As the family relationships deteriorate, all family members, particularly the symptomatic adolescent, experience an increasing sense of isolation.

The more the family members focus on the adolescent's symptomatic behavior, the more they are liable to see the youngster as "the problem," leading him or her to feel misunderstood and increasingly isolated from the rest of the family. As efforts to eliminate the symptom repeatedly fail, the family members feel increasingly helpless and frustrated. In this context of isolation and alienation, symptoms tend to escalate (see Figure 2.1). This "symptomatic cycle," whereby isolation

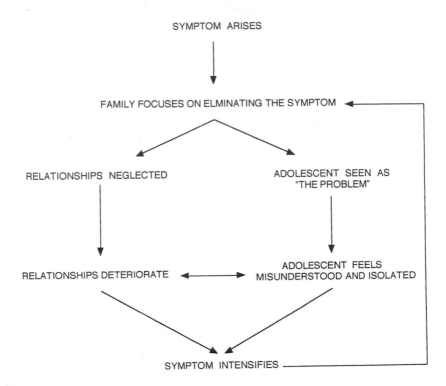

FIGURE 2.1. The symptomatic cycle.

fuels symptoms and symptoms fuel further isolation, constitutes the basic process driving symptomatic behavior (Brendler, Silver, Haber, & Sargent, 1991; Hoffman, 1981).

For example, consider a family with an adolescent boy who exhibits violent temper outbursts. The parents may become so preoccupied with their son's outbursts that they neglect other relationships, such as their relationship with each other, or with their other children. The more the parents focus on managing the boy's violence, the less attention they pay to his other qualities, such as his wit, intelligence, or vulnerability. In response to this myopia, these qualities of the boy begin to fade from view, reinforcing the tendency to see him as "the problem."

The family is now caught in a bind. Labeled as the problem, the boy feels misunderstood by his family, which increases his isolation from them. As the violence intensifies, the other family members find it increasingly difficult to see beyond the violence to the boy's other qualities, and are thus less equipped to help him find alternative ways of handling frustration and hurt. Deprived of his family's guidance, the boy continues to be susceptible to temper outbursts, thus reinforcing the family's focus on his violence.

Symptoms begin as relatively minor alterations in behavior that can be a response to many different factors, such as genetic vulnerability, developmental stress, or traumatic experiences. These minor behavioral changes occur from time to time in all adolescents and are usually transient. Some of the time, however, they evolve into lasting problems that defy solution. The crucial element in problem development is the way in which the family responds to these ubiquitous behavioral changes characteristic of developing adolescents[2] (Minuchin, 1974). Most families adapt to the developmental challenges associated with adolescence and flexibly adjust their responses to provide the adolescent with whatever he or she appears to need from them at that particular time. However, some families can't make these adjustments, or they misread signs that the adolescent is in distress. These families are prone to react in unproductive ways that can contribute to the development of serious symptoms.

There are four common patterns that represent variations on the theme of the symptomatic cycle:

1. Enmeshment. In families where boundaries are too diffuse (so called "enmeshed" families; Minuchin, 1974), even the minor changes associated with the normal transitions in the family life cycle may be experienced as threatening. If a symptom emerges during one of these transitions (such as a child entering adolescence), the family members overreact and focus all energies on eliminating the symptom so they can return to the comfortable status quo. With their attention thus drawn to eliminating the symptom, the family members are distracted from the real task at hand: making the changes necessary to negotiate the developmental transition successfully.

2. Disengagement. When family members are distant and insufficiently involved with one another (so-called "disengaged" families Minuchin, 1974), a symptom may increase in intensity before it reaches a threshold sufficient to attract the family's attention. Perhaps the family members failed to notice that the adolescent needed their help until it was too late. Sometimes, the parents don't realize there's a problem until someone outside the family (e.g., the school or legal authorities) calls their attention to it. Even then, the absence of solid relationships within the family inhibits their efforts to help. The parents become preoccupied with eliminating the symptom and thus distracted from what really needs attention: strengthening their relationships with one another.

3. Unresolved parental conflict. Often families cannot be characterized in absolute terms as either enmeshed or disengaged, but rather contain relationships at various degrees of closeness. A familiar pattern is one in which one parent is overly involved with a child and the other parent is peripheral. From their different vantage points, these parents are likely to react differently when a symptom emerges.

For example, the more involved parent might see a depressed child as a victim, and so respond in an overly protective manner, while the less involved parent may see the child as misbehaving, and so respond in a punitive or demanding manner. Or, the less involved parent (e.g., a peripheral father) might blame an adolescent's oppositional behavior on the disciplinary tactics of the more involved parent. These opposing complementary positions put the parents in conflict with one another. As the conflict intensifies, the parents are less effective in helping the symptomatic child. This process fuels the emergence of more symptomatic behavior.

4. *Misguided efforts to help.* In other families, well-intentioned efforts to help the symptomatic child backfire and make the problem worse. For example, parents who repeatedly rescue their child from the consequences of his actions might think they are being helpful when in fact they are impeding the natural process of learning from one's mistakes. In some families, there may be underlying reasons for this pattern (e.g., the parents need the child to be dependent on them in order to distract them from marital problems), but in other families, the parents might be unwittingly making the problem worse by their sincere efforts to help.

The Multifaceted Self

In a systemic paradigm, an individual's "self" is seen as a fluid concept, changing as the context changes. Salvador Minuchin and Charles Fishman (1981) describe the self as "multifaceted" and maintain that different aspects of the self emerge in different contexts. The context, as it were, pulls particular facets of the self to the fore.

Families who are locked in rigid patterns around symptoms are repeatedly engaging the same facets of each other. These facets exist in complementary and symmetrical relationship, and are typically so pronounced that it is difficult to see beyond them to other, more positive facets.

For example, a father who insists on setting more limits on a symptomatic child might be perceived by the mother and other family members as overbearing and harsh. Other aspects of the father—such as his sensitivity, understanding, and nurturance—are neither activated nor reinforced in such a context. Similarly, to the extent that the father's harshness elicits the mother's overprotectiveness, her other facets, such as her capacity to discipline with gentleness, are not activated. These complementary facets of the parents are mutually activated in such a way that rigid patterns emerge. The therapeutic task is to engage the untapped resources (facets) of each family member and use these newly engaged facets to help stimulate new interactional patterns. By using his or her relationship with each family member, the therapist draws out new facets of each family member. As the family members come to see each other differently, they can begin to interact with each other differently[3] (see Figure 2.2).

Arrested Development

As people develop, they discover more facets to themselves and learn to integrate these facets. The availability of a variety of facets permits optimal adaptation to a constantly changing environment. Families who are caught in symptomatic cycles repeatedly draw upon certain facets of themselves to the exclusion of others, a process that impedes the development of all family members.

While it is the symptomatic adolescent whose development is most obviously impaired, it is important to recognize that the developmental arrest affects all members of the family who participate in the symptomatic cycle. The model of the *family life cycle* (Carter & McGoldrick, 1980) proposes that individual development and family development are inextricably linked and influence each other. As one member of the system develops, others must follow suit or exert pressure on the changing member to revert to more predictable forms of behavior. The family, which is the optimal "matrix" (Minuchin, 1974) or "crucible" (Schnarch, 1991) of human development, becomes instead a prison where the development of all family members is stalemated.

As the symptomatic cycle is disrupted and new facets of each family member emerge, family members are faced with the prospect of change. At this stage of treatment, it may be appropriate to consider individual therapy for one or more family members to help promote the developmental process and to complement the changes occurring in family therapy. Some families oscillate back and forth between reemergence of the symptomatic cycle and developmental progression, which requires relentlessness and patience on the part of the therapist and attention to the needs of all family members. As I discuss later in this chapter, supporting individual development to the exclusion of the relational context of this development runs the risk of reactivating the symptomatic cycle.

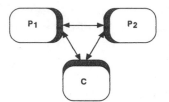

(1) The initial conditions in the family prior to therapy. The sympotmatic cycle repeatedly activates the same facets of the parents (P_1 and P_2) and the symptomatic child (C).

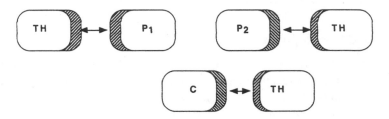

(2) The therapist (TH) engages in interactions with the family members that activate facets of the self that had not been activated by the symptomatic cycle.

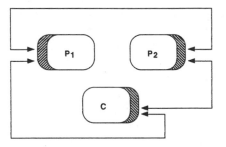

(3) The therapist then induces the family members into new patterns of interaction that activate the facets of the self that had not been activated by the symptomatic cycle.

FIGURE 2.2. Disrupting the symptomatic cycle.

Interlocking Narratives and the Complementarity of Biased Perceptions

Jeff Bogdan (1984) has offered a reconceptualization of family structure (Minuchin, 1974) as an "ecology of ideas." According to this notion, each family member develops particular interpretations and beliefs about events in the family and the behavior of other family members. These beliefs, in turn, influence how the family members interact with one another. The meanings attributed to these interactions will either modify the original beliefs or confirm them. In nonsymptomatic families, the belief system and the interactions mutually evolve and become more complex (and thus more adaptive) over time.

In symptomatic families, narratives are rigidly organized and closed to new information. These closed narratives function as organizing schemas that promote selective attention to information that confirms the schemas. Family members seek out information that proves their preferred view is the "right" one, thus reinforcing the original narrative and decreasing the likelihood that disconfirming information will be noticed. These views form a system of complementary biased perceptions (Micucci, 1995).

For example, the harsher parent selectively notices evidence that the other parent is "too lenient" and interprets this evidence as justification for his or her own harshness. Similarly, the more lenient parent selectively notices evidence that the other parent is "too harsh" thus justifying his or her own leniency. Direct challenges to these beliefs, either by the therapist or by other family members, often have the effect of reinforcing the beliefs, since the family member redoubles his or her selective attention to observations that support the belief in an attempt to defend it (White, 1983). Moreover, each family member might attempt to convince the therapist of the validity of his or her belief about the problem, thus inviting the therapist into a coalition against other family members.

The therapist must break up this web of complementary perceptions in order to disrupt the symptomatic cycle. Generally, the therapist can accomplish this goal in two ways: (1) directly challenging the beliefs by calling attention to disconfirming information, or (2) stimulating new behaviors in the session that can provide the seed around which new beliefs can crystallize. The former approach is advocated by the proponents of solution-focused (de Shazer, 1985) and narrative therapy (e.g., White & Epston, 1990). The latter approach is favored by models that advocate more action-oriented techniques such as enactment[4] (Minuchin & Fishman, 1981). I believe that these approaches complement one another, and both can be useful at different points in the therapy process.

Goals of Treatment

These four concepts—the symptomatic cycle, multifaceted self, arrested development, and interlocking narratives—form the foundations for the treatment model advocated in this book. In its simplest form, treatment follows three basic steps: (1) identifying the symptomatic cycle, (2) contracting and goal setting, and (3) disrupting the symptomatic cycle.

Keep in mind that these steps are not so much distinct stages of therapy as they are general episodes in the course of treatment. Each stage of therapy requires different skills of the therapist and poses certain common pitfalls. These are discussed in the following sections.

IDENTIFYING THE SYMPTOMATIC CYCLE

Three sources of information are useful in identifying the symptomatic cycle: (1) the language used by each family member to describe the problem, (2) the history of the problem, and (3) interpersonal transactions that take place in the therapy room.

Language: How Does Each Family Member View the Problem?

By carefully tracking how each family member talks about the problem and about each other, it is possible to gain insight into the symptomatic cycle and the system of interlocking narratives that supports it. By beginning an initial session with the question, "How do you see the problem?," the therapist can elicit from each family member his or her narrative about the problem and the person with the problem, and his or her relationship to the person with the problem. Thus, the therapist can uncover the unspoken and unquestioned assumptions each family member brings to therapy.

As Jay Haley (1976) recommends, it is important to ask each family member to state his or her view of the problem during the first few minutes of the initial session, before spending too much time pursuing details. This practice permits the therapist to get an overview of family members' perceptions of the problem and of each other, calls attention to "marginalized" or ignored narratives (White, 1993), and avoids the pitfall of induction into a single, monolithic narrative of the problems in the family.

For example, a father said, "My daughter is the problem. She has anorexia. She won't eat and keeps losing weight. There's nothing we can do to get her to eat."

This response implies several hypotheses about the father and his relationship to the problem. He sees the problem as residing within his daughter. He sees the problem as having a name, which he also describes more specifically in behavioral terms ("She won't eat and keeps losing weight"). He expresses impotence and frustration at his failure to help, but the phrase "*get* her" implies that he may be in a power struggle with his daughter.

In contrast, a mother said, "I just hope that she finds the strength within herself to get well. She didn't ask for this disease. She doesn't want it. She just wants to get well."

Like the father, the mother sees the problem as a "disease." She believes that the solution lies within the girl. She also makes several statements that imply that she has access to the girl's private thoughts and feelings. Meanwhile, the girl, Tina, remained silent, thus implying assent, if not agreement, with the mother's assumptions about her.

When asked for her view of the problem, Tina replied, "I don't know; it just happened." When the therapist pushed for more, Tina muttered a few inaudible words, then burst into tears. This behavior only serves to reinforce the mother's view of her as a helpless victim, who lacks the "strength within herself to get well."

In this example, it is clear how these narratives in the family reinforce and complement one another. Father says the girl "won't eat," while Mother implies that she "can't eat." While both the mother and father seem to agree that the solution to the problem resides within the daughter, the father implies that one solution is to "get her" to eat while mother implies that the solution must come from "within herself." As Father intensifies his efforts to "get her" to eat, Mother will undermine these efforts in order to support her view that the girl "can't eat" and that the solution, if it exists, lies "within herself." Tina herself remains noncommittal, though she clearly presents herself as helpless, not only against the "anorexia," but also in the face of the therapist's questions. Her apparent powerlessness is deceptive, however: In her adamant refusal to eat or even to speak, she renders both of her parents helpless.

History of the Problem: What Solutions Have Already Been Tried?

Previous unsuccessful attempts at problem resolution tell the therapist what has not worked and how these solutions may have unwittingly exacerbated the problem. Often, problems crystallize because the family is attempting to solve new problems by repeatedly using methods that might have worked for them at an earlier phase of development (Fisch, Weakland, & Segal, 1982). These attempted solutions do not solve the current problem because they neglect to take into account the need for a qualitative change in family organization. By carefully tracking the sequence of events leading up to the consultation, the therapist can gain insight into the patterns that have congealed around the problem.

For example, the family described in the previous section related that the current consultation was precipitated after the mother, in searching the girl's room, discovered empty bottles of ipecac (an emetic available in most pharmacies). Asked why she was in her daughter's room, the mother could respond only that she "suspected something was not right" and felt compelled to investigate. Noteworthy was the fact that Mother took unilateral action rather than consulting with Father. Asked what happened after Mother found the ipecac bottles, she responded that she confronted the girl, who became very upset. Mother could not calm her, so in desperation she called the father, triangling him into the conflict between her and her daughter. Father then began to attack Mother, who defended herself against Father's attacks, while the girl wept silently in the background. Finally, Mother hung up on Father and called the girl's therapist (another triangulation). Sensing the mother's extreme anxiety and the danger involved in the girl's abuse of ipecac (which the girl had concealed from her therapist), the therapist suggested that the mother contact me for a consultation.

These events suggest the following pattern: Mother feels disconnected from the girl and attempts to connect with her by violating a boundary. Then, she confronts her daughter with the information she discovered, and the girl collapses. Unable to deal directly with the girl, Mother contacts Father, who unhelpfully begins to criticize Mother. Mother and Father get lost in their conflict together, while their daughter's needs are neglected. Finally, Mother rejects Father and seeks out the girl's therapist, who recognizes that the situation has spiraled out of control and recommends a consultation.

This pattern suggests that the mother and daughter are not able to regulate closeness in their relationship without involving a third party. It also suggests that Mother and Father are unsuccessful at working collaboratively as parents to help the girl. Father appears peripheral, which is reinforced by Mother's efforts to distance him, a natural response to his hostility toward her. Father expresses his anxiety by attacking the mother, which only fuels further conflict and keeps the cycle going.

Transactions in the Room: How Do the Family Members Interact?

Often, the pattern that is revealed in the family's account of events leading up to the consultation will be played out in the therapy session itself, either verbally or nonverbally. The therapist can gain insight into the cycle by noticing patterns of speaking, who speaks when about what, who speaks to whom, and what dyadic interactions occur more or less frequently.

For example, in the case just described, Father and Mother ignored each other during the session. When one spoke, the other quickly qualified what was said by offering to the therapist (not to the other parent) his or her point of view on the matter just discussed.

To bring the symptomatic patterns to light, it might be necessary for the therapist to elicit an obscured conflict. Circular questions (Selvini-Palazzoli, Boscolo, Cecchin, & Prata, 1980) can be a useful way of accomplishing this goal. For example, the therapist can ask one person in the family to comment on the relationship between two others in the family. This response will reveal not only the respondent's perception of this relationship, but also the respondent's relationship to the two other parties. Often, the other parent will spontaneously defend or qualify the response, and the therapist can call attention to the ensuing conflict.

For example, the father responded to the question, "How do you see the relationship between Tina and her mom?" with the response, "I can only go by what Tina has said to me. There isn't enough structure. She was a working mother, and she was out a lot." Mother immediately defended herself against this perceived attack, which brought the conflict between the mother and father into the open. The therapist then asked, "How long have you two been fighting like this?" to which they responded almost in unison, "We don't fight, we just ignore each other." The therapist directed their attention away from their argument by pointing out how their pattern of mutual avoidance was related to their unsuccessful efforts to solve the problem of anorexia.

Pitfalls at This Phase

Failing to Recognize the Role of Absent Members

In the initial session, family members might directly or indirectly suggest that absent parties play a key role in the symptomatic cycle. These individuals might be members of the nuclear family, members of the extended family, or individuals outside the family who have engaged in significant interactions with the family around the problem. It might be necessary to prolong the assessment phase of treatment until it is possible to arrange for these absent parties to attend a session.

Failing to recognize the key role of absent members can lead the therapist to an incomplete account of the symptomatic cycle. Conversely, the therapist should not automatically assume that everyone in the family is a participant in the symptomatic cycle. Often, symptomatic cycles involve only a subsystem of the family, and do not include everyone in the household, such as siblings or grandparents. While it is often useful to include these individuals in at least one assessment session to ascertain their role in the cycle, it is rarely useful to insist that they participate on a regular basis.

Overemphasizing Pathology

When families first come to treatment, it is natural for them to emphasize their problems and minimize their strengths. Therapists diligently searching for insights into the symptomatic cycle can become so distracted by this task that they fail to notice the strengths of the family.

Failure to notice the family's strengths has two consequences: (1) therapists can become inducted into the symptomatic cycle by focusing on the symptom, just as the family has been doing, and (2) therapists can miss opportunities to note the unrecognized positive qualities of family members, around which new patterns can be constructed.

For example, the father in the preceeding example betrays several problematic aspects of his relationship with the mother and his daughter, but at the same time he reveals that he is very concerned about his daughter and recognizes the severity of the problem. It is important to avoid the trap of trying to decide what is "the truth" about the father. Is he peripheral, critical, and controlling, *or* is he concerned, sympathetic, and available? Putting questions such as these in either–or terms demeans the father's complexity and fails to recognize the "multiplicity of truths" inherent in any human interaction (Hare-Mustin, 1994; Paré, 1995; Parry, 1991). The father exhibits all of these qualities, and which quality (facet) emerges at any particular time depends upon the interpersonal context and the questions the therapist chooses to ask.

CONTRACTING AND GOAL SETTING

After the therapist has developed a hypothesis about the symptomatic cycle, the next step is to negotiate a treatment contract with the family. While it is possible in some cases to proceed without specifically discussing with the family the goals and terms of treatment, I believe that an explicit contract will help to focus the therapy and prevent it from going off on interesting but ultimately unproductive tangents.

The formulation that the therapist offers the family should provide a unique perspective on the problem, and should link the problem to the relationships in the family. For example, I offered Tina and her parents the following formulation: "Tina is losing weight and can't eat because she feels isolated and alone, unable to express her true feelings to anyone. She is wasting away not only from lack of food but also because of the absence of nurturing and sustaining relationships in her life. This deprives her of the valuable help you both can offer her to grow and become the young adult she is capable of becoming."

This formulation includes the following elements:

- A statement of the problem ("Tina is losing weight and can't eat").
- A hypothesis about why the problem is present ("because she feels isolated and alone, unable to express her true feelings to anyone").
- A link between the problem and the relationships in the family ("She is wasting away not only from lack of food but also because of the absence of nurturing and sustaining relationships in her life").

The formulation that the therapist offers the family should frame the problem in a unique way that deviates from all of the problem definitions circulating in the family. By carefully analyzing the symptomatic cycle in the way just advocated, the therapist will gain insight into the competing narratives in the family and can avoid aligning with any one of them. Rather, the therapist should attempt to link all of the narratives by proposing a frame that is consistent with them all, or propose a formulation of the problem that is entirely new for the family.

For example, in the case described above, Father described the problem as "not eating and losing weight," while Mother emphasized Tina's helplessness in the face of an unwanted disease. The metaphors of growth and sustenance were used to extract a similar theme from both the mother and father's accounts by linking Tina's weight loss to an inability to derive sustenance from the relationships in her life.

After presenting the formulation, the therapist then proposes a plan for solving the problem. It is not necessary to spell out this plan in great detail, but it should state clearly that the goal of treatment will be to change the relationships in the family.

For example, I proposed the following plan to Tina and her parents: "If you are interested, I will work with you all, as a family, to give you the chance to begin building more sustaining relationships, so that Tina may begin to grow again."

This plan is brief but to the point: It states that the goal of therapy will be to change the way the members of the family relate to one another ("to begin building new and more sustaining relationships, so that Tina may begin to grow again"). It does not imply that the primary goal is for Tina to eat or gain weight. Rather, weight gain is linked to improved relationships in the family, consistent with the formulation that Tina was "wasting away . . . because of the absence of nurturing and sustaining relationships in her life."

If a family member asks the therapist to be more specific regarding the number of sessions or who should attend, it is best to say something like, "We'll have to see as we go along, but to start I'd suggest meeting once a week for 50 minutes, at a time when everyone will be able to attend."

Pitfalls and Complications

Lack of Agreement between the Therapist and the Family

Families in crisis might agree to therapy but then fail to follow through when the therapist expects them to comply. It is useful at this stage to review the information that had been gathered during the assessment with family members and allow them to challenge the definition of the problem offered by the therapist. The therapist should enter into these discussions in good faith and without the intent of coercing the family to accept his definition of the problem.

The problem that will be tackled in therapy should be negotiated (O'Hanlon & Wilk, 1987) between the therapist and the family. It is far better to settle for a definition of the problem that the family members are willing to accept than to remain locked in a battle of wills with the family over what the "real" problem is. If the therapist insists on a particular problem definition, he may replicate in his relationship with the family the same power struggles that are going on among the family members. The therapist needs to let go of controlling the outcome, but rather work to influence the therapeutic system to alter its transactional patterns in any way possible.

Lack of Agreement within the Family

Sometimes the family refuses to accept any specific definition of the problem because the polarization between key family members is so great that they cannot agree. At these times, the therapist might suggest the following: "I'd like to continue to meet with you for X more sessions so that I can gain a more complete understanding of your problem.

So, I propose that we delay treatment for a few more sessions until we can determine all of the factors contributing to the problem and which factors we will work on together." This *evaluation frame* removes the pressure from family members to commit to a single problem definition. Rather, it engages them in the process of carefully observing themselves and each other, which in itself could counteract their mutual efforts to control one another.

Therapist Appears to Align with One of the Family Members

Unwittingly, the therapist might have defined the problem in a way that aligns with one of the competing narratives for explaining the problem in the family. Some family members might perceive the therapist's proposed problem definition as an attempt to align with the family member who favors this particular narrative against the other family members, who favor other narratives. I am not referring here to the structural technique of unbalancing (Minuchin & Fishman, 1981), which is a deliberate move on the part of the therapist to alter family structure. Rather, I am referring to those times when the therapist does not realize that she has aligned with a particular family member, a phenomenon that has been termed "induction" (Minuchin & Fishman, 1981).

If the therapist's framing of the problem is already consistent with one of the competing narratives in the family, then the therapist has essentially joined the symptomatic cycle. Change will not occur under these circumstances. Whenever the therapist attempts to "push" her frame, the competitors will assert their opposition.

If, in the course of therapy, the therapist recognizes that the problem definition she had offered the family, and the family had appeared to accept, is actually one of the family's original competing narratives, the therapist must take steps to correct this error. Probably the most straightforward way of doing so is to announce to the family that, after thinking for some time about their problem, the therapist has realized that she has been wrong all along to see the problem in this way. The therapist then apologizes to the family and either offers the "evaluation frame" (discussed earlier) or offers the family another problem definition that is more consistent with the principles outlined in the previous paragraphs.

DISRUPTING THE SYMPTOMATIC CYCLE

Once the specific nature of the symptomatic cycle in the family has been identified and the therapist and family members have agreed on a goal for treatment, therapy then proceeds with interventions to disrupt the cycle. Whenever the therapist induces the family members to interact in a new or different pattern, the symptomatic cycle is momentarily disrupted. In most cases, however, these disruptions are temporary, only to be submerged and often forgotten by the family members when the cycle later reemerges. The cycle must be disrupted repeatedly before the family members begin to experience the new patterns as "natural." In most cases, this process is unlikely to occur until the family members have resolved the conflicts underlying the cycle and struggled with the anxiety aroused when these conflicts are aired.

At times, therapy reaches an impasse requiring creative and sometimes dramatic interventions by the therapist, such as paradox (Madanes, 1981, 1984; Weeks & L'Abate, 1982). In most cases, however, the therapist can get much mileage from the more straightforward techniques described later. The key is not so much finding the "right" intervention as it is maintaining the conviction that the family members can and will change if the therapist persists in relentlessly interrupting the symptomatic cycle whenever it appears.

At various times, the therapist might find any or all of the following methods useful for disrupting the symptomatic cycle:

- Promoting dialogue
- Uncovering hidden conflicts
- Discouraging control
- Encouraging unilateral change
- Identifying and enacting "unique outcomes"
- Constructing new narratives
- Meeting privately with individual family members

Promoting Dialogue

True intimacy is precluded by the symptomatic cycle, where polarized perceptions and conditional terms of acceptance prevail. Real dialogue is virtually impossible, because everything said and heard is filtered through the organizing schemas of the biased perceptions. When the family members attempt to engage in dialogue on their own, they are likely to feel attacked and, in response, defend themselves or counterattack, which aborts the dialogue. The therapist must help the family members accept their differences without attacking one another, or without feeling compelled to reach consensus.

Nonreactive Listening

People in symptomatic families typically respond impulsively to each other in ways that only elicit more of the same. In the language of Bowenian therapy, the family members act as if they are "fused" or poorly differentiated from one another (Kerr & Bowen, 1988). In symptomatic families, people are repeatedly reacting to each other's reactions, a process that fuels anxiety and precludes the discovery of solutions.

The therapist must help the family members modulate their reactions to one another. This goal can be accomplished by reminding the family that (1) listening does not mean agreement, (2) an immediate response is not required of them, (3) the parents should digest what they have heard and discuss it with one another before offering a response to the adolescent, and (4) the parents can be honest with the adolescent about their own feelings, as long as they take responsibility for these feelings and do not blame the adolescent for "making" them have these feelings. If one parent can successfully modulate his or her reactivity to the child's disclosures, then others in the family are likely to follow suit.

"Tell Me/Don't Tell Me"

Symptomatic adolescents often find themselves in a "*Tell me/Don't tell me*" bind. Overwhelmed and anxious about being blamed for the child's problem, the parent gives the youngster a double message: "Open up to me—but be sure not to say anything I don't want to hear." Trying to avoid upsetting the parent, the child withholds information, which only increases the parent's anxiety. For many kids, complete silence is their only defense against this bind.

In this situation, the therapist might meet with the parents alone to help them recognize their own anxiety about what the child might say. In many cases, parents will admit that they are really "not ready" to hear certain things. It is then helpful for the parent to communicate this to the youngster, thereby releasing the child from the bind.

Alternatively, the therapist could meet individually with the adolescent to build a relationship with him or her. Given the protection of confidentiality, many adolescents will confide in the therapist. At this point, many therapists are tempted to abandon family therapy and continue to meet with the youngster individually. Another option, and one likely to be more productive, is to discuss with the adolescent how trust in the parents could be increased. The content of subsequent dialogue in the family sessions then shifts away from the specific information to be disclosed and onto the issue of facilitating trust.

In rare cases, the adolescent will disclose privately to the therapist information that the therapist believes is crucial to communicate immediately to the parent. For example, a girl might disclose that she has been sexually abused by a close family member. If the girl's immediate safety is at stake, it might be necessary for the therapist to disclose the information to the parent even if the adolescent refuses to do so herself. If immediate safety is not the issue, the therapist can meet with the parents alone and confirm their suspicion that their daughter has something serious to tell them, but is afraid to do so because she is afraid of hurting them. The therapist can then work with the parents to help them address their own ambivalence about hearing the adolescent's disclosure, and use the crisis to increase the parents' willingness to tolerate and manage their own anxiety rather than expecting the child to keep them comfortable by withholding information from them.

Uncovering Hidden Conflicts

Conflicts will emerge naturally in the context of a dialogue. Families oversensitized to the disrupting effects of conflict might recoil at this point and engage in conflict-avoidant maneuvers, such as detouring, that is, focusing on a third party to reduce the tension between them (Minuchin, 1974). These processes only reinforce the family members' belief that they are incapable of dealing with conflict. Positive reframing (Minuchin & Fishman, 1981) by the therapist can be helpful. For example, the therapist might reframe a parent's criticism of a child's school performance as an expression of the parent's confidence in the child's ability to excel at school.

It is far more important that a conflict be aired than it be resolved. People in symptomatic families often believe that all conflicts must be resolved immediately. The therapist should discourage this practice and instead point out that premature closure can be a way of avoiding conflict. Conflicts are a necessary part of family life, and family members can actually grow closer to one another by expressing their differences, acknowledging them, and "agreeing to disagree."

Discouraging Control

Edwin Friedman (1987) has written, "The most serious symptoms in family life, e.g., anorexia, schizophrenia, suicide, always show up in families in which people make intense efforts to bend one another to their will" (p. 29). This view is consistent with that of Gregory Bateson (1972), who believed that human preoccupation with conscious control of the ecological balance of nature is responsible for many environmental problems.

Explaining the position known as "second-order cybernetics," Atkinson and Heath (1990) pointed out that systems (such as families) are self-corrective as long as the individual parts (in this case, individual family members) are not intent on imposing their own goals on the other family members. Atkinson and Heath give an example of a father who is locked in a struggle over control with his adolescent son. The more the father attempts to control the boy, the more the boy resists the father's control. A family therapist might approach this situation by encouraging the father to "back off," thus breaking the cycle. Atkinson and Heath, however, point out that the father's *motives* in "backing off" are relevant. If the father backs off because he believes that this move will give him a strategic advantage in the battle for control, then the intervention is not likely to be successful, since the father's "change" has simply been incorporated into the cycle. On the other hand, if the father backs off *and* (either before or after backing off) begins questioning his assumption that the only way for him to be happy is if his son meets his expectations, then a true "second-order change" has occurred and the cycle of control–resistance has been transcended.

In the face of potentially life-threatening behavior, it is natural for family members to resort to methods of controlling one another to prevent the behavior from escalating. Control is the antithesis of true dialogue, where the goal is to understand and accept rather than to force the other person to change. Instead, I encourage family members to substitute *curiosity* for *control*.

Specifically, I encourage family members to (1) ask questions rather than give directives, and (2) take responsibility for one's own reactions rather than trying to change the behavior of others in order to reduce one's own anxiety.

Encouraging Unilateral Change

Family therapists are familiar with the "you-first" phenomenon: Each member of the family is willing to change, as long as someone else in the family goes first. A variation on this theme is the quid pro quo: "I'll change if you'll change." These patterns are examples of paradoxical double binds, whereby change is precluded because it is contingent upon a second change which is contingent on the first.

A therapist can challenge this bind by *advocating unilateral change*.

The therapist places the responsibility for change directly at the feet of a single family member, and challenges that family member to change unconditionally, regardless of the response he or she receives from the other members of the family. If the family member is successful in changing, it will break the impasse and interrupt the symptomatic cycle.

It may seem "unsystemic" for a family therapist to advocate individual change as one route to disrupting a cyclical family process. However, the procedure of working through a single member of the family in order to effect systemic change is well known in the family therapy field. It is the essence of the approach advocated by Bowen (Kerr & Bowen, 1988), whereby the effort of one member of the family to increase his or her level of differentiation has a "ripple effect" that benefits all members of the family. Selvini-Palazzoli and Viaro (1988) described a method of working through an individual to alter the moves in the "family game." The structural technique of "unbalancing" (Minuchin & Fishman, 1981) aims to dissolve an impasse by appearing to side with one person's perceptions about another in order to encourage the latter to change. Nichols (1987) has argued convincingly that *all* changes in family interactions are mediated by changes made by individual family members.

As with most interventions, its true therapeutic effect unfolds as the family struggles with the aftermath. Say, for example, that a father agrees to change unilaterally and unconditionally. Assuming that the change has been defined specifically, and in a way that all could agree on (this is essential), the issue of whether the father "really" changed or not could be discussed in the family. On the other hand, if the father "really did change," then any event that occurred in the family subsequent to this change being noticed could be framed either as support for the father's efforts or as efforts to test father's resolve.

Identifying and Enacting "Unique Outcomes"

Because of their complementary biased perceptions, the family members are often blind to events that do not fit with the symptomatic cycle. Even when these events are called to their attention, they often discount their significance. For example, in Tina's family, neither Father nor Mother could recall incidents when Tina did not appear "helpless," even though Tina was engaged in expertly sketching a profile of the therapist during this conversation.

Michael White (1986) has used the term "unique outcomes" to refer to those times when the problem is less severe or not present at all. The family members' selective attention to information that confirms their biased perceptions makes it difficult for them to notice these "unique outcomes" on their own. Yet, to the extent that unique outcomes go unnoticed, they are less likely to recur, thus setting up the conditions for a "self-fulfilling prophecy" (Rosenthal & Jacobson, 1968). It is useful for the therapist to help the family notice these unique outcomes and then invite them to construct new narratives around them. This process can dissolve the complementary system of biased perceptions by introducing new complexity to the shared family narratives.

Enactments (Minuchin & Fishman, 1981) in the therapy room can provide the seed for these new narratives. Family members can be induced to engage in a new pattern with one another, and then be invited by the therapist to reflect on this experience and construct new meaning around it. The evolving narrative is then reinforced by engaging the family members in another enactment or by giving them an out-of-session task that expands on the change that was observed in the therapy room.

For example, I noted that Tina's father rarely spoke to her directly, but instead addressed her indirectly through the therapist or through her mother. To encourage direct contact between Tina and her father, I drew upon their mutual interest in art to suggest that they spend a day together at the art museum and then talk with each other about their reactions to the paintings they saw. After a number of experiences such as this, in which father and daughter come to know each other better, the relationship between them has grown to be far more complex than it once was: Now, it is *sometimes* distant and *sometimes* close, and there is an opportunity for the father and daughter to build upon the latter "unique outcomes" to create a new narrative about their relationship.

An important corollary to this point is the distinction between *initiating change* and *sustaining change*. Many families (and therapists) claim that they "can't change" even though there are likely to be countless unnoticed examples of small changes (de Shazer, 1985). As noted by the proponents of the model of brief family therapy developed at the Palo Alto Mental Research Institute (MRI), it is often sufficient to assist the family in initiating change, which then "snowballs" on its own to facilitate additional changes (Fisch et al., 1982). Even if one finds it difficult to embrace this optimistic view, it is nevertheless important to draw a distinction between the *first step* toward change and *complete resolution of the problem*. Therapists can unwittingly collude with the family's biased perceptions by minimizing the significance of the first stirrings of change. Perhaps one of the most important contributions of solution-focused therapy (de Shazer, 1985;

O'Hanlon & Wilk, 1987) has been its emphasis on noticing and capitalizing upon what the family is *already doing right.*

Once change has been initiated, the challenge is no longer "getting change to happen" but rather "helping change to continue." The original problem, that the family was "stuck," has "dis-solved" (Anderson & Goolishian, 1988), and is now replaced by a "new" challenge, namely, how to *keep on the road to change.* Pointing out this distinction to the family can instill hope and undermine their biased perceptions.

Constructing New Narratives

The experiences that family members have with one another are encoded in language and linked together in the form of stories or narratives (Bruner, 1987; Parry & Doan, 1994). Michael White and David Epston (1990) have pointed out that families come to therapy with "problem-saturated" narratives that selectively exclude attention to the "unique outcomes," times when the problem is less severe or absent. They have developed a technique that enables the family to deconstruct their problem-saturated narrative and replace it with a new narrative that encourages more attention to the unique outcomes. Toward this end, White and Epston advocate the following steps:

1. Externalizing the problem. The therapist and family give the problem a name, such as "anorexia" or "depression," that distinguishes the problem from the person seen by the family as "being" the problem. This process allows the therapist to talk as if the problem is oppressing the entire family, thus uniting the family in an effort to oppose the problem.

2. Mapping the influence of the problem. The therapist then "maps the influence" of the problem on the family by exploring with the family members in great detail all of the ways that the problem has affected each of them. Typical questions might be: How has the anorexia affected your relationship with your daughter? How have the fears blinded you to your resources? What has the anger gotten you to do that has been against your better judgment? In what situations is the depression most likely to assert itself? How has your marital relationship changed since the mistrust has been part of your lives? (See also Freedman and Combs, 1996.)

3. Searching for unique outcomes. Next, the therapist engages family members in a search for the "unique outcomes," those times when they *could have* "given in" to the problem but did not. The therapist calls attention to the distinction between the "problem narrative" and the narrative constructed around the unique outcomes. The force of this intervention is to highlight that the family members still retain some influence over the effects of the problem and actually at times experience themselves as more powerful than the problem. Typical questions might be: Are there times when the anorexia is less powerful? Have there been times when you have been able to outsmart the fears? Are there times when the anger could have taken over but you have kept it out of the picture? Have you noticed any times when you act in ways different from the ways that depression usually gets you to act? Have you noticed any occasions when you have been able to keep the mistrust out of your marital relationship?

4. *Developing a new narrative.* The therapist then helps the family members weave a new narrative around the unique outcomes and contrasts this new story with the "problem-saturated narrative." The therapist calls attention to times when the problem was not present or not as powerful and helps the family members recognize what they did to assert themselves over the influence of the problem. Typical questions might be: What do you think your being able, from time to time, to resist the demands of anorexia says about you as a person? Were there any events in your past that might have predicted that you would have been able to outsmart the fears? When you were able to keep the anger out of the picture, did you learn anything new about yourself? What was it about yourself that allowed you to act in ways different from the ways that depression usually gets you to act? What did your ability to keep the mistrust out of your marriage say about your relationship as a couple?

5. *Expanding the narrative.* Eventually, by focusing on those times when the problem was not present or less powerful, and elaborating a new narrative around those events, the problem-saturated narrative is replaced by one that is more complex and that incorporates those times when the family members had "solved" the problem without even realizing it. The therapist helps the family members expand this narrative by "recruiting an audience" or projecting the narrative into the future. For example, the therapist might ask: Who in your life might be most surprised to hear that you had sometimes resisted the demands of anorexia? Who in your past might have predicted that you would have been able to outsmart the fears as you did? Who else in your life would be interested to know about the new things you learned about yourself when you were able to keep the anger out of the picture? How do you think you can help other people see the qualities you drew upon to act differently from the way depression usually gets you to act? If you both were more and more successful in keeping the mistrust out of your marriage, how do you think your relationship with each other would develop over the next 5 years?

White and Epston's method challenges family members' unquestioned assumptions about the problem. Essentially, if family members accept the idea that the problem is an external influence on them rather than an attribute of a single family member, then the system of complementary biased perceptions that sustains the symptomatic cycle is altered.

Some therapists might find White's method too cognitively oriented and recoil at the cryptic nature of some of his suggested questions. Some family members might find questions such as these irrelevant, and might feel that the therapist is not taking their problems seriously enough. As with any technique, therapists should not use it unless they feel comfortable with it, believe it can be helpful, and are employing it flexibly as a means toward an end rather than as an end in itself.

One pitfall that must be avoided if this method is used is the possibility that the family members might see the problem as an external force that is *victimizing* the symptomatic person. To avoid this pitfall, the therapist must map the influence of the problem on *all* members of the family, not limiting the inquiry just to the symptomatic member. If the family members can't identify the ways in which the problem has affected them all, then the method should probably not be used. Even in these cases, however, the therapist can point to the unique outcomes and encourage the family members to take note of these, as demonstration of their unacknowledged competency over the problem. In other words, the therapist should invite the family to explore the question: How is it that we are not *worse* than we are?

Meeting Privately with Individual Family Members

Some family therapists insist that the entire family come for every session and refuse to meet with individual family members even when a family member requests a private meeting. I believe, however, that individual sessions can be a useful adjunct to family therapy by helping to complement the work being done in the family sessions. What is important is not who is in the room but what is in the therapist's head (i.e., his hypotheses about the family and his reasons for selecting one method over another at a particular time).

At the beginning of therapy, individual sessions can help the therapist assess the contribution of an individual family member to the symptomatic cycle and facilitate the process of joining with a particular family member. In the middle stages of therapy, while the therapist is focusing efforts on disrupting patterns, individual sessions can be used to challenge a family member to change. In the later stages of therapy, after the symptomatic cycle has been disrupted, individual sessions can help family members meet the challenges associated with the resumption of their developmental process.

Individual Sessions Early in Therapy

It might be helpful to request a private session with a family member to explore in more depth a topic that the therapist believes is not appropriate to discuss in the presence of the entire family. For example, a therapist might learn in the first sessions with the family that the father received a medical discharge from the service for combat-related stress, or that the mother was hospitalized for depression before she was married, and might want to gather more information about these experiences to determine if they are important to the family's current situation.

Individual sessions early in treatment can further the process of joining with a particular family member. As I have emphasized throughout this chapter and the previous one, therapists must utilize their relationships with each member of the family to stimulate new interactional patterns among the family members. Thus, a strong relationship with each member of the family is crucial if the therapist is to engage this person in the process of change.

In some cases, the therapist finds it difficult to join with one or more members of the family in the context of the family session. For example, a peripheral father might reluctantly come to an initial session scheduled by the mother, who proceeds to dominate the session and interrupts whenever the therapist attempts to connect with the father. One possibility is to block the mother's interruptions and persist in trying to engage the father in the family session. This approach, if used in the first few sessions before the therapist has built a solid relationship with the mother, might offend her and may result in her dropping out of therapy. Yet, to ignore the father reinforces his peripheral position in the family. The therapist might decide to request an individual session with the father so that he can concentrate on his relationship with the father, without the distraction of worrying about his relationship with the other members of the family.

Often, an individual session or two early in therapy is necessary to engage an adolescent in treatment. Many (if not most) youngsters come to therapy reluctantly and expect the therapist to take the parents' side. Meeting individually with the adolescent is a good way to communicate that the therapist is interested in him or her as a person and is committed to making therapy a valuable experience for the youngster. If the adolescent is particularly resistant to the idea of participating in therapy, some of the suggestions in Chapter 6 (pp. 184–187) might be helpful.

The Issue of Confidentiality

Before meeting alone with any member of the family, the therapist must decide whether information disclosed in a private meeting will be held in confidence. There are arguments for and against the practice of offering confidentiality to individual family members. Family members (especially adolescents) might be more willing to disclose important information if the therapist promises not to report this information to the other members of the family. On the other hand, a therapist who is told a family secret risks being inducted into a coalition with the family member who revealed the secret and, as a result, may lose the trust of the other members of the family. Family members could get in the habit of holding back in family sessions and instead use confidential individual sessions with the therapist to express feelings or thoughts that the therapist believes should be brought up in the family session.

However the therapist decides to resolve the issue of confidentiality, it is essential that all family members understand the conditions under which information disclosed in individual sessions might be reported to other members of the family. This issue must be discussed explicitly with the entire family before the therapist meets individually with anyone. It is important also to keep in mind that in many jurisdictions, parents have the right to insist that the therapist disclose information obtained in a private session with a minor child. If the therapist believes it is essential to offer confidentiality to a minor, he or she should obtain an explicit agreement to that effect from the parents before meeting with the child.

At the beginning of therapy, I inform the family that there are circumstances in which confidentiality will not apply (e.g., immediate danger to self or others, child abuse) and explain that in these instances, I might unilaterally decide to disclose confidential information in order to protect someone from serious bodily harm. I then discuss the ground rules for individual sessions. I tell the family that keeping important secrets from one another could jeopardize our work together. Whenever I meet alone with a family member, I ask if he or she would permit me to share any information we discuss with the other members of the family if I feel it would be helpful to do so. If family members request confidentiality, I will usually agree, but I tell them in advance that I might encourage them to reveal the confidential disclosure to other members of the family if I decide that keeping the information secret would seriously compromise my ability to help them as a family. I suggest that they not tell me anything that they would absolutely not consider revealing to other family members. If a family member expresses the desire to have confidential sessions on a regular basis, I will first evaluate the validity of this request, and if it appears appropriate, I might refer that person to a colleague while I continue to work with the entire family.

Individual Sessions in the Middle Phase of Therapy

After the therapist has identified the symptomatic cycle and negotiated a goal with the family, the subsequent sessions focus on disrupting the cycle and encouraging new patterns among family members. The therapist uses her relationship with individual family members to encourage them to restrain themselves from their usual ways of responding and instead experiment with new ways of solving problems. While most of this work can and should take place in the family sessions, it is also helpful at times to meet individually with a member of the family.

For example, in working with a family where the father relies on authoritarian methods of discipline and recoils from even gentle challenges in the family sessions, the therapist might meet alone with the father to help him understand that his reactions to the therapist's challenges are making it difficult for the therapist to be helpful to the family. Rather than confronting the father directly, the therapist might frame his aversion to the therapist's challenges as a sign that their relationship is not strong. The individual session can be used to strengthen the relationship with the father and to secure his assurance that he will allow the therapist to challenge him in future family sessions.

Periodically, the therapist should meet individually with the adolescent to maintain his connection with the youngster. Even when the therapist has joined successfully with the adolescent early in treatment, it is prudent to keep checking back in with the youth, especially if the family sessions have focused on supporting the parents' authority.

For example, the therapist might meet alone with an adolescent to coach her in ways of more effectively communicating her opinions to her parents. Or, if the therapist believes that it is necessary to confront the adolescent about something, the therapist might first ask her to decide whether she wants the therapist to be honest with her or whether she prefers the therapist to hold back and not risk offending her feelings. Many adolescents will be more receptive to hearing confrontations when they don't have to risk losing face in front of the other family members, and when they believe that the therapist cares enough about the relationship to be honest, even at the risk of offending them.

I want to stress that the most effective use of these individual sessions during the middle phases of therapy is not to work on issues that the family members identify as personal or private. This work is best delayed until later in treatment (to be discussed). The purpose of these individual sessions is to use the relationships that had been forged during the early phases of therapy to challenge the family member to change in ways that will help disrupt the symptomatic cycle. The best challenge is one that is couched in terms of the relationship with the therapist; that is, the therapist requests a personal commitment from the family member to try something new for the sake of the relationship with the therapist and whether or not another family member changes also. For example, in a private session, the therapist asks an authoritarian father for a personal commitment to try less punitive methods of discipline, a commitment that is not made to anyone but the therapist and that is not contingent upon anyone else in the family changing.

Individual Sessions Late in Treatment

Once the symptomatic cycle has been disrupted, the individual development of each family member is free to resume. Signs that individual development is resuming include the following: (1) the symptomatic person begins to engage in age-appropriate activities at higher frequency; (2) he or she begins to bring up developmentally appropriate issues at family sessions; (3) the parents begin addressing the change in their relationship ensuing from the family life-cycle progression; and (4) suppressed family conflicts rise to the surface.

Families often vacillate between stasis and change. When the cycle is disrupted, development resumes, which creates anxiety and triggers the reemergence of the cycle. The return of the cycle halts the developmental process once again. The therapist returns to disrupting the symptomatic cycle, only for the pattern to repeat. Thus, therapists should postpone addressing issues of individual development until there is convincing evidence that the family has replaced symptomatic patterns with new, more flexible and adaptive patterns.

Individual sessions with the symptomatic person may be beneficial at this point to help address the developmental crisis directly. Once the symptomatic cycle is disrupted, formerly symptomatic adolescents often face challenges that are developmentally normal but for which they are inadequately prepared, because their own developmental process had been delayed by the cycle. These demands generate anxiety that could lead to the reemergence of the symptomatic cycle.

The metaphor of "multiple selves" or "multiple voices," proposed by Richard Schwartz (1987, 1995), can be useful at this juncture. Each part of the person (facet of the self) could be labeled as a "self" or "voice" and the characteristics of this part of the self delineated and explored. Through this process, adolescents learn to reflect on their behavior, which makes them less likely to react impulsively. For example, in the case discussed earlier, Tina was encouraged to get to know the parts of herself that we identified as "anorexia," "bulimia," "the little girl," and "the young adult." In so doing, she embraced the conception of herself as a complex person who could tolerate ambivalence and avoid reacting impulsively to anxiety.

It is important to note that it is not just the symptomatic adolescent who faces developmental challenges. The development of all family members is free to proceed once the symptomatic cycle is disrupted. It would be an error to focus attention strictly on the developmental issues of the postsymptomatic adolescent while neglecting to consider the disorientation that other family members are likely to experience once development resumes. Parents might need help with the complementary developmental challenge of redefining their role as parents of a developing teenager (Steinberg & Steinberg, 1994).

Pitfalls at This Stage

Stalemates

Most family members come to therapy feeling hopeless about their situation. They have tried many ineffective solutions to their problem. They have considered whether they should simply learn to "live with" their problem. They want to be rid of their problem, but they are unsure what the cost (emotional or financial) will be. Family members might try to "bargain" with the therapist. They express willingness to change, but not to the degree necessary to eliminate the problem. Instead, they might dicker about how much change to exchange for how much relief. Some families present the therapist with the paradox, "Rid us of the problem but don't change us" (Selvini-Palazzoli, Boscolo, Cecchin, & Prata, 1978), which places the systemically minded therapist in a double bind.

Many therapists refer to the family's apparent struggle with change as evidence of "resistance." This term, which typically refers to the family's apparent refusal to comply with therapeutic interventions, is a controversial one in family therapy. Proponents of models that describe families as homeostatic systems have no difficulty with the term and define it as the system's efforts to resist change (Hoffman, 1981). Other therapists reject the concept completely, and describe it instead as a mismatch between the expectations of the family and those of the therapist (de Shazer, 1985). Still others view the family members' apparent resistance as their recoil against the anxiety generated by altering the delicate balance of closeness and distance in their relationships (Kerr & Bowen, 1988).

Any of these models can explain why a particular family seems not to respond to the therapist's interventions by changing in expected ways. What is most helpful, however, is for the therapist not to blame the family for the apparent lack of movement in therapy. The therapist should always consider the possibility that he may be contributing to the impasse. For example, has the therapist given up on the family? Is the therapist abdicating her responsibility to challenge the family? Has the therapist lost focus by deviating from the stated goal and contract? Has the therapist allowed herself to be triangled by the family by accepting the role of mediator for family conflicts?

Therapists who are at an impasse with a family might feel anxious, inadequate, incompetent, or angry. To deal with these feelings in a way that will not impede treatment, the therapist must accept these feelings as her own and not blame them on the family. Two ways that therapists often deal unproductively with their feelings of frustration are by *triangling in another professional* or by *abandoning a systemic frame*.

Triangulation of Another Professional

Calling in a consultant (e.g., for medication or psychological testing) at a time when the therapy is stuck runs the risk of triangling the consultant into a conflict between the family and the therapist (Carl & Jurkovic, 1983). According to Kerr and Bowen (1988), when the anxiety in any two-person system cannot be contained within that system, one person in the dyad typically "triangles" in a third person. Similarly, if the therapist and the family have reached an impasse, the anxiety associated with the impasse might be too great to be contained in the therapeutic system. At this point, the family might attempt to triangle in another expert, by requesting a "second opinion" or quoting literature that appears to refute the therapist's approach. The therapist, too, might attempt to discharge the anxiety associated with the impasse by triangling in another party, such as a consultant. The therapist, feeling frustrated and "stuck" with a nonresponsive family, might feel there is no alternative to a consultation. The consultant is in most danger of being triangled when the therapist fails to realize this, and instead defines the reason for the consultation as "for the family" rather than for him- or herself.

Before calling in a consultant, the therapist should examine his or her motives for doing so. Is the therapist attempting to find an ally to join in a coalition against the family? Does the therapist want to terminate therapy but is reluctant to address this issue directly with the family? Does the therapist feel frustrated or angry at family members for their noncompliance and, rather than dealing with these feelings directly, invite a consultant to defuse the conflict?

One of the ways to avoid this pitfall is for the consultant to meet with the therapist in the presence of the family. The roles of the therapist and the consultant should be clearly negotiated, and the family apprised of these roles. The consultant must recognize that his or her role is to dissolve the impasse in the therapeutic system. This will generally require an intervention that changes the way the problem is defined (see Omer, 1994), or changes the pattern of interaction between the therapist and the family. The case discussed in Chapter 7 presents an example of an effective consultation that helps to dissolve a symptomatic cycle involving a therapist and a family.

Abandoning a Systemic Frame

When a family does not seem to be responding to family therapy, the therapist might be induced to join with the nonsymptomatic family members in scapegoating the symptomatic member. The nonsymptomatic family members might interact with the therapist in a way that suggests they see themselves not as patients but as cotherapists trying to "help" the symptomatic person. Gradually, the family sessions begin to focus less on family interactions in the room and more on educating the nonsymptomatic family members about the "right" way to interact with the symptomatic member.

The therapist's approach is reinforced when the nonsymptomatic family members appear to comply with the therapist's instructions. If the symptomatic person fails to improve in response to these interventions, then the therapist could be induced to collude with the family in scapegoating the symptomatic member as "noncompliant" or "suffering from serious psychopathology." At these times, the therapist might be inclined to dismiss the other family members from treatment and work individually with the symptomatic member. The nonsymptomatic family members are only too happy to comply with this suggestion, relieved that the therapist has finally vindicated them. However, once the therapist begins meeting individually with the symptomatic member, little leverage remains for the therapist to intervene directly in family patterns that support the symptom. The symptoms might intensify, and the therapist might interpret this intensity as a sign of increased anxiety in response to "dealing with meaningful material" in the individual therapy sessions. As more material surfaces in the individual sessions, the therapist becomes more convinced that the symptomatic member is indeed severely impaired and that individual therapy is the most appropriate treatment strategy (Haley, 1980). What the therapist has not recognized is that she and the family are now participating in a symptomatic cycle.

Under certain circumstances, it is possible to effect change in the symptomatic cycle by working through a single member of the family. For example, strategic interventions are often directed through a single family member (Haley, 1976; Madanes, 1981). Bowenian therapists target a single individual and work to increase his or her level of differentiation from the other members of the family (Kerr & Bowen, 1988). Szapozknik, Kurtines, Foote, Perez-Vidal, and Heris (1983) have shown success with "one-person family therapy" utilizing structural methods. All of these methods see the individual patient through the lens of the symptomatic cycle. The goal is to alter symptomatic patterns by working through a single person, not to explore intrapsychic dynamics.

There is, of course, another pitfall associated with working with a single family member: The therapist could unwittingly become inducted into a coalition with that family member against the rest of the family. This coalition can be overt or covert. When overt, the therapist might side with the patient in conflicts with the other family members. When covert, the therapist might accept the individual's biased perception of events and conclude that the family is "too dysfunctional" to succeed in family therapy. In either case, the therapist has been inducted into the symptomatic cycle and thereby rendered less effective as an agent of change.

ENDING THERAPY: BEYOND THE SYMPTOMATIC CYCLE

As the symptomatic cycle is disrupted, conflicts previously avoided will often surface. Addressing these conflicts might require the family members to reconsider major decisions about their marriage, living arrangements, custody, finances, or careers. Despite the turmoil that sometimes ensues, the therapist should expect these conflicts to emerge and should avoid intruding unnecessarily on the family members' efforts to find their own solutions.

There are important differences between the uproar accompanying the symptomatic cycle and the natural turmoil associated with the process of conflict resolution. While family members once responded to conflicts with control or flight, they now face conflicts openly and directly. Family members are now less inclined to react impulsively to frustration and more likely to tolerate anxiety while they listen to each other and consider all points of view.

In the final phase of therapy, the role of the therapist becomes more superfluous as the family members utilize the repertoire of skills at their disposal to deal with the issues facing them. Now more than ever, the therapist should allow the family to struggle on its own. In most cases, the therapist need only make minor suggestions or adjustments to the family's way of handling the problem. One key role for the therapist at this stage is to encourage the family members to face their conflicts and persist until they are resolved.

Pitfalls at This Stage

Overreacting

The therapist might overreact to intense affect in the family and assume that the family is responding to a crisis in ways reminiscent of the symptomatic cycle. Once the end phases of therapy are reached, therapists must restrain themselves from intervening prematurely, but rather allow family members to struggle with conflict on their own. Unless there is convincing evidence that the symptomatic cycle is returning, therapists should remain in a supportive role, normalizing any strife, and encouraging family members to utilize their newly discovered resources to handle the conflict.

Premature Disengagement

Though less serious than the previous pitfall, it is also possible that therapists could disengage too quickly from the family. Unless therapy was contracted as time-limited at the start, it is best to allow the family to decide when to terminate therapy. Many therapists feel compelled to advise termination as soon as the family appears to be handling matters well on its own. Often, however, the family needs continued support from the therapist to avoid regressing. Rather than terminating abruptly, it is usually preferable to decrease the frequency of the sessions gradually.

SUMMARY

We have covered much ground in this chapter, so before ending I want to summarize the major points. The approach I am advocating in this book rests on four major concepts:

- *The symptomatic cycle.* By attempting to control or eliminate the symptom, the family members fall into a rigid pattern of interactions that keep them from utilizing parts of themselves that could lead to a resolution of the problem.
- *The multifaceted self.* As Sal Minuchin has said, we are all more complex than we realize. We all have untapped resources that under the right circumstances can be brought to the fore. Family members caught in a symptomatic cycle repeatedly draw upon only a small part of themselves. One of the goals of therapy is to help the family members experience parts of themselves that are not usually evident to them or other family members and then to use these new aspects of themselves to respond differently to one another.
- *Arrested development.* Family members become increasingly constricted as they repeatedly draw upon the parts of themselves that participate in the symptomatic cycle. This process is occurring not only in the symptomatic person but in all participants in the symptomatic cycle.
- *Interlocking narratives and the complementarity of biased perceptions.* Each family member develops beliefs about the problem and about the other members of the family. These beliefs tend to be self-confirming as evidence supporting the beliefs is noticed and evidence refuting the beliefs is ignored. Often, the beliefs that family members have about each other reinforce one another in a complementary fashion.

To help families break free from symptomatic patterns, the therapist must first identify the symptomatic cycle in the family and then use a variety of methods to help disrupt the cycle and introduce the family members to new ways of interacting with one another.

To identify the symptomatic cycle, the therapist attends to the following information:

Language: How do the family members describe the problem?

History: What solutions have already been tried?

Transactions: How do the family members interact with one another?

After constructing a hypothesis about the symptomatic cycle from this information, the therapist then offers the family a formulation of the problem and a contract for treatment. The formulation of the problem must link the symptom to the interactions in the family and provide a unique perspective on the problem that differs from the ways that family members have viewed the problem thus far. The proposed contract focuses on changing the ways that family members interact with one another.

After the family members have agreed to the contract, the therapist then proceeds to disrupt the symptomatic cycle. *The basic principle is this: The therapist uses his or her relationship with each member of the family to encourage change in the ways in which the family members respond to each other.* Some specific methods that might be useful to achieve this goal include: promoting dialogue, uncovering hidden conflicts, discouraging control, encouraging unilateral change, identifying and enacting "unique outcomes," constructing new narratives, and meeting privately with individual family members. Therapy ends as the therapist gradually disengages while the family members utilize their repertoire of new skills to deal with the issues facing them. Now, more than ever, the therapist should allow the family members to struggle on their own and intervene as little as possible.

WHAT COMES NEXT

The following chapters expand on these ideas by showing how they can be applied to common problems facing families with adolescents: eating disorders, depression and suicide, aggression and defiant behavior, psychosis, school-related problems, and problems associated with "leaving home." In Chapter 4, for example, I return to the case of Tina and discuss the process of treatment in more detail. First, however, I examine what developmental psychologists have learned about the second decade of life. In the next chapter, I provide an overview of current research on adolescent development to serve as a backdrop against which the diagnosis and treatment of problems of adolescence should be viewed.

NOTES

1. The relationship between adolescent adjustment and family functioning has been well documented in the literature (e.g., Alexander, 1973; Hauser et al., 1984; Levin & Schonberg, 1987; Offer & Offer, 1975; Plass & Hotaling, 1995; Steinberg, Lamborn, Darling, Mounts, & Dornbusch, 1994). Several studies have supported the efficacy of family therapy for treating problems of adolescents (e.g., Chamberlain & Rosicky, 1995; Gutstein, Rudd, Graham, & Rayha, 1988; Joanning, Quinn, Thomas, & Mullen, 1992; Liddle & Dakoff,

1995; Robin, Siegel, Koepke, Moye, & Tice, 1994; Russell, Szmulker, Dare, & Eisler, 1987; Seelig, Goldman-Hall, & Jerrell, 1992; Tavantzis, Tavantzis, Brown, & Rohrbaugh, 1985; Tolan, Cromwell, & Brasswell, 1986). At least one author has argued that family therapy is the "treatment of choice" for troubled adolescents (Fishman, 1988).

2. The typical challenges faced by youngsters and families during adolescence are discussed in detail in the next chapter.

3. I do not mean to imply that family members first come to see each other differently and then act differently based on these new views. The process is circular and recursive. The therapist elicits new behaviors from each family member in the presence of the others, and seeing this new behavior the other family members have the opportunity to respond differently than they usually do. Alternatively, the therapist can directly encourage the family members to change their views of each other, perhaps by calling attention to previous behaviors they may not have noticed. The latter approach is similar to that of Michael White and David Epston (1990) and is discussed later in this chapter.

4. In carrying out an "enactment," the therapist asks the family members to interact in a particular way in the session. For example, a therapist might ask two parents to arrive at a decision without interruption by the child. The therapist insists that the parents continue their dialogue in the session until they reach a decision and prevents the child from interrupting by moving him or her to another part of the room.

CHAPTER 3

ADOLESCENT DEVELOPMENT

Let's consider six quick vignettes:

Vignette 1: *Jill, age 13, is afraid to go to a party because she thinks everyone will notice the pimple that has just sprouted on her nose.*

Vignette 2: *Sean, age 15, knows that it is dangerous for people to ride their bicycles on an unlit highway at night but frequently does it anyway, because he believes that no harm will come to him.*

Vignette 3: *Rod, age 16, can't seem to decide on a career and vacillates weekly between wanting to be a physician and wanting to study art.*

Vignette 4: *Gloria, age 13, is certain that she wants to be a surgeon like her mother, and has never even considered other careers.*

Vignette 5: *Bonnie, age 14, is flabbergasted when a close friend bursts into tears at a casual remark Bonnie made about her hair.*

Vignette 6: *Rick, age 15, argues that he would not divulge the identity of a friend who has broken into a neighbor's home, because he believes that loyalty to one's friends is his most important value.*

———◆———

It may come as a surprise to many families, but these vignettes all describe typical and developmentally normal adolescent behavior. Many adults, including many mental health professionals, continue to hold the view that adolescent turmoil is a universal phenomenon (Offer, Ostrov, & Howard, 1981). They are wrong. Developmental psychologists long ago abandoned the idea that adolescence is inevitably characterized by emotional turmoil and upheaval. This "storm and stress" view of adolescence was first proposed by G. Stanley Hall (1904) and reinforced by early psychoanalytic thinking (Freud, 1958; Blos, 1962). However, these early notions were based on a biased sample of adolescents who were in treatment. Recent studies, based upon more representative, random samples of adolescents, have failed to find support for widespread turmoil (see Offer & Schonert-Reichl, 1992).

Belief in this erroneous "storm and stress" view of adolescence can have a number of adverse consequences:

1. *Ignoring serious problems.* Families and therapists can underestimate the severity of disturbance in an adolescent who presents for treatment by misinterpreting problematic behavior as developmentally normal. If parents believe that it is typical for an adolescent to be moody, irritable, and sullen, they can aggravate the problem by ignoring it.

2. *Overreacting.* Families and therapists may overreact by assuming that a behavior signals pathology, when in fact it is typical for many adolescents. For example, if Rod's parents conclude that his uncertainty is problematic, they might exert pressure on him to make a decision before he is ready to do so. If Jill's parents interpret her anxiety as evidence of low self-esteem, she may begin seeing herself in this way also.

3. *Self-fulfilling prophecies.* Biased and inaccurate perceptions of adolescents can create self-fulfilling prophecies (Rosenthal & Jacobson, 1968). If Sean's parents interpret his behavior as evidence of irresponsible recklessness, they are apt to respond in a punitive way that could push Sean to exhibit more such behavior in an effort to assert his autonomy. Similarly, since these perceptions reinforce one another (Chapter 2), Sean may begin seeing his parents as controlling and punitive authority figures who do not support his efforts to achieve greater autonomy.

4. *Inhibiting growth by restricting freedom.* Widespread belief that adolescents are by nature out of control can lead institutions to develop restrictive policies that limit the civil rights of adolescents and deprive them of opportunities for growth through exploration (Quadrel, Fischhoff, & Davis, 1993). Ineffective educational practices emphasizing discipline and sanctions can be perpetuated (Eccles et al., 1993). Interactions between adolescents and adults can quickly turn into unproductive power struggles.

Stereotypes about adolescents as wild, rebellious, and disdainful of authority can lead parents to overreact when their child challenges them. Believing that teenagers aren't interested in a relationship with them, many parents back off too quickly, which deprives youngsters of the nurturance and guidance they continue to need (Mackey, 1996). In doing so, parents fail to provide the optimal context for growth during this stage of life. Adolescents need parents who allow them ample room to experience the consequences of their own decisions, but who also provide reasonable limits that mirror the limits the adolescent is likely to encounter in the adult world.

The purpose of this chapter is to review the literature on normal adolescent development so to provide a context for the discussion of problems of adolescents and their families in the subsequent chapters. I shall not attempt to cover all of the voluminous literature on adolescent development but rather highlight information that is most relevant to the practicing clinician. Readers who are interested in a more detailed discussion of normal adolescent development can consult one of the many fine textbooks in the field (e.g., Feldman & Elliott, 1990; Muus, 1996; Steinberg, 1996).

DEVELOPMENTAL ISSUES OF ADOLESCENCE: AN OVERVIEW

We can divide the second decade of life into three general phases, during each of which a particular set of developmental challenges is at the forefront. These stages and the accompanying issues are as follows:

Early adolescence (ages 11–13)

- Adjusting to pubertal changes
- Learning to use new cognitive capacities
- Finding a place among peers
- Dealing with gender-related expectations

Middle adolescence (ages 14–16)

- Handling sexuality
- Making moral decisions
- Developing new relationships with peers
- Balancing autonomy and accountability

Late adolescence (ages 17–19)

- Consolidating an identity
- Experiencing intimacy
- Leaving home

Although the unfolding of these developmental challenges describes the typical pattern for adolescents in our culture, it is also important to keep in mind three considerations:

1. *Context and the definition of normality.* Any discussion of "normality" poses a paradox: How can we describe what is normal without being so inclusive that the description is meaningless, or so restrictive that any deviations from the norm are considered pathological? Needless to say, our ideas of what is normative is influenced by cultural expectations.

Adolescents are often considered troubled when they exhibit behavior that violates the norms of a particular setting, such as home, school, cr community. But all behavior exists in a context. Labeling an individual "troubled" assumes that the problem exists *inside the person* rather than *in the context.* Efforts are then directed to treating the troubled individual rather than trying to understand why his or her behavior does not fit the context. A mismatch between the kid and the context does not necessarily signal a problem with either, but it does suggest that a change in context might be considered instead of, or in addition to, a change in the youth.

To take a dramatic example, one adolescent I saw was determined that school was not relevant to him. He struggled through school, often experiencing debilitating bouts of depression when the workload piled up. Originally, the parents (and I) assumed that the school problems were a result of the boy's depression. However, pharmacology and psychotherapy appeared to relieve the boy's depression but did not improve his motivation at school. Only in the course of several sessions of individual and family therapy did it occur to us that the school problems and depression fed each other: As the boy became more depressed, he could function less well at school. But, also, as the boy felt more and more trapped at school, he became more and more depressed. Finally, in resignation, the parents acceded to the boy's wish to drop out of school after the 10th grade. The boy got a job working at a plant nursery and supplemented his minimum-wage income with a second, part-time job as a janitor. Though the boy was working over 60 hours a week, he was no longer depressed.

This case is perhaps extreme, but other, less dramatic instances can be identified as well. While we can't ignore the potentially negative consequences of "marching to one's own drummer," we shouldn't rule out the possibility that the negative outcomes might not happen, and that the young person might indeed be happy living a "deviant" lifestyle.

2. *Asynchronicity in development.* Consider the case of the 6-foot, 200 pound quarterback who was an "early bloomer" and at age 14 had

essentially completed his physical growth. Now consider his classmate, who at 5'6" and 140 pounds has hardly begun. The divergent physical appearances of these boys can elicit different expectations from adults. Will not the quarterback be expected to act more mature, while less mature behavior will be tolerated from his classmate? Will not adults assume that the quarterback is capable of handling more privileges than his late-blooming classmate?

The course of development is not necessarily linear or coordinated in all areas. An adolescent almost always develops at different rates in different areas. The youngster whose body has not yet physically matured may be capable of sophisticated reasoning, while the adolescent whose body appears similar to an adult's may be unable to appreciate the perspective of another person.

The error of assuming that development proceeds at the same pace in all areas can lead parents to expect too much of a youngster. Just because an adolescent is mature in one area doesn't mean that he or she is mature in other areas as well. Just as the adolescent's body becomes gangly because different parts of it grow at different rates, we can say the same about adolescent development in general. It is a "gangly" time of life, because advances in one area are not necessarily in pace with advances in others.

3. Interaction between adolescent and parental developmental issues. Psychological development continues throughout the lifespan. While our focus will be on adolescent development, we should also keep in mind that parents are facing developmental challenges as well.

In some cases, it is the adolescent's struggle that triggers the complementary struggle in the parent (see Steinberg & Steinberg, 1994). For example, a mother experiencing menopause might feel threatened by her daughter's nascent sexuality, and so responds by attempting to restrict the girl, who reacts by hiding her sexual experimentation from her mother.

In other cases, the adolescent is progressing normally, but it is the parent who is struggling with his or her complementary developmental challenge and projecting this struggle onto the adolescent. A father who is going through a "midlife crisis" of regret over his own achievement might exert pressure on his son to get higher grades in school. The boy responds to his father's pressure by prematurely asserting his decision to forego college and become a construction worker.

Try to recall these three considerations (context and the definition of normality, asynchronicity in development, and the interaction between adolescent and parental developmental issues) as we examine in more detail the events of the three phases of adolescence.

EARLY ADOLESCENCE

Adjusting to Pubertal Changes

What's Happening?

The most public signs of adolescence are the physical changes associated with puberty. While the development of secondary sexual characteristics, such as breasts in girls and facial hair in boys, is the most obvious, the biological changes that initiate puberty start long before evidence of these changes becomes visible (Buchanan, Eccles, & Becker, 1992). Menarche, for example, occurs midway through the process of pubertal development for girls. For boys, first ejaculation, usually experienced between ages 11½ and 14½ during masturbation or nocturnal emission (Stein & Reiser, 1994), occurs only after several other less obvious physical changes have occurred.

The adolescent "growth spurt" is a well-known phenomenon, as is the observation that girls, on the average, experience their growth spurt about 2 years earlier than boys (Marshall, 1978). The gangly appearance of many adolescents seems to be associated with the fact that different parts of the body grow at different rates (Tanner, 1972). It is also well-documented that puberty occurs at an earlier age than in previous centuries. For example, the average age of first menstruation in 1990 was 13, while in 1900, it was 15½. This phenomenon is known as the "secular trend" and seems to be attributable to improved environmental conditions such as wider availability of good nutrition and better health care (Eveleth & Tanner, 1976).

Am I Developing Normally?

Some adolescents worry whether their bodies are developing normally. They become preoccupied with their bodies and overreact to minor somatic symptoms. Education about the typical sequence and tempo of pubertal changes can help to reassure a worried adolescent.

The physical changes of adolescence generally follow a predictable sequence for both boys and girls, though there can be some variability, especially for girls. While the sequence of pubertal changes is more or less predictable, there is far more variability in the timing of these changes. Early-developing girls, for example, can experience first menstruation at age 10, while late-developing girls may not menstruate until age 16. Similarly, for boys, testicular growth may start as early as age 10 or as late as age 13. There is also individual variability in the length of time an adolescent takes to complete the pubertal changes. The interval can range from 1½ to 6 years in girls and from 2 to 5 years in boys. There does not appear to be a relationship between the age at which puberty begins and the rate at which it proceeds (Tanner, 1972).

Raging Hormones?

It is a controversial issue whether the hormonal changes associated with puberty significantly affect an adolescent's mood and behavior. According to one study (Csikszentmihalyi & Larson, 1984), adolescents' moods are more intense and change more frequently and rapidly than do moods of adults. At first glance, this finding seems to confirm the "storm and stress" view of adolescents as moody and unstable. But the authors of this study reported another finding: Adolescents and adults are comparable in the degree to which their moods can be predicted from the environment. According to Csikszentmihalyi and Larson, adolescents may appear to be more moody than adults because "teenagers move from one context to the next more rapidly than adults, and thus their emotions have a greater chance of being affected by situational factors" (p. 123).

Whether hormonal changes play a significant role in influencing these moods is a different issue. While there is some evidence of an association between hormones and mood, the commonly held belief that adolescent mood swings are a result of hormonal changes is not strongly supported by available evidence (Buchanan et al., 1992). Hormonal influences on mood and behavior appear to be far less important than environmental and psychosocial factors.

Psychological Impact of Pubertal Changes

The physical changes associated with puberty, in themselves, have little negative impact on the adolescent's self-image, except in one instance: when the adolescent is going through puberty around the same time she is experiencing other changes in life, such as changing schools (Simmons, Burgeson, Carlton-Ford, & Blyth, 1987). Far more important than the physical changes themselves is the reaction of the social context to the adolescent's physical changes (Brooks-Gunn & Reiter, 1990). Girls, in particular, are at risk for developing eating disorders because of the societal emphasis on thinness (Attie & Brooks-Gunn, 1989). I return to this issue in the next chapter.

Boys who mature early are accorded respect and status among their peers, but not so for girls. Early-maturing girls are often the target of lewd remarks by adolescent boys—an experience that is devastating to many girls (Pipher, 1994). Compared to girls who mature on time or late, an early-maturing girl is more likely to exhibit behavior problems, probably because she is more apt to associate with older peers who introduce her to activities (e.g., sex, substances) that she's not ready to handle (Magnusson, Strattin, & Allen, 1985; Silbereisen, Petersen, Albrecht, & Kracke, 1989).

Early maturation appears to be particularly harmful for girls who exhibit problem behavior prior to puberty. According to a study by Caspi and Moffitt (1991), early maturing girls who do not exhibit behavioral problems prior to puberty are at only slightly higher risk for postpubertal behavior problems than girls who mature on time or late. In contrast, among girls who exhibit behavioral problems prior to puberty, early-maturing girls are more likely to display problem behavior in adolescence than are girls who mature on time or late.

Impact of Puberty on Family Relations

At the onset of puberty, it is common for adolescents and their parents to experience increased distance in their relationship (Steinberg, 1987b). Adolescents seem to become allergic to parental curiosity. Locked doors and hushed phone conversations only serve to make their parents more curious.

This change in family relationship seems to occur regardless of the age at which the adolescent enters puberty, suggesting that it is puberty itself that correlates with increased distance from parents, not simply age. It is likely that a process of mutual withdrawal is taking place. The adolescent prefers more privacy and the parents back off, because they think that they need to give the adolescent "space," or they are simply trying to avoid conflict.

Parents who are threatened by the pubertal adolescent's increased desire for privacy might elicit a backlash from the adolescent, who withdraws even more to avoid parental scrutiny. Parents who have relied on the child to meet their needs might feel personally rejected, and respond by becoming depressed or by rejecting the adolescent in retaliation. In other cases, the parental relationship comes into sharp relief when the adolescent removes him- or herself from the picture. The child who was triangled into a detoured parental conflict, who now removes himself or herself from the triangle, puts the parents squarely in contact with one another and forces them to confront their own unresolved marital issues (Haley, 1980).

Learning to Use New Cognitive Capacities

The Shift to Formal Operational Thought

Adolescents begin to develop more sophisticated modes of thought that include increased ability to think about future possibilities, increased awareness of alternatives, abstract reasoning, and relative thinking. They also become aware that it is possible to think about thinking itself (metacognition). Jean Piaget has identified these cognitive abilities as *formal operational thinking* (Inhelder & Piaget, 1958).

It might come as a surprise to many parents (and therapists) that during adolescence, thinking becomes more sophisticated. To them, adolescents appear rigid, unyielding, unable to foresee alternatives, and unable to reflect on themselves. If anything, it seems more difficult to reason with an adolescent than with a younger child.

It is possible to reconcile these apparently contradictory views. On the one hand, adolescents become capable of more sophisticated modes of thought. On the other hand, they are not yet experienced in the use of these new capabilities. Therefore, they are in transition from the more concrete modes of reasoning characteristic of children to the more sophisticated modes of reasoning associated with adulthood. Furthermore, because they are relatively unskilled in the use of these modes of thought, adolescents are prone to make certain types of cognitive errors.

Egocentricism

David Elkind (1967) has described the phenomenon of *adolescent egocentricism*, a tendency in younger adolescents to become extremely self-absorbed. According to Elkind, there are two aspects to adolescent egocentricism: the *imaginary audience* and the *personal fable*. The former refers to the tendency for many young adolescents to imagine that they are continually "on stage," that their behavior is the focus of everyone else's attention. Jill (Vignette 1) exemplifies this tendency in her angst over going to the party with her new pimple. The personal fable refers to the belief that one's own experiences are unique and therefore impossible for another person to understand. One manifestation of the personal fable is the belief that one is "invulnerable" to the dangerous consequences of risk-taking behavior. The case of Sean (Vignette 2) exemplifies the personal fable. Though he apparently knows the danger involved in riding his bike at night, he believes that he will somehow be exempt from harm.

Although there is some controversy regarding whether these characteristics are universal features of adolescents, or whether they describe only a minority of adolescents (see Quadrel et al., 1993), these concepts can provide parents and clinicians with a helpful framework for understanding the seemingly irrational behavior of some adolescents. Many adults, for example, find it difficult to understand why teenagers place so strong an emphasis on the evaluation of their peers.

Consider the case of Jill (Vignette 1), presented at the beginning of this chapter. Some adults might conclude that Jill's strong identification with her peer group reflects poor self-esteem and low self-reliance. However, the concept of the imaginary audience tells us that it is typical for young teenagers like Jill to worry almost obsessively about what their peers may be thinking about them. Ironically, what does not occur to the adolescent is that his or her peers are similarly concerned. What seems to the youngster to be the real opinions of the peer group are actually manifestations of the imaginary audience.

Adults who point out this irony and attempt to help the teenager gain insight into the workings of the imaginary audience are likely to fail, because they run into the wall of the other manifestation of adolescent egocentricism: the personal fable. The more adults try to convince the youngster that her way of thinking is erroneous, the more she is likely to feel misunderstood and compelled to defend her position more strongly.

The concept of adolescent egocentricism also explains the apparently greater tendency of teenagers to take what adults consider foolhardy risks. Studies of risk taking have shown that the process of weighing benefits over possible losses is very similar in adolescents and adults (Quadrel et al., 1993). However, for youngsters under the gaze of the imaginary audience, the risk of being ridiculed or ostracized by the peer group is far more threatening than many adults can comprehend.

Add to this tendency four other factors and we can understand many of the conflicts between teens and adults. First, adolescents become more facile at arguing, which make them more formidable opponents for adults than are younger children, whose concrete reasoning doesn't stand a chance against an adult's more sophisticated and abstract formal operational thinking (Steinberg, 1996). Second, adolescents have less idealized views of their parents than do younger children and are therefore more likely to question parental perceptions (Steinberg & Silverberg, 1986). The father who was idolized by his 9-year-old daughter experiences an understandable blow to his ego when his daughter, now fourteen, blithely points out all his faults, most of which he secretly acknowledges but tries to hide. Third, parents and teenagers often define issues very differently; in a sense, they live in "separate realities" (Larson & Richards, 1994; Smetana, 1989). Parents often define issues as matters of values and personal accountability while adolescents define the same issues as matters of autonomy or differences in personal taste. A parent might challenge an adolescent's choice of clothing on the grounds that "People just don't dress like that to go to school," while the teenager argues that all of *her* friends dress that way. Fourth, early adolescents are not yet fully capable of adopting the point of view of another person, particularly one whose reasoning seems alien to their own. Robert Selman (1980) has proposed an interesting theory that encompasses this latter tendency.

Taking the Perspective of Another Person

Selman posits that the capacity to take the perspective of another person progresses through a number of stages. Younger teens are just entering the stage when they can imagine what the point of view of another person might be, and so are inept at identifying when others experience a situation differently than they do. Bonnie (Vignette 5) is a case in point. She is surprised at her friend's response to her remark because she is not yet adept at recognizing that other people might experience a situation very differently than she does.

Adolescents like Bonnie are just beginning to adopt what Selman calls the "third-person perspective" that allows them to analyze a conflict between themselves and another person from a more objective and less personalized point of view. It is only later in adolescence (and for some, not until adulthood) that the young person can accurately infer the perspective of another person and also imagine the perspective of a theoretically impartial third party. Two years later, at age 17, Bonnie could say, "I have to be careful what I say to Tracey about her hair because she is very sensitive about it," or, "Tracey and I often get into arguments because we're both so stubborn."

Selman's model provides a framework for understanding how adolescents reason about social situations. It would be futile to expect kids in their early teens to appreciate the merits of points of view different from their own. They realize that the same situation could be viewed differently by different people, but they still remain invested in their own points of view and are likely to designate the others as "wrong."

For example, Gary, a bright 13-year-old, argued doggedly with his mother about the "silliness" of her rule that he lock the door whenever he left the house. "It's a stupid rule," he argued. "We live in a safe neighborhood. No one will come into the house." His mom tried to explain her opinion that the neighborhood was not as safe as Gary seemed to think, offering as evidence that a neighbor's house had been burglarized only a month before. Gary listened politely, but continued to push his point. "Can't you just see it my way?" Gary's mom finally pleaded. "No, I can't," Gary retorted. "You're just making a big deal out of nothing."

It is only later that teenagers can recognize that there are elements of right and wrong in all perspectives, and that compromise is the most prudent course. Gary's 16-year-old-sister agreed with Gary that their neighborhood was relatively safe, but also agreed that it was reasonable for her mother to want the door locked. Many parents, who are presumably adept with more sophisticated reasoning processes, engage head-to-head with the teenager in a futile battle over whose point of view will prevail, losing sight of the importance of achieving a workable compromise that takes into account the adolescent's perception of the situation and the fact that the youngster is likely to have radically different needs and tastes (Larson & Richards, 1994). Although Gary still adamantly held that he was right and his mother was wrong, he and his mother eventually agreed that whenever he left the house, it would be through the back door that locked automatically when it closed.

Finding a Place among Peers

The Importance of Peers

Early adolescence marks a dramatic shift in the importance of the peer group. The prepubertal child has friends but still puts the approval and attention of adults first. After puberty, this balance shifts. The child in his early teens appears to throw himself into his peer group, to the point that many parents feel that they are fighting a losing battle with peers for the adolescent's time and attention. Sometimes, the parents, adolescent, and peers become locked in a triangular struggle: The child uses the peer group as a way of challenging parental authority; the parents blame the peer group for the child's "bad" behavior, and the adolescent bonds with peers through shared contempt of parents.

Despite the attendant frustrations to parents, the peer group nevertheless serves important developmental functions. First, the peer group is a context where young people learn the skills that are the foundation for adult friendships and intimacy. Second, the peer group provides adolescents with a temporary reference point for their emerging sense of identity (Brown, 1990). Through identification with peers, adolescents begin the process of defining who they are and how they differ from their parents. Third, the peer group serves as a "transitional object" that midwives the process of individuation from the family of origin. It becomes a surrogate family that provides a secure context in which the adolescent can begin to experiment with independence. Thus, acceptance by a peer group becomes almost a matter of psychological survival for a young teenager. But the adolescent believes that acceptance requires conformity. Thus, it is during early adolescence that peer conformity is at its height, declining steadily after age 14 (Berndt, 1979).

Peer Pressure?

Parents often blame "peer pressure" when their adolescent misbehaves, but peer cliques simply do not operate in this fashion. An adolescent does not passively respond to peer pressure; peers are actively exerting pressure on *each other*. According to *peer cluster theory* (Oetting & Beauvais, 1987), peer cliques develop their membership and norms through a process of mutual influence. Kids who share values, attitudes, and beliefs are attracted to one another, forming highly homogeneous "peer clusters." Then, each member of the cluster participates in actively shaping the norms and behaviors of that cluster. In other words, both *selection* (choosing a friend who is similar to oneself) and *socialization* (becoming more similar to one's friends) are equally important in the formation and maintenance of adolescent peer groups (Kandel, 1978).

Dealing with Gender-Related Expectations

Gender-Role Intensification

During the early teenage years, both boys and girls experience increased pressure to behave in gender-typical ways, a process that has been termed "gender-role intensification" (Hill & Lynch, 1983). Messages from parents, peers, schools, and the media encourage boys to be strong, assertive, and self-reliant, and girls to be attractive, charming, and compliant. The extent to which the adolescent is successful in conforming to these expectations has a significant impact on his or her self-image. Masculine girls and effeminate boys are likely to be ostracized by peers and consequently experience a blow to their self-image, which can be even more intense if the adolescent is also coming to terms with homosexual feelings.

Androgyny

Earlier conceptions of masculinity and femininity as bipolar opposites have been supplanted by the realization that they are separate dimensions. Many individuals exhibit an equal mix of traditionally masculine and traditionally feminine traits, a characteristic that has been termed "androgyny" (Bem, 1975). An androgynous boy might be one who plays football on his high school team on Saturday afternoon and also enjoys taking care of the toddlers in the Sunday day care center at his church. An androgynous girl risks injury to help her team win the soccer game, then goes home to spend hours getting ready for her date that night.

While there is some evidence to support the idea that androgynous adults are better adjusted than those who are very masculine or very feminine, this does not appear to be the case for adolescents. Among teenagers, it is the masculine component of androgyny that seems to be associated with better adjustment (Markstrom-Adams, 1989). While androgynous girls show higher levels of both peer acceptance and self-acceptance than do very feminine or very masculine girls, very masculine boys show higher levels of peer acceptance and self-acceptance than do androgynous boys (Lau, 1989; Massad, 1981). For boys, "masculinity" is seen as incompatible with behaving in ways that are considered traditionally feminine. Hence, boys are actively encouraged to relinquish feminine traits. For girls, femininity is encouraged, but so are traditional masculine traits such as independence and self-reliance. The absence of masculine traits in girls is actually a disadvantage, both in terms of self-image and peer acceptance.

At first glance, it might seem that the greater tolerance for masculinity in girls places girls at an advantage relative to boys, who are actively discouraged from exhibiting feminine qualities. However, what appears to be social tolerance is often experienced by girls as a bind that takes a toll on their self-concept. Many girls become consumed with worries about not being attractive or popular, characteristics that they assume are hallmarks of success as a woman. At the same time, girls become aware that the feminine traits they are being encouraged to develop are not those that society values most highly. It is not surprising, then, that girls score lower than boys on measures of self-esteem, particularly in the early adolescent years, when they have not yet developed the cognitive sophistication to recognize and challenge these mixed messages about gender (Simmons & Rosenberg, 1975). Some experts have argued that these conflicting cultural messages explain the higher incidence of depression among adolescent and adult females as compared to adolescent and adult males (Petersen et al., 1993). Though less attention has been paid to the impact of gender role pressures on boys, recent scholarship has highlighted such consequences of masculine socialization as decreased capacity for intimacy, increased aggressiveness, and preoccupation with competition (McLean, Carey, & White, 1996).

Table 3.1 summarizes the developmental issues, and typical and atypical behaviors of early adolescence.

MIDDLE ADOLESCENCE

Handling Sexuality

The increased interest in sex and the increased capacity for engaging in sexual activity bring the adolescent face to face with issues of

TABLE 3.1. Early Adolescence (Ages 11–13)

Major developmental issues

- Adjusting to pubertal changes
- Learning to use new cognitive capacities
- Finding a place among peers
- Dealing with gender-related expectations

Typical behaviors

- Increased attention to physical appearance
- Concern about whether their bodies are developing normally
- Increased ability to reason in abstract ways
- A temporary period of extreme self-consciousness
- Idealism (i.e., because things *could* be so, they *should* be so)
- Adolescent invulnerability—apparent disregard for rules of safety ("I know it's not safe, but it won't happen to me.")
- The personal fable—self-dramatization and belief that their experiences are so unique that no one (especially adults) could possibly understand them
- Increased argumentativeness, accompanied by what may seem to be rigid thinking, because they cannot objectively weigh the merits of their own point of view against those of the person with whom they are arguing
- Intense involvement with the peer group, perhaps even to the extent of neglecting other responsibilities
- Increased conformity to peers and concern about acceptance
- Increased attention to differences between "masculine" and "feminine" gender roles and disapproval of gender-atypical behavior in others.

Signs of problems

- Appears unusually and consistently secretive about activities, particularly those that involve peers
- Consistently fails to practice personal hygiene, for example, refuses to bathe or groom
- Has no friends or doesn't seem interested in having any friends
- Gets along well with adults but doesn't relate well to peers

sexuality and sexual orientation. For some, sexual feelings arouse anxiety and result in various avoidance mechanisms that can detour social development. Others lack the capacity to delay gratification, and so may attempt to satisfy sexual needs indiscriminately. Still others recognize that the direction of their sexual interest is toward members of their own gender and experience not only the frustration of being unable to satisfy these needs but also the fear of being discovered and ostracized.

Dealing with adolescent sexuality can awaken conflicts in adults, who might not have adequately resolved their own sexuality issues. Some parents are threatened by their child's sexuality. Younger parents might be envious of the teenager's apparent sexual freedom. For older parents whose own sexual interest and prowess are waning, the adolescent's nascent sexuality can be a harsh reminder of what they have lost (Steinberg & Steinberg, 1994). Some parents follow a policy of benign neglect, grudgingly acknowledging their child's sexuality while refusing to address it directly, rationalizing that a discussion of sex with the adolescent might condone and encourage the behavior. Some parents ignore the issue entirely. Others overreact by imposing strict restrictions on dating.

Adolescent sexual values are influenced by parental values, but are far more influenced by the prevailing peer norms (Moore, Peterson, & Furstenberg, 1986; Newcomer & Udry, 1984; Treboux & Busch-Rossnagel, 1990). The availability of sexual partners in the peer group and the manner in which the peer group accords status to sexual activity are more influential than prohibitions issued by adults. There is nevertheless evidence that close relationships with parents are associated with later onset of intercourse, and that adolescents who perceive their communication with parents as poor are more likely to initiate sex early (Inazu & Fox, 1980; Jessor & Jessor, 1977). Parents who are too intent on pushing their values on the child in order to prevent early sexual activity may undermine their own efforts if the adolescent's resistance to these values leads to family conflict and communication breakdown.

Gay and Lesbian Adolescents

During middle adolescence, a boy or girl might become aware of sexual feelings toward members of the same sex. Even with increased societal tolerance for homosexuality, it is almost universal that these first stirrings of homoerotic feelings are experienced by the adolescent as undesirable or frightening. Kids who are suspected of being gay or lesbian are subject to harassment by peers, which might account for the higher incidence of suicide, running away, and school problems among gay and lesbian youth (Remafedi, 1994; Savin-Williams, 1994). As aptly noted by Janet Fontaine and Nancy Hammond (1996), "Compared to the 'development' of a heterosexual identity, a norm requiring little conscious thought or effort, the attempt to develop a healthy and viable bi- or homosexual identity is a draining, secreting, anxiety-producing, and lonely task for adolescents" (p. 819).

Cass (1979) has identified six stages in the process of forming a gay or lesbian identity. In Stage 1, *identity confusion*, a young person first becomes aware of same-sex attraction and begins to wonder (or worry) if he or she might be gay or lesbian. Denial is common at this stage. In Stage 2, *identity comparison*, denial no longer serves to suppress the sexual feelings, but the adolescent might rationalize the feelings as situational (à "phase") or might attempt to intensify heterosexual feelings. In Stage 3, *tolerance*, the individual begins to recognize the futility of denying his or her same-sex attractions. At this point, he or she might seek out the company of other homosexuals for companionship, though sexual contact, if present at all, is fraught with anxiety and secrecy. By Stage 4, *identity acceptance*, the individual increases contact with other homosexuals and begins to disclose his or her sexual orientation to others. In Stage 5, *pride*, the individual becomes more assertive about the validity of a gay or lesbian identity, might experience anger at heterosexuals, and militantly opposes prejudice or discrimination. Finally, at Stage 6, *synthesis*, the individual abandons the "militant" role, reestablishes relationships with supportive heterosexuals, and shifts emphasis to other aspects of identity development, such as career or family roles.

Although, for obvious reasons, there are no empirical data to support this model, it seems probable that gay or lesbian adolescents will be struggling with Stage 1 or 2 issues, and that a few might have successfully transitioned into Stage 3 or even Stage 4. Fontaine and Hammond (1996) provide useful guidelines for counseling adolescents at each of the six stages. One of their most important points is that the counselor must maintain an attitude of acceptance toward homosexuality without pressuring adolescents at Stage 1 or 2 to "accept" their homosexual identity. Many teenagers experience transient attractions toward members of the same sex and may even act on these attractions (Kinsey, Pomeroy, & Martin, 1948), but later identify themselves as heterosexual. In helping adolescents explore their sexuality, it is important to consider many factors, including their history of sexual attractions, fantasies, and the content of sexual dreams (Coleman, 1990).

Some other points to keep in mind when counseling gay and lesbian teens are listed in Table 3.2.

Making Moral Decisions

With increased independence and exposure to new experiences, adolescents face the challenge of deciding between "right" and "wrong." Expanding upon Piaget's theory, Lawrence Kohlberg (1963) presented a model for understanding how individuals at different ages and developmental stages make moral decisions. Kohlberg proposed that moral decision making progresses sequentially through six stages. Each stage is characterized by the principal rationale for making a particular moral decision. These stages are as follows:

TABLE 3.2. Guidelines for Counseling Gay and Lesbian Adolescents

- Avoid communicating disapproval of gay or lesbian sexuality.
- Don't pressure the adolescent to reach a decision about his or her sexual orientation.
- Provide education to dispel stereotypes about gays and lesbians.
- If the adolescent is sexually active, discuss "safe sex" and the risk of sexually transmitted diseases.
- Try to separate the issue of sexual orientation (being gay or lesbian) from sexual behavior. Some adolescents might use their sexual orientation as justification for promiscuity, prostitution, or sexual involvement with adults. Don't back down if the adolescent accuses you of homophobia if you raise questions about these behaviors. Help adolescents realize that being gay or lesbian does not exempt them from having to make responsible choices about sexual behavior. Education about the diversity of lifestyles among gay men and lesbians can help.
- Explore the role of the adolescent's family, but do not pressure the adolescent to "come out" to family members.
- Remain neutral on the issue of heterosexual experimentation—neither encourage nor discourage it. Explore the adolescent's motives for seeking out heterosexual experiences.
- Help the adolescent handle the reactions of other people to his or her sexual orientation.

Stage 1: To avoid punishment

Stage 2: To earn rewards for oneself

Stage 3: To receive approval from significant others

Stage 4: To obey rules and laws

Stage 5: To preserve the common good

Stage 6: To comply with universal and abstract ethical principles

Although Kohlberg's theory has been criticized as more applicable to boys than girls (Gilligan, 1982), his framework can be useful for assessing the sophistication with which an adolescent makes moral choices. For example, a boy who is primarily at Stage 2 will base decisions of "right and wrong" on whatever will earn him the better outcome. He'll return a lost wallet if there is a chance he'll get a reward; otherwise, he'd be inclined to keep it.

Because moral development progresses sequentially through these six stages, it would be futile to try to persuade this boy with arguments based on the common good ("We all need to help one another if we're going to live together in society") or universal moral principles ("Relieving the owner's anxiety over the lost wallet takes precedence over the inconvenience you would incur from trying to locate him"). A more realistic goal might be to help this boy move to Stage 3. One way to do so might be to help him see that the approval he'd receive from the wallet's owner is reason enough to return the wallet, even if no monetary reward were offered.

Many arguments between teenagers and parents regarding moral issues reach an impasse because a parent is using Stage 5 arguments to persuade an adolescent who is at Stage 2 or 3. By using Kohlberg's framework to assess how an adolescent thinks about issues of right and wrong, a clinician can more effectively help families through these impasses.

Studies using Kohlberg's framework with adolescents have shown that very few adolescents are at Stage 4, and virtually none are at Stage 5. Colby, Kohlberg, Gibbs, and Lieberman (1983) found that only about 8% of 14-year-olds and 21% of 18-year-olds were at Stage 4. Their sample of 14-year-olds was about evenly split between Stages 2 and 3, with a very small percentage at Stages 1 and 4. About 60% of 16-year-olds were at Stage 3, though a sizable minority (30%) were still at Stage 2 and a smaller minority (15%) were at Stage 4. By age 18, over 50% are still at Stage 3, and the rest are about evenly divided between Stages 2 and 4. Rick's (Vignette 6) justification for not "ratting" on a friend seems to place him in transition between Stages 3 and 4, which is typical for a boy his age.

What these data imply is that it is not particularly unusual for a 14-year-old to cite tangible or social rewards as the prime determinant of what is the "right" thing to do. Young adolescents will voice opinions that they believe will earn them the most approval, and since young adolescents are more oriented toward their peers than toward their parents, the approval of the peer group will weigh most heavily. Thus, Rick (Vignette 6) argues that loyalty to his friend dictates his choice not to report his friend's crime. However, in referring to loyalty as "a value" Rick is displaying a characteristic associated with Stage 4 reasoning, where one's choices come under the influence of rules and laws.

In many cases, the norms of the peer group are close enough to those of the family to prevent major clashes over issues of right and wrong. In some cases, however, affiliation with a peer group whose norms diverge significantly from those of the family can lead to uproar. Two courses of action are available to assist families in this situation. Therapists can attempt to foster greater attachment to the family, so that earning the approval of the family will take on more significance for the youngster. Alternatively, therapists can try to nudge the teenager toward Stage 4 reasoning by enlisting the youth's participation in establishing rules for himself to which he would be willing to pledge allegiance.

Patience will be necessary if either alternative is chosen. Depending upon the level of alienation in the family, the prospects for developing stronger attachments between the child and parents may seem dim. Likewise, adolescents who are comfortably at Stage 3 may need time to realize the disadvantages of this stage and the advantages of establishing rules by which they will voluntarily govern their own behavior. Meanwhile, therapists can block futile clashes between Stage 3 adolescents and parents who are utilizing arguments more appropriate to a higher stage.

Developing New Relationships with Peers

During the early years of adolescence, a boy or girl socializes primarily with small cliques of same-sex peers, and interaction between the sexes is usually limited to large-group activities. By middle adolescence, the composition of the peer group has shifted. At this age, the original same-sex peer cliques are breaking up as many boys and girls are pairing off into couples (Dunphy, 1963).

Along with this change in the way social time is spent, adolescents are also beginning to experience themselves as more differentiated from the peer group. During early adolescence, the peer group functions almost as an extension of the self. Eleven- to 13-year-olds have difficulty distinguishing what they think or feel from what (they believe) their friends think or feel. By age 14 or 15, teenagers begin to distinguish their own beliefs and feelings from those of their friends, and begin to feel more comfortable acting on their own beliefs and feelings. Since the youngster's peers are also going through the same process, the middle years of adolescence herald greater tolerance among the members of the peer group, and less anxiety over being seen as "different" by one's associates.

Kegan's "Evolving Self"

Robert Kegan (1982) has proposed a model that helps to explain the shift in the teenager's relationship to the peer group during midadolescence. According to Kegan, an individual develops through successive stages characterized by increasing complexity and sophistication in the way the person differentiates self from the world. The "self" is continually evolving as one gradually recognizes that experiences that were once considered part of the self can be differentiated from the self and taken by the self as an object of perception:

> Subject–object relations emerge out of a lifelong process of development: a succession of qualitative differentiations of the self from the

> world, with a qualitatively more extensive object with which to be in
> relation created each time; a natural history of qualitatively better
> guarantees to the world of its distinctness; successive triumphs of
> "relationship to" rather than "embeddedness in." (p. 77)

According to Kegan, infants in the first 2 years of life (the "incorporative" stage) have difficulty differentiating self from the environment—what is "self," and what is "other" is often confused in the mind of the very young child. Gradually, as children learn to differentiate self from the environment more accurately, they enter the "impulsive" stage, when they are bound to their own perceptions and see themselves as equivalent to their impulses rather than "having" these impulses. The 3-year-old wants what he wants when he wants it, and there are no other options.

As children gradually differentiate themselves from their impulses, so that they can observe these impulses as an object rather than as equivalent to the self, they enter the "imperial" stage. This stage, which corresponds to Piaget's stage of concrete operations, is characterized by an embeddedness in one's own needs and perceptions and an inability to appreciate that others might experience situations differently from oneself. The 8-year-old can wait patiently for her father to take her to the playground but can't appreciate that her dad may not find the experience as enjoyable as she does.

According to Kegan, the early years of adolescence are characterized by a transition from the imperial stage to the "interpersonal" stage. During this transition, teenagers gradually become aware of the limits of the "imperial" way of making sense of the world through interactions with other people who expect their needs to be taken into account. However, at this stage, adolescents have difficulty distinguishing their own needs, wishes, or interests from those of the group.

In the early teen years, Kegan claims, kids have trouble telling the difference between who they really are and how they are seen by their peers, and this confusion explains their intense preoccupation with the opinions of the peer group. It is not that teenagers are putting their own needs and wishes aside in favor of what the group is prescribing in order to be "accepted." Rather, according to Kegan, young teens have not yet developed the cognitive capability to differentiate their own thoughts and feelings from those of the group. In other words, the sense of self, the sense of who I am, what I want, what I like to do, is defined by my membership and participation in the interpersonal community (the peer group) and has a feeble existence apart from the group. A young teenager's sense of self is so tied up with the perceived expectations of the group that he's unsure where the group ends and he begins. The 13-year-old really doesn't even consider whether he likes hard rock music because it appeals to him, or because his friends think it's "cool."

The emergence of a separate self that can evaluate more objectively the perceived norms and expectations of the group begins in the middle years of adolescence and is often not complete until well into young adulthood. At this point, the young person enters the "institutional" stage, when a clearer sense of personal identity is crystallizing. The 16-year-old acknowledges with some pride that her passion for 1950s jazz music sets her apart from her friends, who are more interested in contemporary popular music.

Kegan's model is compatible with the constructivist position that reality is never perceived directly, but rather is continually constructed by the person's efforts to make meaning out of sensory data (Rosen & Kuehlwein, 1996). Kegan adds to the constructivist position a developmental perspective. He proposes that infants, young children, preadolescents, adolescents, young adults, and older adults have characteristic ways of perceiving the world, and that the sense of self (and other) is inextricably intertwined with this process of meaning making.

Adolescents view themselves and other people in a way that is qualitatively different from the way adults (i.e., their parents) do. Teenagers and adults exist in "divergent realities" (Larson & Richards, 1994). Beyond a simple problem in "communication," adolescents and adults interpret the world in radically different terms. Take, for example, the case of Rick (Vignette 6) at the beginning of this chapter. He defines the issue of divulging the identity of a friend who has committed a crime as one of loyalty to one's peers, while his parents are likely to define the same issue as one of deference to social authority.

Kegan posits that the transition from one stage to the next is often associated with a repudiation of the meaning-making style of the stage that is being left behind. This observation can provide insight into the struggles that often erupt between parents and teenagers. Parents who are in transition between the interpersonal and institutional stages might react vigorously against an adolescent's embeddedness in the interpersonal stage, because they themselves are in the process of rejecting the "old self" that was interpersonally embedded. The teen's interpersonal embeddedness represents for the parent the way of making sense of the world that they themselves are repudiating in favor of the new institutional balance. Based on Kegan's model, we might expect that parents who are comfortably situated in the institutional stage or beyond would experience less difficulty empathizing with adolescents and moderating their reaction to them. It would seem, then, that the resolution of cyclical, escalating conflicts in some families might require a developmental shift in the parents rather than, or in addition to, a developmental shift on the part of the adolescent. Although Kegan does not explicitly recommend it, family therapy seems the ideal context for facilitating the simultaneous and coordinated development of both teenager and parents.

Balancing Autonomy and Accountability

"So I skipped school again today. So what? Why do you care? I don't want you to care."
                    –A 15-year-old boy defending his truancy to his mother

Adults and teenagers often disagree on the definition of "autonomy." Parents emphasize that autonomy requires responsibility, while kids define autonomy as freedom from adult authority. Many adults believe that teenagers are merely puppets of the peer group, but this belief is not supported by the available evidence. As I pointed out earlier, peer conformity peaks in early adolescence (ages 12–14), but then declines (Berndt, 1979).

While adolescents are strongly influenced by peers in matters of dress, music, and choice of leisure activities, most young people defer to adults in those areas in which adults are perceived as having expertise, such as career choices and financial decisions (Young & Ferguson, 1979). But adolescents view their parents less idealistically and more realistically than their younger siblings (Steinberg & Silverberg, 1986). They no longer see their parents as the all-powerful and all-knowing authority figures of childhood. Teenagers can see their parents' flaws with remarkable clarity and are often not particularly tactful in calling attention to them.

Autonomy must expand in proportion to accountability. As adolescents exercise more freedom in making their own decisions, they also must experience the impact of these decisions on themselves and others. Consider the following case:

A family came to therapy with a familiar complaint: A 15-year-old son was not responding to his parents' limits. Whenever the parents attempted to restrict the boy's freedom in any way, such as setting a curfew, he'd simply do what he wanted anyway, and then challenge his parents to react. The parents were afraid that they had lost all influence over their son. To make matters worse, at the end of the first session, the boy announced that he would not return for another session. After futile attempts to convince the boy to continue in family therapy, the parents gave up, resigned to their son's adamant refusal to participate.

I agreed with the parents that they could not force their son to attend therapy, but I disagreed that this meant that they had to forego therapy for themselves. I suggested that they tell the boy that they intended to continue therapy themselves, and that while he was invited and encouraged to attend, his refusal to do so would not prevent them from continuing in therapy to work on their goal of decreasing the level of tension in the household. I informed the boy that I would be more likely to be fair if he attended and presented his point of view. However, if he chose not to do so, I would still work with his parents. If so, he should realize that I could not help but see things from their point of view.

Though many kids will reconsider at this point, this boy remained adamant. The parents came alone to the next session, where they related their most recent clash with their son. The boy had called to ask permission to sleep over at a friend's house. When they refused, he informed them that he was going to do so anyway. The parents proceeded to engage him in an argument, which ended in the parents shouting at the boy and him hanging up. The parents alternated between rage at the boy and guilt over how they had handled the conflict.

I suggested to the parents that rather than arguing with the boy, they should simply point out the obvious: that they can't control what he does. If he chooses to stay out, he is doing so without their permission. They should avoid reacting to his attempts to engage them in an argument. The next day, after the boy returned home, they should inform him calmly how hurt and disappointed they felt. If the boy attempted to convince them to change their feelings, they should not do so, announcing, "I can't change my feelings so quickly. I'm sure I'll get over it, but it might take a while." The parents carried out my suggestion and reported that relationships in the home were improving, and the boy was being more cooperative.

This case illustrates a key concept in working with adolescents: *Avoid reacting to their reactivity.* To the extent that the parents attempted to restrict or argue with the boy, they were impeding the process of differentiation. The struggle for these parents, as for most, was to relinquish responsibility for the adolescent's choices while at the same time remaining connected to him. This can occur only if the parents let go of the urge to control the adolescent and instead focus on strengthening the relationship with him.

When the parents could get past their anger at the adolescent for defying their authority, they got in touch with their feelings of grief and hurt at the way their son was treating them. By communicating these feelings to the boy, by exposing to him their vulnerability and acknowledging his power to hurt them deeply, they were confronting him with the unintended social consequences of his relentless pursuit of freedom and providing him with an opportunity to consider ways of balancing his desire for autonomy with his accountability to the important relationships in his life.

The Independent Rebel?

Many adolescents confuse rebellion with autonomy. In fact, rebellion is simply another form of dependency, since it requires having someone or something to rebel *against.* In the terminology of Kerr and Bowen (1988), chronically rebellious adolescents and their parents are likely to be poorly differentiated from each other. By reacting punitively to the adolescent's rebellion, parents are unwittingly fueling the process of fusion and mutual reactivity that underlies the rebellion.

A study by Fulgini and Eccles (1993) supports this idea: Adolescents who were most dependent on peer-group approval were those from the most authoritarian homes. Adolescents from homes in which parents encouraged independent decision making actually were less oriented toward peers. The parents' attempt to limit the adolescent's autonomy simply pushed the adolescent closer to the peer group, which only increased the parental attempts to control, in a pattern that could erupt into a full-blown symptomatic cycle.

Erin's family presented an example of this cycle. Dressed in torn jeans, a dirty T-shirt and with hair wildly unkempt, 15-year-old Erin presented an amusing contrast to her father, an attorney, dressed conservatively in a polo shirt and khaki pants. Almost immediately, Erin's father launched into the predictable litany of complaint about Erin's clothing, choice of friends, room decor, and insufficient commitment to academics. On cue, Erin spat back slogans about her "individuality" and accused her father of trying to deprive her of her right to be herself. I wondered if Erin could tell the difference between being herself and being the opposite of what her father wanted her to be.

It was clear that Erin and her father shared many similarities: the same rusty blond hair, the piercing blue eyes, the articulate manner in which they precisely sculpted words to express their positions. Perhaps it was these similarities that made Erin so cautious about adopting as her own anything endorsed by her father, who so clearly saw himself as being on the right side of any argument.

Two sessions later, I felt connected enough with Erin to ask her the question that had been on my mind since our first meeting: "How do you know when you are doing something because you really want to or because your father doesn't want you to do it?" Erin looked at me quizzically. I could tell that she knew that I was on to something. She didn't know the difference, and she seemed almost relieved that I knew she didn't know. We could now begin exploring who Erin really was. Her father would have to help by refraining from being such an easy target.

Authoritative Parenting

The parenting style that is most supportive of adolescent autonomy and individuation has been termed "authoritative" or "enabling." According to Steinberg (1996):

> Authoritative parents are warm but firm. They set standards for the child's conduct but form expectations that are consistent with the child's developing needs and capabilities. They place a high value on the development of autonomy and self-direction but assume the ultimate responsibility for their child's behavior. Authoritative parents deal with their child in a rational, issue-oriented manner, frequently engaging in discussion and explanation with their children over matters of discipline. (p. 162)

Authoritative parenting must be distinguished from *authoritarian* parenting (laying down the law with little input from the child), and *laissez-faire* parenting (imposing few, if any, restrictions on the kid's behavior). A large body of literature has supported the correlation between authoritative parenting and positive outcomes for adolescents, leading to the conclusion that authoritative parenting is best for adolescents (see Steinberg, 1996).

Authoritative parents are not permissive. They have standards and expectations, and communicate these clearly to the adolescent. They set limits, but are open to negotiation. They avoid unnecessary power struggles and refrain from taking the adolescent's apparently irrational behavior as a personal affront. Authoritative parents freely offer guidance when asked but try to avoid protecting adolescents from the consequences of their own choices. Only when these natural consequences are likely to be severe or irreversible do the parents intervene with more immediate and ultimately less devastating consequences of their own.

> Ann and Vince Rossi were examples of authoritative parents. When 15-year-old Frank announced that he was taking a part-time job after school, Ann and Vince discussed with him their concerns about the impact of the job on his schoolwork. Because they had laid the foundation of a strong and mutually respectful relation-

ship over the years, Frank listened patiently, but in the end decided to take the job.

Ann and Vince were anxious, but decided to step back and allow Frank to see for himself if the job would interfere with his other responsibilities. Though tempted to do so, they did not gloat or pontificate when Frank sheepishly showed them his next report card, where his average had dropped from a B+ to a C+. Before expressing their own opinions about his grades, they asked Frank what he thought about his report card. Frank was a nice kid but not perfect: A bit arrogantly, he dismissed the C+ as unimportant and stated that he could bring his grades back up without quitting his job. Ann and Vince told him that they weren't as confident as he was, and said that they would let him know their decision in a few days, after they had time to discuss it between themselves.

Three days later, Ann and Vince again asked Frank if he had reconsidered his position about his job. He had not. Ann and Vince then calmly told him their decision: They expected him to cut down his hours at work immediately. If he could bring his average up by the next report card, they would consider allowing him to increase his time at work. If his average failed to go up, then Ann and Vince would insist that he quit his job.

Frank argued with his parents. They remained firm. On his next report card, his average had increased to a B. He insisted that this was the best he could do. Ann and Vince met with Frank and his teachers. The teachers unanimously agreed that Frank was capable of earning higher grades if he spent more time on his studies. Frank reminded his parents that they had stated that he would have to quit his job only if his average failed to increase.

Ann and Vince offered a compromise: Frank could choose whether to cut back his hours at work, or he could spend one evening each weekend studying rather than going out with his friends. Not without some blustering, Frank chose the latter. By the next report card, Frank's average had increased slightly but had not returned to the level it was prior to his taking the job. What had become clear to Ann and Vince in the interim was that Frank was really comfortable with his academic performance and seemed to realize its potential impact on his future. They acknowledged that Frank was still performing above average and that his goal to attend the state university was still realistic. They admitted that foregoing a job in order to get higher grades was a value to which they were strongly committed, but that Frank was not.

In the end, Ann and Vince decided to stick to their original stand: As long as Frank was able to keep his average above C+, he could keep his job. Frank ended the year with a B− average, but earned several hundred dollars that he applied to purchasing car insurance. He also appeared more mature and confident, which he attributed to his experiences on the job. Most important, perhaps, he and his parents had maintained their warm and mutually respectful relationship, and in some ways had even grown closer.

Some caveats are in order. First, some research has separated authoritative parenting into its components: warmth, structure, and support of autonomy (Steinberg, 1990). A finer gradation of parenting style based upon the relative strength of these three components might ultimately prove to be a more beneficial way of characterizing parenting practices.

Second, the whole notion that parenting can be categorized into a style can be criticized. Most parents use a variety of methods in disciplining their children, and to characterize a style may be too limiting. The Rossis did their share of yelling, but not too often. In the final analysis, what characterizes authoritative parents is an attitude about their relationship with their child rather than a particular set of skills (see Darling & Steinberg, 1993).

Third, the family's ethnic and cultural background must be taken into account. Authoritative parenting is not common among all ethnic groups (Steinberg, Lamborn, Dornbusch, & Darling, 1992). For example, African American parents are more likely to use physical rather than verbal punishment, but they are also more demonstrative in expressing affection for children (Staples, 1992). Authoritarian methods are also more common among Hispanic and Asian families (McGoldrick, Pearce, & Giordano, 1982).

Furthermore, the advantages of authoritative parenting may be applicable only to white, middle-class families (Dornbusch, Ritter, Leiderman, Roberts, & Fraleigh, 1987). The apparent adverse effects of authoritarian parenting found among white, middle-class families may not apply to families from other ethnic backgrounds. While *laissez-faire* and neglectful parenting appears to be detrimental to children regardless of culture, the relative advantage of authoritative parenting compared to authoritarian parenting appears to depend on the family's cultural background (Steinberg, Lamborn, Darling, Mounts, & Dornbusch, 1994). Parental control might be viewed differently by youngsters in different cultural contexts. Rohner and Pettengill (1985), for example, reported that Korean youths perceived parents as showing more warmth toward them when the parents are more (rather than less) controlling.

One reason for these findings might lie in the way researches have defined "parental control." Lau and Cheung (1987) pointed out that parental control that is restrictive, dominating, and intrusive can be differentiated from a style of parental control that is focused on maintaining organization and order in the family. Ruth Chao (1994) argued that the concepts of authoritative and authoritarian parenting are ethnocentric and do not capture the important features of child rearing in Asian cultures, where strict limit setting coexists with strong family ties, physical closeness, and intense investment in the child's success. Thus, in minority families, what might be most relevant is not the degree of independence given to children but rather the amount of warmth children experience in their relationships with parents.

Table 3.3 summarizes the developmental issues, and typical and atypical behaviors of middle adolescence.

TABLE 3.3 Middle Adolescence (Ages 14–16)

Major developmental issues

- Handling sexuality
- Making moral decisions
- Developing new relationships with peers
- Balancing autonomy and accountability

Typical behaviors

- Greater awareness of the needs of others and a greater willingness to compromise
- In making decisions about right and wrong, less emphasis on obtaining tangible rewards and more interest in gaining the approval of significant others
- Increased interest in sex and curiosity about sex
- Shifting in peer associations, formation of couples
- Increased differentiation from the peer group; more tolerant of differences and more supportive of expressing one's own individuality
- Increased emphasis on being independent and free from parental rule
- The beginning of the moratorium—increased attention to defining one's identity, which includes exploration and experimentation in a variety of areas

Signs of problems

- By age 15 or 16, still seems to show many of the characteristics typical of the younger teenager (ages 11–13)
- Seems preoccupied with sex (e.g., a copy of *Playboy* tucked under the mattress is to be expected, but a cache of hard-core pornography might signal a problem)
- Sexual promiscuity–although many (perhaps most) adolescents at this age are sexually active, indiscriminate choice of sexual partners is not common
- Unusually anxious about sex (e.g., becomes nervous whenever sexual issues are discussed, claims to have no interest in sex)
- Doesn't seem to feel guilty when he or she does something that is clearly wrong or that hurts another person
- Has a very narrow range of activities (e.g., seems interested in little else but "hanging out" with same-sex peers)
- Appears to be a "loner," has no friends and doesn't seem interested in associating with peers
- Associates exclusively with peers, avoids the company of adults, even those (e.g., teachers, coaches, employers) who have taken a personal interest in him or her

LATE ADOLESCENCE

Consolidating an Identity

If asked to identify the major developmental task of adolescence, most clinicians would probably say that adolescents are struggling to establish an identity. This point of view is derived from the writings of Erik Erikson (1959, 1968), who identified adolescence as the fifth of his "eight stages of man," characterized by the task of establishing an identity. It is during adolescence that one must explore and eventually define who one is, and thus be equipped move into the next stage, which poses the challenge of establishing an intimate relationship with another person.

Marcia's Identity Statuses

James Marcia (1966, 1976) developed a method of identifying an adolescent's position or "status" in the process of defining an identity. Marcia identified four possible "identity statuses" that are defined by the intersection of two dimensions. The first dimension describes how much exploration the adolescent has engaged in prior to reaching a decision. The second dimension describes the strength of the adolescent's commitment to the decision. The resulting four statuses are depicted in Figure 3.1.

An example of an adolescent in Diffusion might be one who shows little concern about the future and is focused almost entirely on immediate gratification. A boy who shows no interest in academics, sports, or the arts, who hasn't even a hazy dream about a future career, and who spends all his free time "hanging out" with peers who seem similarly adrift exemplifies the Diffusion status. Gloria (Vignette 4) is an example of an adolescent in Foreclosure. She is certain about her career choice and has never considered other alternatives. Rod (Vignette 3) is an example of an adolescent in Moratorium. He has not decided on a direction for his future and is actively considering alternatives. After a few painful years of this process, Rod will probably settle on a choice and will then have attained the Achievement status.

Research using Marcia's model (see Adams, Gullotta, & Montemayor, 1992) has revealed that the adolescents who are most likely to exhibit problematic behavior are those in the category of Identity Diffusion. These are the youngsters who have not committed themselves to an identity definition, and who seem uninterested in doing so. These young people are most susceptible to negative peer influence and are unlikely to exhibit much motivation in school or other

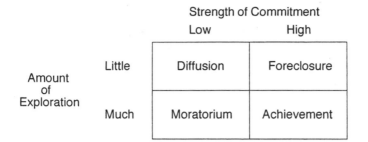

FIGURE 3.1. Marcia's four identity statuses.

achievement-related areas. According to Erikson's framework, these adolescents might have failed to resolve one or more of the earlier developmental crises. For example, prior to adolescence, children must successfully establish a sense of industry, a sense that they are "good" at something. Those children who fail to do so, by virtue of, for example, learning disability or severe parental neglect, are ill equipped to deal with the issue of identity, and so often fall into the Diffusion status.

Adolescents in the Foreclosure status, those who seem to have committed themselves to a decision without a period of exploration or experimentation, are generally well adjusted but are likely to be relatively constricted and conservative about taking risks. Often they were reared in authoritarian households with parents who were probably themselves foreclosed. They are apt to identify strongly with parental values. Other foreclosed adolescents reject parental values but borrow an identity by affiliating with a deviant peer group (Muus, 1996).

The optimal position, according to Erikson and Marcia, is Moratorium. Adolescents in Moratorium are in the process of exploring who they are but defer a final decision until all evident alternatives are explored. These adolescents eventually emerge with a clearly defined identity, at which time they would be classified in the Achievement category. Research has indicated, as predicted, that the number of adolescents in the Achievement category increases with age (Meilman, 1979).

Critiques of Erikson's and Marcia's Models

While Erikson's and Marcia's models provide useful frameworks for understanding the process of identity development, there have nevertheless been some criticisms. Some have argued that the models do not apply to girls, whose sense of identity is typically intertwined with competency in relationships (Gallatin, 1975; Josselson, 1987). For girls, the process of identity development and the establishment of intimacy might coincide or overlap. The period of moratorium might therefore be longer for girls, since the successful establishment of an intimate relationship, for heterosexual girls at least, is contingent upon the boys catching up to them in their capacity for intimacy, which for boys is thought to emerge after an identity has been established.

The other concern about Erikson's and Marcia's model is the manner in which the establishment of an "identity" is characterized as a "task" to be completed or achieved. Recent scholarship on social constructionism would take issue with this idea, claiming instead that our sense of ourselves is constantly evolving and changing (e.g., Markus & Nurius, 1986).

Furthermore, it is important to keep in mind that identity is not a single "thing." Rather, there are multiple aspects to identity, such as occupational identity, religious–value identity, gender identity, ethnic identity, and political identity. The process of establishing a position in each of these areas can follow different time frames and trajectories (Archer, 1989). For example, a young person who is gay or lesbian might not "come out" until well into their 20s, though their identity might be secure in other areas. Similarly, it is conceivable that an adolescent might be in Moratorium on some issues, Foreclosure on others, and in Diffusion on still others, such as the high school junior who is actively exploring career options (Moratorium), but has unquestioningly adopted his family's religious beliefs (Foreclosure) and seems uninterested and unconcerned about politics (Diffusion). Thus, the model shouldn't be used to categorize adolescents, but rather to assess how young persons are dealing with important life decisions.

The Role of Parents in Adolescent Identity Development

One of the challenges facing parents is their position regarding their adolescent's exploration of identity. Many parents are uneasy with a prolonged Moratorium, and so exert pressure on the young person to decide on a course of action. As a result, the adolescent prematurely forecloses on a decision, or becomes distracted from the task of Moratorium by engaging in battles with the parents over autonomy. Many parents mistakenly believe that adolescents should have a clear idea of their future career goals by the time they leave for college.

Research, however, has indicated that less than 10% of high school seniors have reached the Achievement status (Meilman, 1979).

Sometimes, an adolescent has reached Achievement, but the parents don't like the choice he or she has made. Parents are brought face to face with their own value systems and might experience clashes not only between each other but within themselves and the extended family. More sophisticated parents may try to hide their disappointment when their honor student decides to become a motorcycle mechanic, thinking that any expression of disapproval could unhinge their relationship with the adolescent. Instead, they suffer in silence, though the tension in the relationships is palpable.

If therapists are consulted on issues such as these, the Erikson and Marcia models can provide some guidance. Young teenagers (such as Gloria in Vignette 4) who appear to have decided on a direction for their lives might be encouraged not necessarily to drop this direction, but to learn more about it and related fields. Parental opposition can be reframed as an opportunity for the teen to explore whether he or she is indeed committed to the decision.

In the case of older adolescents who genuinely have settled on a direction after a period of exploration, a different approach is indicated. Here, the young person has passed through a period of Moratorium and has decided on what is best for him- or herself despite parental objection. To encourage the youth to explore other alternatives could encourage a developmental regression. Rather, it is better to help the parents understand the process by which the young person has made the decision, and help the young person understand that one of the consequences of the decision is conflict with her parents. Similarly, the therapist should point out to the parents that the very fact that the adolescent has made a decision despite their objections shows that the young person has integrity, a characteristic that they no doubt have encouraged. Therapists can help parents understand that, just as the adolescent was faced with the difficult decision to follow his or her own compass, they, too, are now faced with the difficult decision of working to keep a relationship with their child or deciding that the relationship must be sacrificed. The very process of working through conflicts such as this will facilitate a process of differentiation of self (Kerr & Bowen, 1988) in both parents and adolescents.

What about adolescents in Diffusion? First of all, the clinician should assess all aspects of identity, for the adolescent might not be in Diffusion in all areas. Sometimes, adolescents who appear to be in Diffusion in one area (e.g., career goals) are in Moratorium in other areas (e.g., personal values). In these cases, therapists might try to move the young person from Diffusion to Moratorium by asking questions about the area in which the adolescent appears to be in Diffusion. For example, if the youngster is in Diffusion in the area of career goals, therapists might ask questions such as the following: Where do you want to be in 5 years? How much money do you want to make? How do you see yourself spending your time? Which adults in your life seem to be happy about the career choice they have made? Which adults seem to be unhappy with their careers?

If there are apparently no areas in which the adolescent appears to be in any status but Diffusion, then therapists might explore whether the adolescent could be engaged in a process of moratorium on at least one issue. If this approach is not successful, then it is possible that the adolescent has been arrested at an earlier developmental stage. For example, the adolescent might not have resolved the "industry versus inferiority" (Erikson, 1950) dilemma; that is, he might feel that he's not good at anything. If so, a therapist could help the youngster increase his sense of industry in an area of interest.

For example, an adolescent who has struggled in elementary and middle school might have abandoned any hope of academic success by high school. Not perceiving any alternatives and reacting to parental demands for more commitment to academics, the adolescent simply avoids thinking about his future. In this case, the therapist might help the adolescent identify and develop talents in areas other than academics, such as mechanics or art.

Of course, following Erikson's framework, if the youngster has not resolved the "industry" crisis, it is possible that there have been problems at earlier developmental stages as well. Thus, therapists should start with the "industry versus inferiority" stage, and, if unable to make headway, proceed backwards through the earlier stages to explore where the youngster might be stuck.

Experiencing Intimacy

Intimacy with Parents

Early scholarship emphasized the need for adolescents to sever their emotional ties with parents, a process that has been termed "detachment" (Freud, 1958). Adolescents were expected to repudiate their "infantile dependence" by rebelling against parental authority and rejecting their attachment to their parents. Teenagers who remained close to their parents were considered immature and fearful of growing up. Parents were advised to discourage an overly warm relationship with the teen, lest they impede the process of separation.

Later, this notion was replaced by the idea that adolescents are faced with a more complex challenge: retaining their relationship with the significant adults in their lives while at the same time transforming these relationships to include a greater sense of personal autonomy. This process has been termed "individuation" (Blos, 1967). For girls, especially, the need to remain emotionally connected to parents remains strong, even as they challenge their parents to acknowledge their individuality and respect their choices (Apter, 1990; Kaplan, Klein, & Gleason, 1991). Boys, too, continue to need their parents, but it is harder for them to accept, let alone express, this need because our culture encourages boys to be independent and discourages overt requests for emotional support (Silverstein & Rashbaum, 1994).

Many parents feel that their child has abandoned them in favor of their peers. Parents might feel that the adolescent doesn't love them or need them any more. But peers do not supplant parents as objects of affection and intimacy. While the importance of relationships with peers certainly increases in adolescence, intimacy with parents declines only slightly (Hunter & Youniss, 1982). Parents might feel less emotionally close to their adolescent children, but most adolescents still feel close to their parents. What has changed is that intimacy and involvement with peers have increased, so that parents are no longer the exclusive object of the adolescent's affections.

What occurs during adolescence is the *transformation* of the nature of the relationship between children and parents. The relationship changes from one that is asymmetrical to one that is more symmetrical in terms of interpersonal power and authority (Eccles et al., 1993). Older adolescents want a relationship with their parents, but expect parents to treat them more like equals, less like children who need protection and guidance. From the parents' perspective, showing respect for the older adolescent or young adult means knowing when to step back, and refraining from asking questions, or offering unsolicited opinions. It also means being honest with the adolescent about how he or she is coming across to the parent, and expecting the adolescent to put energy into the relationship as well.

Some parents and older adolescents get stuck in the classic *pursuer–distancer* pattern (Kerr & Bowen, 1988): The more the parent pursues the adolescent, the more the adolescent distances from the parents. This pattern was present in the family of Ken, an 18-year-old college freshman. Ken's parents complained that he never returned their phone messages, never wrote, never phoned, and discouraged them from visiting him at college. Yet, they continued to phone him several times a week, sometimes in the wee hours of the morning in a vain attempt to reach him. Ken, who, incidentally, was doing well academically and socially at college, eventually admitted that he had turned off the ringer of his telephone because his parents were leaving him too many messages! We were able to work out a compromise that broke the cycle of pursuit and flight. Ken would call his parents at a specific time each week, the call would last no longer than 30 minutes, and his parents would refrain from calling him as long as he kept his promise to phone them weekly.

Intimacy with Peers

Peer relationships have been changing and expanding throughout adolescence. In early adolescence, the peer group functions almost as an extension of the adolescent's self, serving as a substitute family and a temporary referent for his or her emerging identity. In the middle years of adolescence, the peer crowd starts to break up as adolescents pair off into couples or smaller cliques. As adolescence wanes into young adulthood, the importance of establishing an intimate bond with a peer increases. Erikson (1959) had placed the "identity crisis" before the "intimacy crisis," claiming that persons must know who they are before they can be truly intimate with another person. Feminist scholars such as Ruthellen Josselson (1987) have challenged this idea, arguing that women often consolidate their identity in the context of an intimate relationship with another person, typically a romantic partner. Rather than being seen as two distinct processes, the tasks of consolidating an identity and developing the capacity for intimacy go hand in hand, strengthening one another in a process that extends well beyond adolescence into adulthood.

It is commonly believed that intimacy is valued more highly by girls than boys (Maccoby, 1990), but it is important to note that boys and girls may experience intimacy differently. While girls experience intimacy through mutual self-disclosure, boys experience intimacy with other boys through shared activity and time spent together (Buhrmester & Furman, 1987). Many (heterosexual) boys withdraw from intimacy with other boys because of fear of being seen as homosexual (Kite, 1984). It is easier for girls to be intimate with other girls, and thus girls, overall, are more comfortable expressing intimacy and are more experienced than boys in moving relationships to a more intimate level. Girls originally learn how to be emotionally intimate with same-sex friends but opposite-sex relationships are more important for the development of intimacy in boys (Buhrmester & Furman, 1987).

Although an intimate relationship need not be sexual, for many adolescents, sexual activity is a way to express and experience intimacy. By age 18, 67% of boys and 44% of girls have experienced sexual intercourse, and by age 20, these figures go up to 80% for males and 70% for females (Katchadourian, 1990). It is reasonable to assume that even higher percentages of adolescents have engaged in sexual activity, even if they haven't gone "all the way."

Despite the so-called "sexual revolution," a double standard in sexuality still holds. Parents and even adolescents themselves are more tolerant of sexual activity by boys than by girls (Gordon & Gilgun, 1987). Boys who have sex are accorded prestige by their peers,. while sexually active girls receive a more mixed reaction. Boys are likely to view their sexual experiences in terms of achievement, as proof of their masculinity and maturity. Girls are more ambivalent: They may want the closeness that sex seems to offer, but deep down they realize that boys don't want the same thing. For girls, sexual involvement is inextricably linked to intimacy and closeness.

The majority of heterosexual adolescents have experienced a "steady" relationship with romantic overtones by the end of high school (Steinberg, 1996). Nearly half of these high school romances end during the first year of college (Shaver, Furman, & Buhrmester, 1985). The breakup is more likely to be initiated by the girl, but, regardless of who initiated the breakup, girls adjust to the end of the relationship better than do boys (Steinberg, 1996). Perhaps for this reason, boys are four times more likely than girls to report feeling lonely during the first year of college (Savin-Williams & Berndt, 1990). Because it is easier (and more socially acceptable) for girls to experience intimacy in same-sex friendships, heterosexual boys tend to depend more on opposite-sex relationships for experiencing intimacy and emotional closeness (Buhrmester & Furman, 1987). Thus, boys are more bereft when an emotionally intimate relationship with a girl ends.

Leaving Home

In our culture, high school graduation is about as close to a "rite of passage" as we come. Graduating from high school marks the point at which the adolescent is expected to loosen ties to the family of origin and step into more independence, whether it be going to college, working full time, or enlisting in the military. This transition is sometimes fraught with turmoil for both the adolescent and the family. In Chapter 9, I discuss in more detail the problems associated with leaving home, and here I want to highlight only a few points.

The crisis of "leaving home" is not restricted to the period following high school graduation. It begins during the senior year of high school, when the end is in sight and the pressure to make post-high school plans mounts. Often, problems that emerge during the senior year of high school are linked to rough spots in the process of leaving home. Adolescents might not express their anxieties about leaving home, perhaps because of actual or imagined expectations on the part of parents and teachers. Thus, they show their reluctance to leave in other ways, such as "forgetting" college application deadlines, neglecting their schoolwork, or developing symptoms.

Whatever the specific nature of the problem presented to the therapist, it is important to inquire about the process of leaving home and invite the adolescent and other family members to express their feelings about the transition. When it becomes clear that the young person is simply not ready to leave, then the therapist must take the lead in helping the family find concrete ways to ease the transition, such as part-time employment, reduced college course load, or a precollege transitional year of schooling.

How do we know whether an adolescent is really "not ready" to leave home or whether he or she simply needs encouragement? The only way to make this distinction is to listen carefully to the adolescent and to the other family members. The boy or girl who has been making steady progress toward college, but who begins to fall behind in senior year, might simply need encouragement. On the other hand, the young person who seems to falter at any obstacle, or who repeatedly creates obstacles that could easily be avoided, is probably not ready to leave. The therapist, of course, does not take the position that development should come to a standstill, but rather that the process of preparing to leave home needs to be prolonged. Much of the work will involve coaching the parents to be supportive of these efforts without being overly protective or too impatient. In Chapter 9 other suggestions for handling problems at this stage will be discussed.

Table 3.4 summarizes the developmental issues, and typical and atypical behaviors of late adolescence.

SUMMARY

We have covered a lot of ground in this chapter, so I want to close by emphasizing what I believe are the most important points for a therapist to keep in mind:

• Adolescence is not a time of inevitable turmoil. Serious or prolonged moodiness, withdrawal, aggression, appetite disturbance, or oppositional behavior should be taken very seriously. Even if at first

TABLE 3.4. Late Adolescence (Ages 17–19)

Major developmental issues

- Consolidating an identity
- Experiencing intimacy
- Leaving home

Typical behaviors

- Begins to narrow down choices for the future to a few options.
- Increased capacity for intimacy; girls may seem more mature than boys in this area (see text)
- High-school romances may be breaking up
- Fewer arguments with parents; daily struggles over rules and freedom have subsided, but adolescents at this age expect parents to show respect for their choices and their individuality
- Getting ready to leave home (e.g., college, job, military)

Signs of problems

- No plans for the future, and little interest in making them
- Still (or again) seems as moody and unpredictable as during the early years of adolescence
- Has no shown no interest in dating (this could also be a sign that the adolescent is struggling with his or her sexual orientation)
- Avoids making postgraduation plans and bristles whenever parents bring up this topic
- Expresses the desire to go to college but is not taking the necessary steps (e.g., filing applications, taking SATs)

glance it appears that a family is grappling with normal developmental issues, it is far less risky to take a few sessions to get to know the family before offering reassurance.

- Although adolescence is not tumultuous as a rule, there are nevertheless a series of normal developmental challenges that are encountered during the second decade of life.
- During early adolescence (ages 11–13), the boy or girl faces the challenge of coming to terms with the physical changes associated with puberty and dealing with the reactions of others to his or her physical appearance. They are beginning to develop the capacity to think and reason more abstractly, and, lacking experience with these new tools, they are apt to apply them clumsily. Thus, for many adolescents, this period is one of intense self-consciousness. Self-esteem tends to drop at this age, especially for girls who experience for the first time the need to suppress parts of themselves in order to be accepted by others (Brown & Gilligan, 1992). Finding a place among the peer group is of upmost importance at this age. For early adolescents, peers provide a reference point for their budding sense of identity and allow a smooth

transition away from the emotional security of the family home. However, peer conformity is high at this age, because young teenagers are not yet able to distinguish their own thoughts and feelings from those of their peers. Temporary intensification of pressure to behave in culturally prescribed "masculine" or "feminine" ways provokes the process of gender-identity development and creates difficulties for kids who don't conform to cultural gender stereotypes.

• During the middle years of adolescence (ages 14–16), the boy or girl must make important decisions about how to express sexuality and how to decide between right and wrong. At this age, they are beginning to differentiate themselves from the peer group and are more willing to deviate from actual or perceived peer conformity. The same-sex peer clique is disintegrating as the members pair off into opposite-sex couples. As adolescents at this age become more independent, they must learn to balance autonomy with responsibility and accountability to others. This balance is fostered by parents who follow an "authoritative" style of parenting: warm, supportive, but firm in setting limits that are negotiated with the child.

• During late adolescence (ages 17–19), the consolidation of an identity becomes the primary challenge, along with the refinement of the capacity to experience and express intimacy. As high school graduation approaches, so does the transition to "leaving home," which for many young people and their families can be a stressful time.

So, in a nutshell, these are the major developmental milestones of adolescence. Keeping them in mind can help us hold realistic expectations of adolescents and provide reassurance to worried families. Some families, however, are not simply muddling through normal developmental issues. It is these families that we therapists are usually called upon to aid, and it is to these families that we turn in the following chapters.

CHAPTER 4

EATING DISORDERS

Frail and bird-like, Tina reminded me of the little waif on the posters for the musical *Les Misérables*. Carrying only 83 pounds on her 5'4'' frame, Tina looked much younger than her 16 years. She clutched a sketch pad under her left arm and a pencil dangled from her right hand. Her hair, with the wispy, thinned quality often seen in young women with anorexia, hung forlornly over her face. Her eyes had the vacant look of a young woman trying to numb some unbearable pain.

Rose, Tina's mother, sat at her right. Her close-cropped red hair framed a face marked with worry for her daughter. Her eyes were glued on Tina, and she sat as if poised to spring up at any moment to defend her daughter from unseen dangers. Her left hand clutched the right arm of Tina's chair. Though I knew that Rose worked full time as an elementary school teacher and had raised two children with no assistance from their father or from other family members, I could see no sign of this competence in her hopeless face. She moved as if checking every motion, restraining herself from gesturing too broadly or calling attention to herself. Her voice, hesitant, tremulous, always on the verge of a sob, told me she was suffering, though her words were never about herself, only Tina.

At Tina's left sat her father, Bill, who had only recently resumed seeing her after 10 years of infrequent and sporadic contact. In his face, I read frustration and mistrust. This was a man who "didn't believe in therapy." He didn't have to tell me (although he did, immediately upon meeting me); I could guess. He warily entered the room, well behind Tina and Rose, then perched on the edge of the seat on Tina's left, grasping the right arm of her chair in a gesture that appeared more desperate than supportive. Tina squeezed into the center of her seat as if shrinking from contact with her parents, who almost literally seemed to be pulling her in opposite directions.

I already knew part of their story from the phone call with Rose[1] that preceded our session. Tina had been losing weight for the past 18 months and was now on the brink of medical crisis. Tina and Rose had been living alone for the past 2 months, since Tina's older brother, Jeff, had moved to California to pursue a career in film making. Three years previously, Rose's second marriage ended when her husband of 5 years left her. Ten years previously, Rose and Bill divorced after 8 years of a marriage that was miserably unhappy for both of them. Less than a year after the divorce, Bill remarried and now had a son by his second marriage.

Bill did not challenge Rose's bid for custody of the children. After 2 years of gradually decreasing contact, the children stopped visiting Bill, aside from the occasional weekend during summer and winter vacations. They had not communicated until 6 months ago, when Rose contacted Bill out of desperation when Tina's pediatrician told Rose that Tina had anorexia. Bill began calling Tina, and for 2 weeks, Tina lived with Bill until she pleaded with her father to send her home because she missed her friends. Bill reluctantly agreed when Tina promised that she would gain 10 pounds if he let her return home.

Following the advice of the pediatrician, Rose immediately sought therapy for Tina. She saw her therapist individually twice a week, but she continued to lose weight. Eventually, she stopped going. Bill phoned Rose several times a week, berating her for allowing the problem to get out of hand. One week before our meeting, Bill threatened to drive to Rose's house, seize Tina, and handcuff her to his wrist until she gained weight. Then Rose panicked when she found empty bottles of ipecac serum in Tina's room. She phoned Bill, who lambasted her for "mishandling" the situation. After an argument that ended with Rose hanging up on Bill, she turned in desperation to Tina's former therapist, who suggested that Rose contact me.

—————◆————

Few symptoms are as terrifying and frustrating as anorexia. The solution seems so simple—just eat, gain weight, and you will be fine. Yet, the girl[2] with anorexia remains steadfast, displaying almost super-human self-control over the most basic of urges to take in nourishment. The more those around her cajole her to eat, the more she resists. Her body, emaciated and ugly to others, always looks too fat to her. She is ruled by the numbers on the scale and by the image of herself that exists not so much in the mirror as in her own mind's eye.

Most parents of girls like Tina are terrified and helpless. The media depictions of eating disorders have taught them that the stakes are high. If she continues to starve herself (as she often does, even with therapy), she could die. For some parents, denial works for a while but eventually shatters as their child grows increasingly skeletal. Pleading, demanding, compromising, arguing, backing off—none of these methods works. Their daughter continues to refuse to eat, continues to lose weight, dying by degrees.

PERSPECTIVES ON EATING DISORDERS

Psychodynamic Perspectives

Early psychoanalytic accounts viewed anorexia as a defense against the threatening sexual impulses reawakened by puberty (Waller, Kaufman, & Deutsch, 1940). Later accounts emphasized two themes in the development of eating disorders: fears of maturity and struggles over autonomy.

Arthur Crisp (1983), for example, believed that anorectics unconsciously equated physical maturity with rejection and abandonment. Hilde Bruch (1982, 1988), on the other hand, described the girl with anorexia as engaged in a struggle to assert herself in a stifling family context. According to Bruch, the future anorectic's mother does not empathically understand the needs of her infant. Thus, the mother responds to the child based not so much on the child's needs as on her own. As a result, the child fails to discriminate among her own perceptions of bodily sensations and emotional states.[3] The mother, also very dependent upon the child's attachment, discourages autonomy. Eventually, the child embodies what she believe others expect of her rather than how she herself feels. Bruch recommends a modification of the psychoanalytic process, away from an emphasis on insight into the symbolic significance of the symptom and toward helping these patients discover their true selves: "They need to face their problems of living in the present, reconstruct what had gone on during the preillness period, and understand how their experiences interfered with their developing a sense of self and competence" (Bruch, 1982, p. 1536).

Feminist Psychodynamic Perspectives

Feminist psychodynamic theorists have challenged the emphasis on autonomy in traditional psychoanalytic theory and argue that eating disorders arise when young girls are confronted with social pressure to reject a way of life based on relatedness in favor of one based on independence, which for many girls is equated with isolation (Steiner-Adair, 1990). Janet Surrey (1991) associated eating disorders with the "loss of voice" experienced by young girls when they reach adolescence and are faced with the demand to conceal their real needs to preserve relationships with others.

Some feminist theorists have also challenged traditional psychodynamic theory's emphasis on the mother as primarily responsible for the development of eating disorders in the child. These theorists point out that the mothers themselves were often recipients of poor parenting in their own families, which diminished their capacity to care for their own children. In addition, feminist theorists point out that the relationship between the father and the mother influences the mother's relationship with the infant. Marital distress can distract the mother and make her less emotionally available to the infant. Eating disorder, then, should be viewed not so much as emerging from the mother–child relationship system as from the triadic relationship system involving both parents and the child.[4]

Sociocultural Perspectives

Since over 90% of those with eating disorders are female (Frasciello & Willard, 1995), it has been argued that women are more likely than men to be exposed to risk factors for eating disorders, particularly those that originate in cultural gender-role definitions (Halmi, 1995). Gilbert and Thompson (1996) have identified four theories that have been proposed to account for the higher incidence of eating disorders among women:

1. *Culture of thinness.* By extolling thinness as essential to happiness and promoting images of emaciated women, patriarchal society seeks to control women by rendering them powerless.

2. *Weight as power and control.* Women submit to cultural pressures to focus on their appearance in order to achieve a greater sense of control over their lives.

3. *Anxieties about female achievement.* Eating disorders represent attempts by successful women to escape from the negative stigma associated with women's achievement by adopting compensatory mea-

sures that will make them look more "feminine." Alternatively, some women focus on weight control as the only area in which they feel competent.

4. *Eating disorders as self-definition*. Traditional sex roles engender an underdeveloped sense of self in women and thus make them more vulnerable to social expectations regarding their appearance. A related perspective is the idea that a young woman's desire for nurturance evokes guilt that is expressed in the form of an eating disorder.

Therapists who subscribe to these notions aim to expose the covert social messages that contribute to the eating disorder and help the young woman find more suitable ways to satisfy her needs.

Family Systems Perspectives

Minuchin's Model of the Psychosomatic Family

Advocates of a family systems approach to eating disorder have focused on the here-and-now transactional patterns in the family rather than on early mother–infant interactions. Minuchin et al. (1978) proposed that families with anorexia commonly manifested four characteristics:

1. *Enmeshment*. Relationships in these families are characterized by a lack of appropriate emotional distance and overinvolvement in each other's lives. Families exhibiting this pattern often engage in "mind reading" (e.g., when a mother says what her daughter is thinking without the daughter having spoken) or "mediating" (e.g., when a mother serves as a go-between for a father and daughter who have little direct interaction with each other).

2. *Overprotectiveness*. Members of families with anorexia are overly protective and solicitous of one another. They are scrupulous about hurting each other's feelings and may go to great lengths to avoid overt conflict. These families are so sensitive to signals of distress in each other that they intervene too quickly to alleviate tension, thus impeding the capacity of the affected family member to learn how to handle stress on her own. As a result, the autonomy of each family member is compromised, and the interdependence of the family members on each other is reinforced.

3. *Rigidity*. These families are committed to maintaining the status quo. They find change threatening and often deny the need for change. Adolescence poses a particular challenge for these families, since they are unable to modify the family structure to permit increasing autonomy for the adolescent.

4. Involvement of the symptomatic adolescent in parental conflict. One of the ways that parents in anorectic families avoid overt conflict with each other is by detouring the conflict through the symptomatic adolescent. They divert attention away from their own conflicts in order to devote more energy to taking care of their daughter, who encourages this pattern by appearing helpless and emaciated. They submerge their own conflict in attacks on the daughter, who is defined as the only problem in the family. Or the daughter can be triangulated between her parents in such a way that she is unable to express herself without being perceived as taking the side of one parent against the other.

Although there has been inconsistent empirical support for the notion that these characteristics are typical of anorectic families (e.g., Blair, Freeman, & Cull, 1995), there has been support for the efficacy of family therapy for treating eating disorders in adolescents (e.g., Robin et al., 1994; Russell et al., 1987). Minuchin et al. (1978) reported on a sample of 50 anorectic families treated with structural family therapy ranging in duration from 2 to 12 months. At follow-up (ranging from 1½ to 7 years), 86% of the cases had recovered normal eating patterns, stabilized body weight within the normal limits for height and age, and had satisfactory adjustment in family, school, work, and peer relationships.

Anorexia as Maintaining Family Homeostasis

Other family systems theories claim that anorexia arises in families as a way of preserving a rigid family homeostasis. Peggy Papp (1983) recommended that therapists first identify the ways in which the anorexia functions to stabilize the family and then utilize paradoxical interventions to provoke change. The Milan School (Selvini-Palazzoli et al., 1978) takes a similar approach in assigning a "positive connotation" to the symptom and paradoxically restraining the family against change. Later, Selvini-Palazzoli and Viaro (1988) identified the "family game" that presumably leads to the development of the eating disorder. From this perspective, the symptom is seen as a strategic move on the part of the patient to achieve more power, but at the same time, the patient becomes a pawn in the game and is used by other family members to their own strategic advantage. Selvini-Palazzoli and Viaro recommend working individually with the patient to help her extricate herself from the game.

A Family Developmental Model

Proposing an integration of psychodynamic and family systems theories, Stern, Whitaker, Hagemann, Anderson, and Bargman (1981) linked anorexia to problems of separation and individuation, but noted that all members of the anorectic family, not just the patient, are developmentally arrested. They recommended that the therapists or treatment team function as surrogate parents to the anorectic family in order to create the optimal "holding environment" that will facilitate the process of separation and individuation. Specifically, the therapists must take leadership in setting the conditions for therapy, thus communicating that they will not allow the patient to act self-destructively, and then within this context challenge the family to accept initiative in taking the risks involved in change.

Narrative Approaches

Recently, interventions derived from the narrative approach to family therapy have been attracting much interest. An early version of this model was Michael White's (1983) exploration of the role of rigid family belief systems in anorexia. White claimed that girls develop anorexia in response to rigid beliefs and role prescriptions that exert tight constraints not just on the girl with anorexia but on all family members. He proposed that successful treatment requires the therapist to challenge the constraining influences of these beliefs by rendering them and their consequences explicit to the family.

Later, White (1987) proposed a process of detailed questioning that was designed to free the family from the constraining effects of their beliefs and open up new possibilities for viewing self and others. Ultimately, White (1993) evolved the technique of "externalizing the problem" that led to exploration of the ways in which "anorexia" had taken over the patient's and family's life ("mapping the influence of the problem"), searching for times when the patient or family were able to resist the problem ("unique outcomes"), and then building upon these unique outcomes to create new narratives about self and others ("reauthoring").[5] White's colleague, David Epston, helped to found the "Anti-Anorexia League," an archive of personal accounts from persons who had been treated for anorexia and who had discovered ways of subverting the effects of the "knowledge and practices upon which the anorexia nervosa depends" (White, 1993, p. 27).

PRINCIPLES OF TREATMENT

All of these theories might at one time or another provide the therapist with insight into the nature and treatment of anorexia. My approach borrows from many of these ideas, but I emphasize a particular theme: In my view, treatment of families with anorexia must be informed by the awareness that profound isolation and disconnection lie beneath the apparent enmeshment in the family (Sargent, 1987a). Although the family members appear to love and care for one another, their acceptance of each other is highly conditional. Each individual is constrained within narrow limits of acceptable behavior, with rejection, guilt, or abandonment being the price for moving beyond these limits. Only certain facets of the self may be presented to other family members, since the emergence of new facets of the self threaten the bond of enmeshment. Facets of the self that do not fit into these prescribed patterns must be hidden or denounced. As a result, all family members become frozen in the process of development.

Isolation and conditional acceptance were apparent in Tina's family. Though each parent hovered over her during the session, Tina avoided direct contact with them. Rose spoke for Tina as if she could read her daughter's mind, while Tina passively encouraged her mother by remaining silent. Her tiny body was in the room, but there appeared to be no soul. Rose described their relationship as close, and I believed that she genuinely experienced it as such, but I wondered how Tina could become so emaciated, and how she could have engaged in secret purging if she and her mother were really as close as Rose described.

Any change in the relationship, especially the changes that accompany adolescence, threatens the family and leads to efforts to counteract these changes. As a result, control substitutes for genuine connections. Fearful of losing the rigidly enmeshed attachment to which they had become accustomed, the family members rely on overt and covert methods of controlling one another. Ironically, the efforts at control only contribute to further isolation and disconnection, as the family members attempt to avoid each other's efforts to control them. Direct requests for change are not possible because of the threat of conflict these requests pose.

As discussed earlier, some theorists have described anorexia as an extreme effort to assert self-control in a system where normal autonomy is discouraged. While there is validity to this assertion, it is also true that the anorectic exerts a powerful influence over the other family members through her symptom. It was tempting to view Tina as a victim of controlling parents. However, this view had to be balanced by the awareness that Tina, in her apparent helplessness, was controlling her parents as well. One had just to look at the pained expression on Rose's face to see just how much Tina's self-starvation had worn her down. Pain and fear also lay not far below Bill's hostile demeanor. He knew that Tina could die, and he was terrified because he had no idea how to prevent it. As he poignantly declaimed in the first session, "First she wasn't happy at 103. Then she wasn't happy at 101, then she had to be 99, then 95, then 90, then 85. Now it's 80. At this rate, the optimum weight is death!"

The Symptomatic Cycle

The cycle begins when a girl starts to use eating as a way to manage the stresses connected with the developmental transition into adolescence. Perhaps she is uncomfortable with the way her body looks, perhaps she is fearful of sexuality, perhaps she is struggling to earn the acceptance of peers. Whatever the specific nature of the stress, because of the injunction against change and conflict in the family, she submerges her true feelings and distracts herself by becoming preoccupied with food and weight. By restricting her food intake, she slows down and eventually reverses the physical changes associated with puberty. She loses her curves and her menses stop. She has managed to hold back the hands of time, and, at first, it appears that the family is calmer. No longer are the family members faced with the need to adjust their relationships to accommodate the new adolescent in the family. Yet they eventually begin to notice that something is wrong.

Their daughter is not eating, and she is beginning to look very thin. At first, the parents and other family members may try indirect methods to encourage the girl to eat, such as preparing special dinners or finding excuses to be with her during meals. These approaches don't work for three very good reasons. First, by focusing on the girl's eating, they fail to address the constricting processes in the family that contributed to the problem in the first place. Second, by approaching the problem indirectly, they are reinforcing the very process of conflict avoidance that gave rise to the symptom. Third, the intense focus on the girl's eating habits distracts the other family members from issues and conflicts of their own.

Eventually, the parents abandon the indirect approach and confront the girl on her eating habits. Then, the battle shifts to a struggle over food and weight. The parents demand that she eat. She refuses, partly because she has now experienced one arena in which she can maintain control, partly because she has no alternative way of managing her stress.

Some parents try to get their daughter to open up to them, to share with them the terrible feelings that must be behind such a terrifying symptom. But in the process the parents only reinforce the "tell me/don't tell me" bind (see Chapter 2). They really don't want to hear anything that will upset them. They want to be reassured. On some level, the girl knows this and denies that she has any problems, or distracts her parents by raising trivial issues. In some cases, the girl herself may have lost access to her true feelings, having submerged them for so long.

The family is now stuck in a full-blown symptomatic cycle. The more control the parents exert over the girl's eating habits, the more she resists. The more earnest their pursuit, the more she shrinks from them, fearful that they might discover something about her that could devastate them. The parents might divert attention from other conflictual issues in order to focus on the girl's condition. Or, as in Tina's family, conflicts between the parents might now be detoured through the symptomatic child. As the girl loses more weight, the parents' arguments about how best to help her intensify. As each parent focuses on winning the conflict and thus exonerating him- or herself, the girl loses more weight, which only fuels more parental conflict.

The Symptomatic Cycle in Tina's Family

This symptomatic cycle was evident in Tina's family (see Figure 4.1). At first, Rose tried to handle Tina's eating problems on her own. She had read about anorexia and believed that it reflected underlying problems that could not be expressed any other way. Rose began to badger Tina to confide in her, anxiously reassuring Tina that she could handle whatever Tina might say. Rose did not realize that she was putting Tina in a "tell me/don't tell me" bind.

Already depressed as a result of her second failed marriage, Rose was not enthusiastic about Tina's growing up. She herself had a stormy adolescence marked by intense conflict with both of her parents. Tina had learned to read her mother very well over the years of their enmeshed relationship. She knew that Rose really couldn't handle hearing that she was angry at her for not taking better care of herself, for working too hard and then rationalizing her constricted life as a gift of love for her children. Tina noticed how much more unhappy her mother appeared when Tina began to spend more time with her friends and less time at home. What would be the point of talking about these things? So, when her mother asked her why she wasn't eating, Tina would mollify her mother with vague answers and divert attention away from her eating patterns.

As Tina lost more and more weight, Rose, in desperation, called Bill, hoping that he might know what to do. Bill had had virtually no contact with Tina or Rose over the past several years. When Rose explained that she was trying to help Tina by being supportive and caring, Bill interpreted her behavior as overly indulgent. He berated Rose for being too soft and blamed her for "allowing" Tina to get so thin.

Rose had forgotten how furious she felt when Bill criticized her. The anger, submerged all these years, returned and she counterattacked, blaming Bill for not being more involved in Tina's life, accusing him of being the cause of her problem. As the battle of mutual blame raged on, Tina continued to lose weight. As is typical, this unproductive process continued until a crisis was reached. In this case, Rose discov-

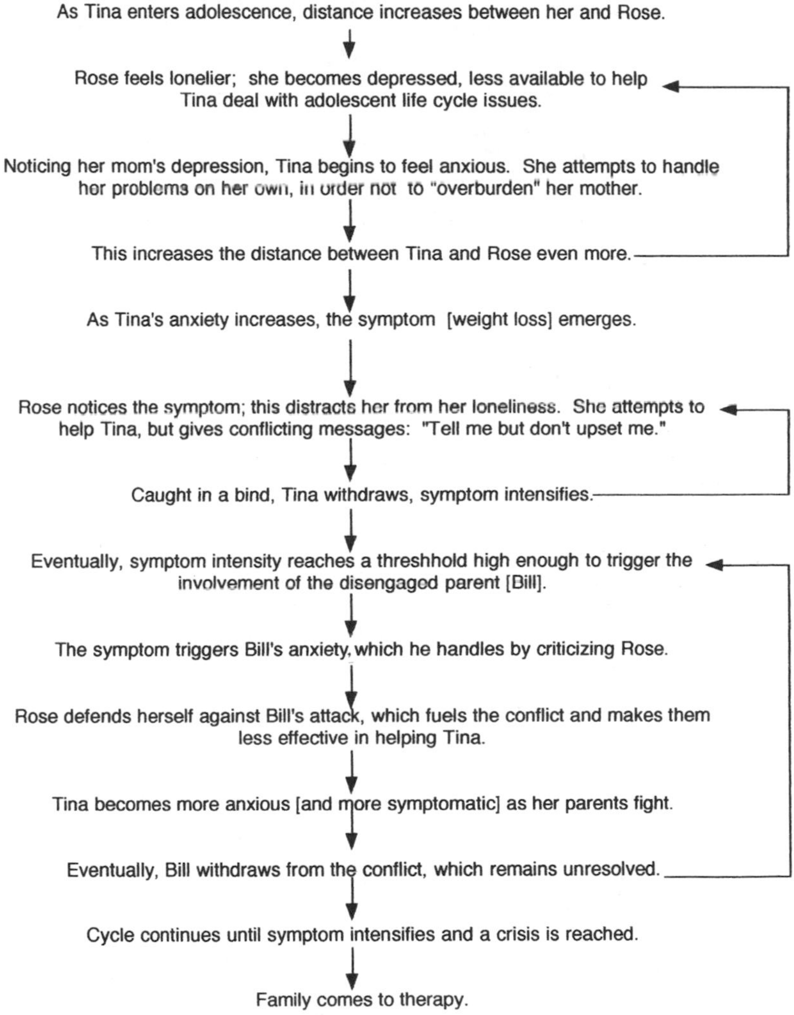

As Tina enters adolescence, distance increases between her and Rose.

Rose feels lonelier; she becomes depressed, less available to help Tina deal with adolescent life cycle issues.

Noticing her mom's depression, Tina begins to feel anxious. She attempts to handle her problems on her own, in order not to "overburden" her mother.

This increases the distance between Tina and Rose even more.

As Tina's anxiety increases, the symptom [weight loss] emerges.

Rose notices the symptom; this distracts her from her loneliness. She attempts to help Tina, but gives conflicting messages: "Tell me but don't upset me."

Caught in a bind, Tina withdraws, symptom intensifies.

Eventually, symptom intensity reaches a threshhold high enough to trigger the involvement of the disengaged parent [Bill].

The symptom triggers Bill's anxiety, which he handles by criticizing Rose.

Rose defends herself against Bill's attack, which fuels the conflict and makes them less effective in helping Tina.

Tina becomes more anxious [and more symptomatic] as her parents fight.

Eventually, Bill withdraws from the conflict, which remains unresolved.

Cycle continues until symptom intensifies and a crisis is reached.

Family comes to therapy.

FIGURE 4.1. The process of symptom development in Tina's family.

ered that Tina had been vomiting, and then, on searching her room, discovered ipecac. Bill threatened to handcuff Tina to his wrist and force her to eat. Conflict had reached explosive proportions.

It is at this point that families will often seek a first or a new therapist, ostensibly because the crisis had escalated beyond control, but actually to repeat the pattern of triangulation that characterizes their typical response to conflict. When there is no one in the family left to triangle, families will often turn to a therapist. What seems to be a good thing (seeking professional help) might actually be yet another attempt on the part of one of the parents to secure an ally in the struggle against the other.

In her first phone call to me, Rose made a point of emphasizing that Bill was reluctant to come to therapy and warned me in advance that he might be "difficult." Yet I also sensed that Rose was reaching out for someone to empathize with her desperation over Tina's condition, since Bill had done nothing but criticize her. I had to find a way of supporting Rose without alienating Bill, and without allowing myself to be triangled into the conflict between them.

Overview of the Treatment Process

Medical Backup Is Important

Before initiating family therapy, it is essential to arrange for a thorough physical examination by a physician who has experience treating patients with eating disorders. The patient might have a medical condition such as Crohn's Disease or colitis that has been misdiagnosed as anorexia, or that could complicate the treatment of a coexisting eating disorder. Once medical reasons for the weight loss have been ruled out, the role of the physician is to monitor the girl's weight and if necessary to hospitalize her if her weight drops below a medically safe level.

I recommend that the minimum weight specified by the monitoring physician be a condition for continuation of outpatient therapy. Should the girl drop below this weight, the physician hospitalizes her on a medical unit and keeps her there until she gains enough weight to be safely discharged. In some cases, hospitalization in a specialized eating disorders unit or psychiatric unit might be necessary, but the general principles of treatment remain the same. Hospitalization might be necessary to jump-start the weight gain, but hospital stays are rarely long enough to allow the full course of treatment to be completed.

Steps in Treatment

Family therapy for anorexia then proceeds through the following steps:

1. Negotiating a treatment contract. The first step is to negotiate a contract with the family that directs the family's attention away from trying to control or eliminate the symptom to changing their relationships with one another.

2. Encouraging parental collaboration. After the contract has been negotiated, the next step is to encourage the parents to work together to help the girl to gain weight. It is important to note the distinction between *helping* the girl gain weight and *controlling* her food intake. The girl's weight is an issue between her and her physician. The parents are not responsible for the girl's weight gain or loss.

The therapist helps the parents to recognize this distinction and to understand how their conflicts with each other have undermined their efforts to help their daughter. The therapist's focus is on stimulating a more productive collaborative process between the parents rather than getting drawn in to address specific issues of content. As a means toward this end, the therapist might give the parents the task of deciding on a (reasonable) weight goal for the girl and a consequence if she fails to achieve it. However, the purpose of this task is not to use behavioral management techniques to control the girl's weight but rather to provide the parents with a concrete issue around which their style of dealing with conflicts can emerge.

3. Addressing unresolved conflicts. As soon as possible, the therapist should begin work on uncovering and addressing unresolved conflicts in the family. One of the purposes of arranging medical backup is to give the therapist space to direct attention away from the girl's weight and onto the relationships in the family. The process of improving relationships between family members requires the therapist to establish a strong relationship with each family member individually, and then build on these relationships to encourage them to take risks and experiment with new ways of relating to one another.

4. Handling relapses. In many cases, as a result of the process of negotiating the contract and encouraging parental collaboration, the girl will gain weight. However, after a while, it often happens that she stops gaining weight or loses some of the weight she had gained. This "relapse" is an important juncture in the treatment process. The therapist must respond to the relapse in a way that discourages the reemergence of the symptomatic cycle and instead keeps the focus on the relationships in the family.

5. *Supporting individual development.* After a period of time, during which the therapist works with the family to disrupt the symptomatic cycle, the cycle weakens and a new phase of treatment begins. Now, freed from the cycle, the development of the family members resumes. At this stage, individual sessions with the symptomatic adolescent and/or other family members can be helpful.

6. *Supporting the transformation.* In the final phase, the therapist becomes less central and takes the role of supporting family members' efforts to resolve their own difficulties. By now, family members have acquired more flexible ways of dealing with problems and interact with one another in qualitatively different ways.

STEP 1: NEGOTIATING THE CONTRACT

How Do the Family Members See the Problem?

Each parent is likely to come to therapy with a very different view of the problem and its solution. As we saw in Chapter 2, Bill believed that Tina was using anorexia as a way to get his attention. Consequently, he expected that Tina would resume eating when he started spending more time with her. When this didn't happen, he revised his hypothesis: Tina was a victim of inadequate parenting by Rose. If Rose had taken charge, as a parent should, Tina would never have lost so much weight. His threat—to handcuff her to his wrist—vividly expressed his view that the solution to the problem was taking control of Tina.

Rose, on the other hand, viewed Tina as a victim of a disease that she never wanted: "She didn't ask for this illness." Rose was convinced that Tina wanted nothing more than to be "happy and healthy." For Rose, the solution was for Tina to find "the strength to heal herself." Rose was not sure how Tina might find this strength, but she definitely did not believe that forcing Tina to eat was the answer. In fact, she believed that girls often fell prey to anorexia if they felt that their autonomy was being taken from them, as would be the case if Bill attempted to force her to eat.

There are certain common elements in each parent's account of the problem. First, both parents saw the problem as inside Tina, and neither parent saw him- or herself as part of the problem. Second, both parents seemed convinced that the problem was that Tina was not eating, and that the solution to the problem required that Tina eat normally and gain weight. Third, each parent believed that Tina was a victim of something that had now escalated out of control, so that she needed help from someone to regain control over herself.

However, each parent also had diametrically opposed ideas for solving the problem: Bill believed that Tina needed more structure, such as he could provide if she were handcuffed to him; Rose believed that Tina needed more space, more opportunity to discover who she was and thereby "heal herself." The more Bill insisted on structure, the more Rose blocked his efforts, since in her opinion, Bill's approach would only make the problem worse. From Bill's perspective, Rose's attempts to undermine his efforts to take charge represented the root of the problem: Rose was too weak and too dependent upon Tina's approval to exercise the necessary authority as a parent. Because these positions were complementary, they reinforced one another in an endlessly repeating cycle (Figure 4.2).

Tracking the Process

During the first session, Rose and Bill each tried to convince me of the validity of their view of the problem, thus inviting me into a coalition against the other parent. When I asked them to reach consensus about how to help Tina, they promptly resorted to shouting at one another. One way that families attempt to triangle a therapist is by engaging in heated arguments during the therapy session. Each parent remains rigidly committed to a position, and the power struggle over which position will prevail reaches such volcanic proportions that the therapist feels compelled to mediate.

Instead of intervening as mediator, I interrupted their argument with a question about the process: "How long have you two been fighting like this?" The purpose of this question was to direct the parents' attention away from the content of their conflict and to put the responsibility for resolution of their impasse back onto them. They answered almost in unison: "We don't fight. We just don't talk to one another."

Defining the Problem

It is important to define the problem in a way that expands the focus of concern beyond food and weight. While the severity and potential lethality of the symptom must be acknowledged, the symptom must be linked to the interactions in the family. Each person in the family (including the symptomatic adolescent) must acknowledge responsibility for having helped to create the problem and accept a role in the solution.

Some approaches to family therapy (e.g., narrative or solution-focused) advocate less directness and eschew confrontation. A narrative

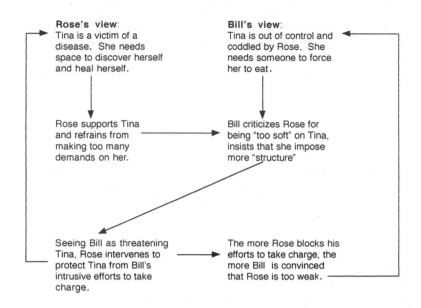

FIGURE 4.2. The system of complementary perceptions in Tina's family.

therapist, for example, might personify the problem as "anorexia" that has infiltrated the family and then work to unite the family members against this invader that has oppressed them all. A solution-focused therapist might divert attention away from those times when family members feel frustrated with one another and instead concentrate on those occasions when they feel satisfied with their relationships with one another.

In contrast to these approaches, I agree with Minuchin et al. (1978) that one of the primary factors contributing to anorexia is the pursuit of harmony through conflict avoidance. Narrative and solution-focused approaches could reinforce the family members' fear of conflict by discouraging "problem-focused" discussions. I believe that therapy should expose underlying conflicts in order to help family members recognize and alter their patterns of conflict avoidance. I accomplish this by utilizing untapped strengths in order to expand the family's capacity for dealing with problems.

The therapist's willingness to address conflicts in the family communicates to family members that the therapist has faith in their ability to survive the painful struggle to find a solution. Insisting that family members take responsibility for the problem and for its solution does not mean blaming the parents for the child's symptom. It means that each member of the family accepts responsibility for his or her *own* role in the creation and maintenance of the problem and refuses to accept responsibility that is shared or rightfully belongs elsewhere.

For example, toward the end of our first session together, I offered Tina's family the following formulation:

> "Tina is losing weight and can't eat because she feels isolated and alone, unable to express her true feelings to anyone. She is wasting away not only from lack of food but also because of the absence of nurturing and sustaining relationships in her life. This deprives her of the valuable help you both can offer her to grow and become the young adult she is capable of becoming. If you are interested, I will work with you all, as a family, to give you the chance to begin building more sustaining relationships, so that Tina may begin to grow again."

I waited for a response. Would the family members accept this formulation? Would they acknowledge that their relationships had deteriorated? Would they agree that the state of their relationships had contributed to Tina's weight loss? The therapist must listen carefully for rejection of the formulation masking as passive acquiescence.

After a few seconds of silence, Bill spoke up: "Yeah, that's what I've been saying. Tina needs to tell her mother what's been bothering her all these years."

Before Rose could defend herself, I responded, "Yes, that will be part of what will need to happen. But, Bill, how do you think that your relationships with Tina and Rose could change?" With irritation in his voice, Bill replied, "I'm willing to do anything to help Tina."

"Do you have any specific ideas about how you could be more helpful to her?" I asked.

He answered, almost predictably, "No, that's why I'm here. You're the expert. You tell me what she needs."

Not taking the bait, I asked, "Why do you think that Tina can't tell you what she needs from you?"

Bill squirmed, then shot back, "I don't think there's a problem between Tina and me. I think the problem is between Tina and her mother."

I had no right to expect that this would be easy. Bill was giving me the message that I shouldn't expect too much of him. If I pursued him too vigorously, he might leave and not come back, just as he had done years ago, when he cut himself off from Rose and the kids. I decided to take a less confrontive tack.

"Well, maybe you're right," I said. "Maybe there really isn't a major problem between you and Tina, though I wonder if she wishes that you and her mom wouldn't fight so much. Anyway, would you be willing to come to family sessions to see if perhaps there is something that you and Tina could work on together, or if there might be something that you could do to help Tina and Rose improve their relationship?"

I wasn't really surprised when Bill replied, "Well, I don't know how often I can come. I work full time, and I have a wife and kid, you know. My wife Ginny loves Tina, and she would do anything for her, but I've got to think of Billy; he's only 4, he needs me at home."

"I understand. So how often do you think you could come to sessions? Would you be able to come twice a week for a while?"

Sounding more annoyed now, Bill replied, "Look, I told you that I have other obligations. I'll tell you what. I'll come when I can."

Trying to get some kind of commitment from Bill, I suggested, "OK, let's look at our schedules and see what we can come up with."

In the end, Bill agreed to return for a family session in one week.

Rose, on the other hand, would have come every day if I had suggested it. I could already tell from the look in her eyes that she saw me as a lifeline. I turned to her next: "Rose, do you have any ideas about how you and Tina need to change your relationship?"

She looked at Tina, then back at me: "I only wish I knew. I only wish she could tell me."

I took this as an opening: "Then let's begin there next time. Tina [she raised her eyes halfway from the floor], would you think about that question so that we could talk about it next session? Would you think about ways in which you would like your relationship with your mom to change?" I took Tina's trembling nod as consent, then moved on to the next step.

STEP 2: ENCOURAGING PARENTAL COLLABORATION

After finalizing a contract with the family around the goal of working on relationships, the next step is to request the parents to agree on a target weight for the next family session.

After making a point of expanding the focus of the problem beyond food and weight, it might seem contradictory to bring weight back into the picture. This, indeed, would be the case if the therapist were treating the target weight as the primary goal of treatment. But this is not the purpose of the therapist's request. Instead, it is the *process* of negotiating the target weight, the involvement (or lack thereof) of the girl in the negotiation, and the development of consequences that are the focus of the therapist's concern. The setting of the target weight is simply a way of utilizing the symptom as a "hook" to engage the family in new ways of relating to one another (Brendler et al., 1991).

I presented this idea to the family in this way:

> "I have found it helpful if parents could make it clear in a very concrete way that they expect their daughter to do her part if they are going to do their part. One way of doing this is to set a target weight. It's Tina's job to gain the weight, and it's your job to help her by working on your relationships. From my experience, I've found that a gain of 2 or 3 pounds a week is realistic. Rose and Bill, I'd like the two of you to decide how much weight you would like Tina to gain by our family session next week."

Most parents are relieved that the therapist hasn't forgotten why they came to therapy in the first place. They usually don't take long to arrive at a target weight. In this case, it was Bill who suggested that they set 2 pounds as the goal: "I'd be happy with that. At least it's a step in the right direction, and I think she could do it." Rose agreed.

I moved on: "Now, can you both tell Tina that you expect her to gain 2 pounds by next week, and that the two of you will help her do this any way you can?"

They complied, first Bill, then Rose. Tina remained silent, eyes downcast. I expected the next question, and it was Rose who asked it: "What if she doesn't gain 2 pounds?"

"That's a good question," I replied. "Why don't you talk with Bill about what will happen if Tina doesn't reach the target weight."

Rose turned toward Bill, and he responded before she could ask him his opinion: "I think there should be some kind of consequence, like maybe she would have to be grounded." Admittedly, this was not a very creative idea, but I remained silent. Without responding to Bill, Rose looked at me for my reaction.

"If you like that idea, Rose, could you talk with Bill about how long she would be grounded?" I suggested.

Bill jumped in again. "I think she should be grounded for the whole weekend, and she should have to stay in her room, in bed even, so that she doesn't work off calories."

Rose retorted, "And how am I going to make sure that she does that?"

More agreeable than I had expected, Bill answered, "We'll just have to see. If she doesn't do what we tell her, you and I will have to talk about what to do next."

With this glimmer of hope that Bill might be willing to collaborate with Rose, I punctuated their agreement and moved on, setting up a time to meet with Rose and Tina in 2 days.

My intent here is not to try to force weight gain through a "behavior modification" procedure of rewards and punishments. My aim is to use a concrete goal that is directly related to the presenting symptom to challenge the parents to relate differently to one another, to collaborate rather than fight. It is an effort to move the family into a new structure, with the parents in charge and supportive of their daughter. In future sessions, the girl's success or failure in achieving the target weight can be related back to the success or failure of the family members in achieving the goal of renegotiating their relationships with each other.

STEP 3: ADDRESSING UNRESOLVED CONFLICTS

Once the parents have agreed on a weight goal, the basic structure of treatment has been set. The next step is *to disrupt the symptomatic cycle by challenging the conflict avoidance that lies at the root of the cycle*. The therapist accomplishes this goal by connecting individually with each member of the family and then building upon these relationships to encourage the family members to take risks with each other that can open up new possibilities for growth and change (Sargent, Liebman, & Silver, 1985).

Conditional Acceptance and the Symptomatic Cycle

The symptomatic cycle is especially likely to take hold in an interpersonal atmosphere where conditional acceptance prevails. Because their relationships are so tenuous in the first place, each family member must operate within a narrowly prescribed range of acceptable behavior lest conflict erupt. Family members are imposing these constraints on each other: No one is victim, no one is villain. As as result, the family members lose access to those parts of themselves that could allow them to initiate new ways of relating to each other, as I saw in the next session when I met with Rose and Tina to begin addressing their conflicts with one another.

Pushing Past the Limits

We began where we had ended our first session: Rose would talk with Tina about how their relationship needed to change. I reminded Tina that I had asked her to think about this question in our first session.

Rose began: "OK, honey, how would you like things to change between us?"

Tina, looking only a little less forlorn than in the first session, spoke in her characteristic whisper, "I don't know."

I silently gave Rose credit for persisting. "Come on, now, honey," Rose pleaded, "I really want to know. Please, tell me. Come on."

This time Tina didn't even bother to reply. She simply pulled her legs up to her chest and kept her eyes glued to the floor. Rose looked at me helplessly. I didn't say anything and Rose got the message that she should persist.

More frantically now, she demanded, "Tell me, tell me, tell me! What did I do? Or didn't do? Or should have done? Tell me, damn it!"

Tina simply whimpered in reply. Rose turned to me, "Give me the bag for my head."

I was puzzled: "What do you mean?"

"She can't look me in the eye to tell me how I failed her as a mother," Rose said, "so I'll wear a bag over my head, so that she doesn't have to look at me."

Though the idea was absurd, and I wasn't really sure that Rose was serious, it did speak to the lengths that Rose would go to help Tina.

I responded, perhaps a bit too firmly, "She has to look at your face while she tells you this."

Once again, Rose turned toward Tina. "Come on now, Tina," she begged. "We've been through this so many times."

Perhaps to rescue her mother from me, Tina found her voice: "I know, I know, I guess it was all those rules."

Given a crumb of content, Rose jumped on it. "What rules? Tell me, what rules? To make your bed? To do your homework? What rules? I want to know. What rules didn't you like?"

I interjected, "Rose, try to listen."

Stronger than I had seen her before, Rose contradicted me: "Yeah, but I don't want generalities, I want specifics. What rules, Tina?"

For the first time, Tina came alive, if only for a moment, "That's what I mean! You talk too much, and all you had to say was, like, one word!"

"OK, then, I'm listening," Rose assured Tina, with only a little less tension in her voice. "Come on then, I'm listening."

Tina retreated again, burying her face in her knees. Rose, unable to go on, burst into tears: "I can't do this anymore."

Here, we see a rigid pattern I assumed was enacted between Tina and Rose over and over again. As Rose became more anxious about finding a way to connect with Tina, Tina became more withdrawn, which intensified Rose's anxiety. Organized by Tina's symptom and her own anxiety about it, Rose drew more and more on the protective parts of herself. When she tried to be more assertive, Tina rebuffed her, withdrew, or expressed anger in an immature way. Experiencing both Tina's rejection of her competent self and a resurgence of anxiety at the prospect of losing Tina, Rose submerged the competent part of herself and reverted to the role of protector who enabled Tina to stay immature and helpless. To break free of this cycle, Rose needed to tap the competent parts of herself to engage Tina in an age-appropriate relationship.

It is essential to keep in mind that the more competent aspects of Rose (and Tina) are not missing; they are simply untapped. It is not that Rose and Tina lack these qualities, that they are deficient in some way, but rather that they have lost access to them. Salvador Minuchin would say to families, "You are richer than you know," communicating his belief that family members have within them untapped resources for growth and change (Minuchin & Nichols, 1993). The therapist must see beyond the immediate behavior of each family member to strengths that are not readily apparent, and must help to create a context in which these strengths will emerge. Once this happens—once a family member experiences an aspect of him- or herself that had previously been inaccessible and invisible to both self and the other family members—an opening is created for new patterns to replace the old. These new patterns can elicit from other family members untapped parts of themselves, thus leading to the creation of new ways of interacting that eventually replace the symptomatic cycle.

A Caveat

Therapists who are too intent on changing families or eliminating symptoms run the risk of implying to family members that certain aspects of themselves are unacceptable and should be suppressed. To disrupt the symptomatic cycle in a way that leads Rose or Tina to feel blamed or attacked would participate in the same culture of conditional acceptance that prevails in the family.

By pursuing change too vigorously, I could inadvertently contribute to the cycle by giving Rose or Tina the message that some aspects of themselves are unacceptable to me. They might act differently merely to satisfy me, not because they want to change. This pattern replicates what has been going on in the family: Each family member has felt compelled to suppress or deny certain aspects of him- or herself in order to remain in relationship with other family members. This conditional acceptance leads not only to isolation and distance, but also contributes to unexpressed fury at the outrage of being put in this position. The way out of this dilemma is to focus not so much on changing people, but rather on engaging them in relationships, with the goal of uncovering strengths that they may have forgotten they had.

I decided that the next step would require me to establish individual connections with Rose and Tina, so that I could use my relationship with each of them to bring about a change in the way they related to one another. For the next session, I decided to meet first with Rose alone, and then with Tina alone, to try to reach those parts of them that were hidden from each other. Then, I would use myself as a catalyst to stimulate a new relationship between them.

Building Connections: Eliciting Competence

To elicit Rose's competence, I decided to approach her as an authority on her daughter and request her assistance in helping me understand Tina. This request served a twofold purpose: first, it communicated respect for Rose as a parent; second, it framed the purpose of our meeting not as "therapy" for Rose, but rather as an invitation to collaborate with me to help Tina. To respond to my request for a consultation, Rose would have to draw upon her competence as a parent. In doing so, she would experience an underdeveloped aspect of herself that was absent from the symptomatic cycle.

As I anticipated, Rose initially related to me in the same anxious, insecure manner that characterized her behavior in the family sessions. I had to remind myself that my goal was not to change Rose, not to repudiate these parts of her, but rather to see beyond them to her hidden strengths.

Through the session, Rose spoke frantically with a pleading tone in her voice, a poignant demonstration that she was starving for a connection with someone who was willing to listen to her. At first, she focused on Tina as a helpless victim of anorexia and fear: "Tina has always been afraid of expressing her feelings. She can't help it."

I encouraged Rose to see beyond Tina's helplessness: "How do you think we can help her take the risk to open up?" The "we" was deliberate. It was intended to reassure Rose that she would not have to do it alone, that I would be there to help her.

Rose looked thoughtful, then tentatively said that she could understand why Tina was so fearful—because of the conflicts in the family.

I prodded, "And her silence contributes to the conflicts, too."

A glimmer of recognition flashed in Rose's eyes as she slowly began to realize that many of her fights with Bill revolved around disagreements over what would be "best" for Tina, who rarely spoke up to express what she thought. Rose recognized that, unwittingly, with the best of intentions, she had neglected to listen to Tina. She had become so distracted by keeping Bill at bay, so intent on convincing Bill that her view of Tina was more accurate than his, that she had never really heard Tina's voice. Rose came to this realization slowly, but without self-reproach. As she talked, her voice became calmer, and she appeared to relax. Her tired, worn look was replaced by a hopeful smile. The competent, secure part of Rose had come to the fore.

Finally, I asked, "So what does all of this have to do with the present?" The purpose of this question was to connect the experience Rose was having with me back to her relationship with Tina.

Rose took off her glasses, as if to ponder this question. Then, a flash of insight: "You mean, right now, today? I guess, I guess I need to *listen* to her, don't I? I really need to listen and not talk so much. I have to let her know that no matter what she has to say, I can hear it, I can take it."

Acknowledging the Adolescent's Pain

My next task was to coax Tina to emerge from her cocoon and express her feelings more directly. Once this had been achieved, I would bring Rose and Tina together and utilize my relationship with each of them to help them have a more productive conversation than the one they had had in the previous session.

So constricted in her immature, withdrawn self, Tina was not easy to engage. I felt myself getting frustrated with her and thought to myself, "This is how Bill must feel."

Tina decided to use the opportunity to be alone with me to plead her case. She talked about her desire to be thin, since it made her feel more attractive. She expressed anger at her parents for insisting that she gain weight, and anger at me for implying that there was anything wrong with her family. Her only problem was that she felt "controlled" by her family, because they would not allow her to decide when or what to eat.

Mustering my patience, I listened for a while, and then, out of the blue, I remarked to Tina that I felt so sorry for her because she looked so unhappy.

Tina burst into tears: "I'm miserable."

I pursued: "And about what besides having to gain weight? Is there anything else that is making you so miserable?"

Over the next several minutes, through her tears, Tina expressed her frustration that her parents "fought all the time," her anger at her father for the way he treated her mother, and her worries about her mother, because she seemed so unhappy since her brother had left home.

Finally, Tina cried, "I wish she would stop worrying about me and worry about herself for a change."

Though I was tempted to hear this statement as another ploy on Tina's part to be left alone to lose weight, I instead chose to hear it as Tina's suggestion for what needed to change in her relationship with Rose: "So I guess there are things that need to change in your relationship. Let's talk about that, so that you'll be prepared for the session tomorrow, when we get back to that conversation between you and your mom."

I sensed that we had just touched the tip of the iceberg, but at least it was a start. We talked for another 20 minutes, during which Tina began to formulate some ideas for her conversation with Rose.

Helping Mother and Daughter to Connect

In the next session, we got right down to business. Reminding Rose of our conversation the day before, I suggested that she again ask Tina to talk with her about what was upsetting her, and what needed to change in their relationship. I reminded Tina to respond to her mother with the mature voice she had discovered in our session the day before.

During the ensuing conversation, whenever Rose's or Tina's newly discovered voices receded, I intervened to elicit them again. In so doing, I hoped to facilitate a connection between Rose and Tina that was grounded in competence and maturity rather than helplessness and immaturity. Initially, Tina needed coaching to tell her mother about her worries, and I needed to remind Rose to listen and accept Tina's fears without responding protectively or defensively, without feeling compelled to soothe Tina or solve her problems for her. Gradually, as Rose and Tina grew more confident in this new pattern of interaction, I found that I could take a less central role.

Interestingly, during this session, Tina repeatedly emphasized how upset "yelling" made her. At one point, she stated rather emphatically, "I hate things to be upset, I hate it when people argue. I have to have things calm, peaceful!"

Though I was tempted to intervene to point out the folly of this position, I restrained myself. My goal was not to challenge Tina's stated policy of conflict avoidance, but rather to facilitate a dialogue between Tina and Rose. This dialogue was progressing very nicely, with Tina speaking up (at one point, she "shushed" her mother when Rose interrupted her) and Rose listening without defending herself or rushing in to protect Tina. By jumping in to challenge Tina's "irrational belief" about conflict, or even by inciting Rose to do so, I could derail the process that was going on between Rose and Tina that we had worked so hard to initiate.

STEP 4: HANDLING RELAPSES

Relapses are inevitable in the treatment of anorexia. After the weight gain has been jump-started in response to the parents' joining forces, a period usually follows when the girl gains weight. Eventually, however, she tests the limit by stopping or reversing the weight gain. How will the family handle this relapse? Will they revert to old patterns, or will they respond differently than in the past?

Relapses test the resolve of both family members and the therapist. Will the therapist abandon the contract? Will the therapist desert the family? Will the therapist reduce her own anxiety by referring the girl for individual therapy or hospitalization? Will the therapist shift the focus back to the symptom and away from the family relationships?

Framing the Relapse

An essential principle in responding to relapses is *to resist the temptation to focus on the symptom.* Rather, the relapse should be linked to interactions in the family. When the contract was originally negotiated, the symptom was connected to the disturbed family interactions. In the case of Tina, her weight loss was framed as a response to the absence of nurturing relationships with her parents. The relapse, then, must be framed in a way that connects it to these same family relationship issues.

The manner in which the therapist frames the relapse depends on whether the girl loses weight, remains the same, or gains weight but fails to gain the amount the parents had specified.

Loss of weight is obviously the most serious. If the girl loses some of the weight she had gained over the previous weeks, it is important to ask what, if anything, was different in the current week that might have contributed to the weight loss. Evidence of regression in relationships in the family should be given the most significance, and the weight loss should be connected to these regressions. If the family relationships have changed, then the weight loss could be framed as an expression of the girl's fear that the change in the relationships could have unwanted consequences for her or for the other family members. These negative consequences can be explicitly discussed, with the girl encouraged to express her feelings about them verbally rather than through the indirect medium of refusing to eat.

If *the girl neither gains nor loses weight*, the simplest way of framing this occurrence is to suggest that she is testing how her parents will respond. Will they recognize that it is not as bad as a weight loss, while still acknowledging that she did not meet the goal? Many parents will fail to differentiate between a failure to gain weight and a loss of weight, though, in fact, the latter is more significant. The split between the parents, with one taking a more permissive stance and the other a more punitive stance, will often be brought into sharp relief at these times. The therapist must challenge the parents to respond to the failure to gain weight in a way that respects each other's position while at the same time not undermining each other or failing to acknowledge that the girl did not meet the goal.

The therapist might frame the failure to gain weight as a sign that the girl is beginning to assert herself. The appropriate framing depends upon the stage of treatment. Early in treatment, when little net weight has been gained, the girl's failure to gain weight should be interpreted as an inappropriate expression of autonomy, and the parents should be supported in treating it as such. Later in treatment, when the girl has demonstrated that she can gain weight and the parents have demonstrated that they can respond appropriately, the therapist might lend more support to the girl and encourage her to speak up in favor of her own freedom of choice rather than use her weight to convey the message to her parents.

A third possibility is that *the girl gains some weight, but less than the amount specified by the parents*. Assuming that the parents had set a realistic weight goal, the girl must be given credit for having gained some weight, while, at the same time, her failure to reach the goal must be acknowledged. The therapist should encourage the parents to discuss how to handle this situation, after they have listened to the girl's side of the story. The therapist should monitor closely the process that unfolds between the parents, intervening as necessary to block intrusions by the girl or attempts by either parent to triangle the girl into the conflict between them.

Failure to gain the full amount of weight can be framed as ambivalence on the girl's part. On the one hand, she feels safe enough to gain some weight, which means that the family has demonstrated some changes. On the other hand, she is afraid to trust her parents completely. Acknowledging this dilemma could lead to a fruitful discussion about power issues in the family and the girl's sense of her own boundaries.

On the other hand, the girl may say that she failed to gain the full amount of weight because she was "afraid of getting fat." This claim could be handled in the same way. Why did the girl choose this method of handling her fear, rather than turning to her parents for support?

For example, Tina met the goal of 2 pounds of weight gain by the date her parents had specified. I framed this apparent success as evidence that the family relationships, particularly those between Tina and Rose, had begun to change, and that Tina was eager to do her part to convince her parents that they were on the right track. At the end of the session, I again asked the parents to decide how much weight Tina should gain over the next week, and they decided that 2 more pounds would be appropriate.

By the next session, however, Tina had gained only 1 pound. I asked Rose and Bill to talk with one another and decide how to handle this situation.

Rose began by explaining to Bill that Tina had been working hard, and that she thought they should acknowledge her efforts. Noticing that Bill was seething, probably viewing Rose's idea as another example of her overprotectiveness, I jumped in before Bill could respond and suggested that it might be helpful if the two of them talked with Tina about her reasons for failing to gain the weight. They did, and Tina explained that she didn't know why she had not gained the required 2 pounds and insisted that she was eating "a lot." Rose appeared willing to accept this explanation, but Bill was not.

I pointed out that Tina's failure to gain 2 pounds was a test of Rose's and Bill's willingness to listen to each other and find a different way of responding to Tina rather than protecting her, as Rose was wont to do, or criticizing Tina and Rose, as Bill was wont to do. I suggested that Tina might indeed not know why she did not gain the weight, and that, in fact, it wasn't really necessary to know the reason why she failed to meet the goal. I reminded them that she began to lose weight in the first place because of the absence of sustaining relationships in her life. The fact that she gained 1 pound might mean that she was cautiously optimistic about the changes that her parents had made, but that she was giving them the message that the changes were not enough. We would need to discuss this issue in more depth, but first, it was important for Rose and Bill to decide how they wanted to respond to Tina's failure to gain the required 2 pounds.

Since this was the first time we were dealing with an incident like this, I decided to go a step further and suggest to them that an appropriate response on their part should acknowledge three things: (1) Tina had gained some weight this week; (2) she had failed to meet the goal her parents had specified; and (3) her weight fluctuations were related to the amount of progress the family members were making in changing their ways of relating to one another.

Developing a Plan Based on the Frame

Rose and Bill listened patiently to my little speech. Bill suggested that rather than grounding Tina for the entire weekend (the original consequence for failing to gain weight), she should be grounded for 1 day, and that Tina could select the day.

Rose looked doubtful. I sensed that she felt that this was too harsh a consequence. I also suspected that underneath Rose's apparent caution were feelings of anger at Bill—after all, she was coming three times a week, he was coming only once; Tina lived with her and she was responsible for monitoring her eating patterns. On the other hand, I thought that Bill's compromise sounded reasonable. I debated whether to intervene to support Bill or whether to allow Rose and Bill to continue struggling together. I decided on the former, since I felt that my relationship with Bill needed to be stronger, and perhaps by supporting him I could bolster our connection.

I stated that I believed that Bill's suggestion was a good one, and that it addressed the first two points I had made. I wondered if we could also address the third point. I asked Bill if he would be willing to spend some time alone with Tina, perhaps on the day that Tina would otherwise be grounded. Anticipating an objection, I immediately reminded him that the grounding was not really a punishment, but rather a way of communicating to Tina that they as parents were serious about holding the line on their agreements.

Bill responded that he thought it was a good idea to spend a day alone with Tina, but he wanted her to be grounded as well—he apparently felt that some punishment was still necessary. After some discussion, we finally agreed that Tina would spend the afternoon of the "grounding" day with Bill and then return home and not be allowed to go out that evening.

Deciding not to push it, I encouraged the family to go with this plan, congratulating them on arriving at a reasonable compromise, and then pointing out that we had successfully addressed all three of my points. Since Tina and Rose had made progress on their relationship, I believed that the failure to gain weight could be interpreted as a message that Tina and Bill needed to work on their relationship. By agreeing to spend time alone together, it would help to strengthen the connection between them and perhaps help Tina feel safer about gaining weight the following week.

STEP 5: SUPPORTING INDIVIDUAL DEVELOPMENT

Development, which is a process of differentiation and expansion of self, is arrested by the symptomatic cycle. As I discussed in Chapter 2, certain aspects of each family member are repeatedly activated, while other aspects are underdeveloped. Once the symptomatic cycle has been disrupted, development resumes, but in a context different from the one in which it would naturally have occurred had the cycle never been present. Emotionally, the adolescent may be profoundly immature for her chronological age. Though therapy can accelerate the process of catching up, it is nevertheless painful.

On Monday morning following Tina's weekend visit with her father, I met with her privately to talk about her experiences over the weekend and to give her an opportunity to express any concerns she had about her relationship with her parents.

For the first time since I had met her, Tina was relaxed and smiling. She stated that she felt that she was "over anorexia" because she had gained weight over the weekend and was not feeling "guilty." Speaking quickly and perhaps a bit too anxiously, she went on to describe her time with her father, emphasizing how much she enjoyed spending the day with him, particularly since they had not had any arguments. At the beginning of the visit, Bill had apologized to Tina for all the times he had blown up at her, and Tina readily accepted his apology. The matter was then dropped, and they spent the rest of the day wandering separately through the art museum. At the end of the day, they met in the lobby. Bill drove Tina home, and dropped her off in front of Rose's house without walking her to the door.

A Dilemma

Hearing this, I was faced with a dilemma. Obviously, Tina was experiencing success over the changes she has made and excitement about the potential she now saw in the relationship with her father. She appeared more relaxed, more animated, more like a typical 16 year-old. She had gained weight and was talking about anorexia as if it were no longer the most significant aspect of herself. I wanted to share Tina's joy, congratulate her on her efforts, and celebrate with her.

However, I noticed that some important things were missing from Tina's account of the weekend. She had neglected to mention whether she and Bill had carried out the task to talk about their relationship, so I suspected that they had not done the task. Rather, it appeared that Tina and Bill had tacitly agreed to avoid conflicts in order to have a "nice" day together. Furthermore, Tina's statement that she was "over anorexia" because she had gained 2 pounds seemed naive, to say the least.

Embracing the Anxiety

I decided to challenge Tina. I asked her to explain exactly what changes had occurred in her relationship with her father. Tina evaded my question. She hastened to reassure me that she was certain that her father now "totally" supported her, but I persisted, repeating my question four times in the course of the conversation. Eventually, unable to answer and unsuccessful in distracting me from my question, Tina burst into sobs.

The anxiety that Tina was experiencing derived from my pushing her to define herself, to declare her feelings, and to justify her point of view. Although I sympathized with the depth of her pain, I interpreted what was happening as a positive sign. Perhaps for the first time, Tina was experiencing directly the anxiety associated with defining herself, an anxiety that is entirely age appropriate.

Freed from the symptomatic cycle, Tina's development is now unblocked, leaving her not free of pain, but rather subject to the discomfort and uncertainty associated with the developmental changes all adolescents must experience. However, rather than submerging her pain and confusion or expressing it symptomatically, she was experiencing it and expressing it directly and verbally, in a way that could lead to new possibilities for resolution. Growth is not without turmoil, particularly growth that has been so long delayed.

A Helpful Metaphor

I decided to stimulate Tina's process of self-exploration by introducing the metaphor of "internal voices," similar to that proposed by Richard Schwartz (1987, 1995). Throughout development, significant people in one's life become represented as different "voices" that can influence one's feelings and behaviors. Over time, myriad voices become internalized, those of parents, teachers, friends, colleagues, and supervisors. Meanwhile, complementary aspects of the self emerge as separate voices that carry on a silent dialogue with the internalized voices of significant others.

The process of putting words to the internalized voices reinforces the differentiation of the voices from each other and stimulates the development of an aspect of the self that can view these voices objectively—an "observing ego," if you will. Implicit in this notion is the idea that one can gain more control over these voices (i.e., impulses, urges, demands), but not by silencing them. Rather, one begins to experience a greater sense of personal agency only when one listens to the voices without feeling pulled to react to them.

The process I was encouraging in my work with Tina paralleled the one that had taken place within the family. Just as I had encouraged the family members to listen nonreactively, to hear and respect one another, I was now encouraging Tina to hear and respect the voices within her. Just as I was attempting to promote greater empathy among family members, here I was attempting to stimulate greater "self-empathy" (Jordan, 1991). One of my goals was to help the family members experience new aspects of their relationships, to become more tolerant of conflict and uncertainty. Similarly, in helping Tina to experience new voices within herself, I was hoping to increase her own tolerance for conflict and uncertainty, which would allow her to soothe herself without resorting to anorexia.

I met with Tina several times individually to explore her different voices. She came to label these voices "The Anorectic," "The Bulimic," "The Little Girl," and "The New Part," the latter being the young adult that she discovered she was becoming. As do many adolescents who are just beginning to experience freedom from their symptoms, Tina initially wanted to stifle the anorectic and bulimic voices, which had been so powerful in the past. However, to give in to this temptation, to stifle these voices, to exterminate these aspects of herself runs the risk of subjecting herself to the culture of conditional acceptance that had helped to sustain the symptomatic cycle.

Held securely in relationship with me, Tina could listen to these voices without feeling pulled to react to them. In turn, I was careful to remain in relationship with that aspect of Tina that could remain differentiated from these voices. In so doing, I wanted to help Tina to view these voices objectively, to hear them without reacting to them, without allowing them to rule her. I hoped that Tina might eventually discover that these voices had something important to say to her that could help her define herself in a more complete and, ultimately, more realistic way.

Constructing Tasks to Further Self-Understanding

To amplify the process of exploring the "inner voices," it is helpful to arrange experiences outside of the sessions that are geared to discovering and strengthening new aspects of the self. For example, I encouraged Tina to develop her artistic talent in a way that could lead her to connect with others, rather than as a way of putting distance between herself and other people, as she so often did. I suggested that she volunteer to give art lessons to young children at her local community center. I also pointed out that she could use her artwork, rather than her symptoms, to express her inner pain, and that through her art, she could make more concrete her newly discovered voices.

Psychological testing can be another resource to help adolescents become acquainted with their many voices. Unlike the traditional model of psychological testing, in which the psychologist administers tests to uncover hidden pathology, I advocate the use of psychological testing to uncover hidden strengths and to advance the course of therapy. Properly timed, a referral for psychological testing can be a powerful intervention (Ziffer, 1985).

In Tina's case, I arranged for a psychological consultation as a way to engage her more actively in the process of self-exploration. The psychologist administered a battery of standard psychological tests (Minnesota Multiphasic Personality Inventory, Rorschach, Thematic Apperception Test), but rather than interpreting the test results as an "expert" on Tina, she engaged Tina in the process of exploring what her test responses might tell her about herself. To expand on this process, the psychologist was invited to a family session to help Tina explain to her parents what she had learned about herself from the psychological testing.

A Question of Timing

As I pointed out in Chapter 2, it is important to postpone work on developmental issues until there is convincing evidence that the symptomatic cycle has been disrupted. Working prematurely on developmental issues can frustrate both the therapist and the adolescent, since each developmental step the adolescent takes can feed back into the cycle and reactivate it. In Tina's case, I could have made this error if I had neglected to consider the symptomatic cycle and had agreed to work individually with Tina to explore the issues she defined as personal or private. This pitfall can be avoided if the therapist remains attentive to the family context, whether or not the family members are physically present in the therapy sessions, and delays working on individual developmental issues until the relationships in the family have begun to change.

In practice, it is prudent not to make an abrupt transition from family work to individual work but rather gradually spend more time alone with the adolescent while still continuing to meet with the family. In many cases, it was precisely the stresses associated with the developmental transition into adolescence that initiated the symptomatic cycle. Thus, developmental movement on the part of any family member could provoke a reactivation of the symptomatic cycle. This point is demonstrated more explicitly in the case of Jamal, discussed in Chapter 7.

To facilitate the process of transformation in the family, it is helpful to weave conjoint family sessions with individual sessions with the adolescent and other family members. As the symptom recedes and the young person begins to struggle with developmental challenges, parents might require sessions to help them adjust to these changes.

Using Complementarity

In the case of Tina's family, as I met with Tina to help her get acquainted with the many aspects of herself, I also met separately with Rose to explore the facets of her new role as the mother of a 16-year-old girl. In one of these meetings, Rose discovered an aspect of herself that she described as "the part of me that cherishes the little girl." At first, she was tempted to deny this part of herself out of fear that she might discourage Tina from growing up. However, just as I had discouraged Tina from silencing any of her voices, I discouraged Rose from silencing this voice. I encouraged Rose to accept this aspect of herself as the part of her that could remind her that Tina was no longer a "little girl" and could help her find new ways of nurturing Tina that were appropriate for a 16-year-old.

By now, Tina had come to recognize that she might not always be aware of which voice was speaking at a particular time. Her new resolve to gain weight could be prompted either by the new "young adult" voice, or it could be a camouflaged deception of her "little girl" voice, which had decided to abandon anorexia because it no longer elicited the expected protective responses from others. Through this process, I helped Tina and Rose see that no behavior could be understood out of context. Most importantly, they were gradually coming to recognize that problematic behavior of any kind, expressed by either of them, was a cue that something was awry in their relationship.

STEP 6: SUPPORTING THE TRANSFORMATION

In a few short weeks, Tina and Rose had undergone a remarkable transformation. Tina's transformation was evident in her body: she had gained 15 pounds, had styled her hair, and dressed in designer clothes rather than the baggy sweat suits she used to wear to our early sessions. Rose appeared more confident and began to display an engaging sense of humor. Though Bill attended sessions infrequently, he maintained regular contact with Rose and Tina.

Rather than dismissing conflicts, as in the past, the family members persisted until they arrived at more lasting solutions. For example, in a session with Tina and Rose 3 months after beginning therapy, Tina burst into tears as she related an incident in which her father yelled at her over the telephone after she told him that she was reconsidering her decision to attend college. As Rose listened, I noted that she restrained herself from protectively soothing Tina or taking this opportunity to attack Bill. Instead, Rose willingly responded to my suggestion that, after listening to Tina's hurt and angry feelings, she support Tina in phoning Bill to discuss the incident. A week later, Bill accompanied Rose and Tina to the session and expressed his surprise at Tina's "mature" response to their argument. Tina had phoned Bill, told him she didn't like it when he shouted at her, and asked him to meet her for lunch over the weekend so they could discuss her college plans more calmly.

The key at this stage of treatment is for the therapist to calibrate carefully his degree of involvement in the family discussions. By now, the family members have developed their abilities to resolve conflicts on their own, and the therapist should remain peripheral, entering only to give the family members a gentle nudge in the right direction. As noted in Chapter 2, the therapist must avoid the pitfall of overreacting to emotional upset in the family and jumping in too quickly to soothe hurt feelings or minimize conflicts. By committing this error, the therapist stunts the family's capacity for growth by distracting them from the conflicts that have been unaddressed while they were preoccupied with the symptomatic cycle.

I continued to meet weekly with Tina and Rose. Tina visited her father, stepmother, and stepbrother every other weekend. Bill attended family sessions about once a month. He seemed content with his relationship with Tina and Rose, and they seemed satisfied with their relationship with him. Tina continued to gain weight, and finally stabilized at 115 pounds, which was well within the normal range for her age and build.

In one of our early sessions, Tina had asked me when she would know that she was "over anorexia." I had responded, "When you have your period. That will mean that you are finally ready to face young adulthood." One day, 6 months after our first session, Tina proudly announced that she had her first period in almost 3 years. Recalling our earlier conversation, Tina declared that she was "not an anorectic any more" and was ready to face the challenges of "being grown up." Tina and Rose agreed with my suggestion that the focus of our sessions shift to helping them recognize and negotiate the pitfalls associated with young adulthood.

We continued to meet at increasing intervals for the next 6 months, and then Tina stated that she did not feel a need to continue coming for regular sessions. Rose and Bill agreed with her. By now, at 17, Tina was a healthy young woman on the threshold of adulthood. Though she did not have a steady boyfriend, she dated regularly and had an active social life. She had decided to apply to college and major in art. Rose had also grown. She had begun to think about dating again and had attended a few community dances.

PITFALLS AND COMPLICATIONS

Though the process described in this chapter will fit for the majority of families, there are times when complications arise. For example, the girl might lose weight despite apparently successful efforts on the part of the family members to change their relationships. At other times, the family members are so rigidly entrenched in their patterns that they are not successful in making changes at all.

It is important that the therapist not conclude prematurely that the family is unable to benefit from persistence in applying the suggestions proposed in this chapter. The model advocated in this book rests on the goal of discovering hidden strengths and utilizing these strengths to forge relationships that foster better communication and healthy development. If a therapist is plumbing the depths for strengths and fails to find any, then the problem may rest with the context, not the family. Perhaps individual sessions with family members could help the therapist strengthen the alliance with each of them and bring their strengths to the fore.

There are, however, some complicating factors that could make the approach in this chapter initially unsuccessful and that therefore might necessitate some modification of the approach.

Subtle Undermining by One of the Parents

Although it might appear that the parents are working as a team, the girl does not gain weight. The possibility that one of the parents might be subtly undermining the other should be considered. For example, one of the parents (typically the father) remains peripheral and by default relegates the other parent (typically the mother) to the role of supervising the girl's eating. The girl resists when her mother tries to help her to eat. In desperation, the mother might modify the original expectation, and the girl might then eat, which reinforces the mother for having made the modification. However, since the girl is not taking in the required number of calories, she fails to gain weight. The mother does not tell the father or the therapist that she had modified the plan, for fear of being criticized.

The therapist might test whether this process is occurring by working out with the family a detailed and specific plan for helping the girl to meet the weight goal. For example, if the therapist suspects that father is not sufficiently involved, she might suggest that father take primary responsibility for helping the girl to eat. A family "lunch session" (Minuchin et al., 1978) is another way to assess the subtle dynamics among the family members. By bringing food right into the session, the parents can enact before the therapist the unsuccessful ways in which they have been trying to help the girl eat, and the therapist can intervene to change these patterns.

Subtle Undermining by Another Family Member

Occasionally, another family member who has not been an active participant in family sessions might be undermining the efforts of the parents to take charge.

For example, a grandmother might be in a cross-generational coalition with the girl and take her side against the parents. A sibling might collude with the girl in helping her deceive her parents about her eating. Sometimes, someone outside the family is undermining the parents. For example, a boyfriend might enable the girl to continue losing weight or undermine efforts to reestablish connections with the parents by monopolizing the girl's time. It is even possible for another member of the professional team to undermine the parents either overtly (by giving the girl advice without consulting with the parents) or covertly (by communicating disdain of the parents or the primary therapist).

In these cases, it is necessary to expand the understanding of the symptomatic cycle to include these other participants. If possible, they should be invited to participate in the sessions so that the therapist can directly intervene in the patterns of undermining. When it is not possible to insist on participation from someone outside the family, the therapist should draw upon his or her understanding of the expanded symptomatic cycle to coach the family on ways to recognize the influence of the external party and to block their interference.

Weak Alliance with the Adolescent

In attempting to support parental collaboration and authority, the therapist can err on the side of neglecting his or her relationship with the adolescent. When this happens, the abandonment dynamic is reenacted and the adolescent might respond by refusing to comply with treatment.

Developing an alliance with the adolescent does not mean entering into a coalition with her against the parents. Rather, it means entering into a relationship with her as a person in her own right. The adolescent must feel that the therapist is interested in understanding her, not simply aligning with the parents to control her. Therapeutic skill is required to communicate acceptance and understanding without feeling compelled to control the adolescent on the one hand, or support the symptomatic behavior on the other. One of the reasons for medical backup is to give the therapist space to focus on relationships while the physician monitors the girl's weight.

Subtle Methods of Control Are Still Being Used

In the case of severe, life-threatening symptoms such as anorexia, it might be very difficult for parents to give up their desire to control the girl. As Bill said in the first session, "The optimum weight is death!" Yet, the more the parents try to control the girl, either overtly or covertly, the more she is likely to resist.

Supporting the parents' efforts to *help* the girl must not be construed as supporting their efforts to *control* the girl. The therapist must be careful not to imply that the parents are being "taught a technique" that will "get" the girl to eat. Rather, the aim is for the parents to put aside their differences and collaborate in helping the girl.

The therapist must have a relationship with each member of the family, and each member of the family must have a goal that he or she is working on for him- or herself. As I pointed out in Chapter 2, one of the common pitfalls in family therapy is that family members are waiting for each other to change. This pitfall can be avoided if each family member adopts a personal goal that is independent of efforts (or the lack thereof) of other family members to change. Whenever the therapist begins to suspect that the parents are focusing too much on the girl's eating habits, the therapist can redirect their attention to their own personal goals, reminding them that the purpose is not to change the girl, but to change themselves in relation to the girl.

Sometimes the parents are unable to let go. The more the therapist encourages letting go, the tighter the parents hold on. In this case, it might be necessary to refer the parent to another therapist for a course of individual psychotherapy, but, again, the family work should continue. If individual work with the parent is not possible or appropriate, the therapist might consider utilizing a paradoxical intervention. Bartholomew (1984) reported a case in which the parents were overly involved with the girl and thereby stifled her attempts to establish a separate self. The impasse was broken by defining the anorexia as "chronic" and the goal of treatment as not to "cure" the anorexia but rather to help the parents learn to live with chronic anorexia without allowing it to take over their lives. In complying with this suggestion, the parents' attention was diverted from "saving" the girl and redirected to their relationships with one another.

When the weight loss is not life threatening, a paradoxical intervention similar to the one utilized by Peggy Papp (1983) might be considered. Papp told the anorectic daughter that the only way she could effectively say "no" to her parents (whom she desperately wanted to please) would be to maintain her symptom and to be as miserable as possible. Since her parents apparently wanted her to get well, the only way the girl could prove to them that she was no longer willing to do what they wanted would be to do the opposite—stay sick and helpless. Eventually, the girl rebelled against this directive and began to gain weight.

Severe Parental Psychopathology

Although a systems lens attempts to substitute descriptions based on interpersonal dynamics for those based on intrapsychic dynamics or individual pathology, it is important to consider the possibility that one of the parents might have an undiagnosed disorder, such as psychosis, paranoia, substance abuse, bipolar disorder, or chronic depression. Sometimes another family member, frequently the mother, also has symptoms of an eating disorder.

It is important to consider these factors, because the therapeutic interventions might be filtered through a meaning system that distorts them and so renders their effect different from what the therapist intended. For example, interventions directed to facilitate collaboration between the parents might be thwarted by paranoid misinterpretations or erratic behaviors associated with substance use or bipolar disorder. Extreme rigidity might be a sign that the parent is attempting to ward off potential disorganization. As the therapist attempts to introduce greater flexibility into the system, the parents might either undermine the interventions or begin to decompensate.

A strengths-based approach helps but does not completely solve this problem. The therapist searches for and connects with strengths in the parents, but if she ignores the psychopathology, she runs the risk of making the problem worse. This is particularly true if the therapist subscribes to the notion that the anorectic's symptoms served the function of keeping more serious pathology at bay. When the parents' pathology emerges, the therapist might feel vindicated in this belief and so redouble efforts to disrupt the family's "dysfunctional homeostasis."

While it might indeed be true that the family has arrived at a compromise through the girl's symptom, the therapist who remains ignorant of what the family members have been attempting to avoid runs the risk of exacerbating the problem. For example, the girl might begin gaining weight and moving away from her parents, who then begin experiencing marital difficulty. No problem, as long as the parents are able to work on their marital conflict. But it might also happen that one of the parents begins to decompensate when the girl begins to differentiate. The other parent does not understand what is going on, and supports the girl's attempts at differentiation by pulling the decompensating parent closer. This move does not help, because it was the parent's symbiosis with the girl that stabilized the marriage. As this symbiosis is threatened, marital impasses can arise. The girl might respond by taking back her symptom, thus restabilizing the family. Or, the girl might revert to another symptom (substance abuse) that has the same effect but maintains the illusion that she has been "cured" of anorexia.

Situations such as this are very complex and can be managed only by a therapist who is familiar with both systems thinking and individual psychopathology. The therapist must proceed slowly, reading carefully the system's response to any interventions. Obtaining history about each parent is essential. While the therapist amplifies the family's strengths, he must also be cognizant of the family's weaknesses so as not to exacerbate a weakness inadvertently by capitalizing on a strength. To use an analogy, if a person whose left arm is paralyzed is taught only to develop the strength in his right arm, the possibility of recovering some function in the left arm is neglected. Training for both arms leads to the most successful outcome.

When the therapist becomes aware of severe psychopathology in the family, it is critical to proceed cautiously. Referral of that family member for individual therapy and/or medication might be indicated. Whether it is the family therapist who provides these services or another professional is engaged depends upon the case, though it is usually better to refer to a colleague who specializes in individual work but who thinks systemically and can therefore work collaboratively with the therapist. Whenever another member is added to the team, efforts must be made to avoid triangulation.

Another possibility to consider when there is severe pathology on the part of one of the parents is to focus interventions through another member of the family who is more intact. This, of course, assumes that the therapist has made a thorough assessment of all family members so that she does not erroneously assume that the parent who appears intact is in fact the most resilient family member. While family sessions should still continue, the therapist who selects this option can also conduct individual sessions with the intact member, enlisting him or her as "cotherapist" in the family.

Sometimes it is the anorectic girl who is the most intact member of the family. In this case, the therapist might choose to work individually with the girl while maintaining a focus on the systemic dynamics in the family. The approach advocated by Selvini-Palazzoli and Viaro (1988) might be appropriate. According to this approach, the therapist works individually with the anorectic girl but attempts to alter the systemic dynamics through her.

The dilemma, of course, is whether helping one member of the family risks harming another. Working individually with one family member runs the risk of ignoring the disruptive impact of that family member's improvement on the other family members. This risk is minimized if other family members are also in individual therapy, though this is not always feasible. The therapist, in the end, might conclude that a psychoeducational approach is the best alternative, helping the girl to avoid the more destructive implications of anorexia, until she has matured enough to begin the process of differentiating from the family. In very, very rare cases, removing the girl from the family might be the only alternative, especially if the girl is in danger of dying, while the pathology in the other family members is not life threatening.

SUMMARY

In this chapter, I have proposed the following steps for treating families with eating disorders:

- Arrange for a physician to monitor the girl's weight so that the therapy can focus on family relationships rather than on developing strategies to force the girl to gain weight.
- Negotiate a treatment contract that directs attention away from food and onto family relationships.
- Encourage parental collaboration to help the girl to gain weight, by, for example, giving the parents the task to decide on a weight goal for the girl.

• Address unresolved conflicts in the family. The therapist forges strong relationships with each family member and then uses these relationships to encourage changes in the way the family members relate to one another.

• Handle relapses by keeping the focus on family relationships.

• Once the symptomatic cycle has been broken, work to support the unblocked developmental process of each family member.

• Support the transformation in the family by taking a less central role and gradually disengaging as the family members struggle to resolve their difficulties.

NOTES

1. I usually address parents as "Mr." and "Mrs." when I first meet them, and only later switch to addressing them by their first names. In this and subsequent case narratives, however, I refer to parents by their first names for the sake of clarity and consistency.
2. I refer to the patient as female throughout this chapter, because the vast majority of patients with anorexia are female. There is very little written on eating disorders in males, but there seems to be agreement that the individual and family dynamics that contribute to the eating disorder are similar for boys and girls. For discussions of anorexia in males, see Carlat, Camargo, and Herzog (1997); Frasciello and Willard (1995); Hamlett and Curry (1990); Lowenstein (1994); Romeo (1994); and Steiger (1989).
3. According to Bruch (1988), anorectics suffer from a "perceptual flaw" that makes it impossible for them to distinguish hunger from other feeling states. Some empirical research has found support for this notion. A tendency known as "poor interoceptive awareness" has been found to be associated with the development of eating problems in girls (Leon, Fulkerson, Perry, & Early-Zald, 1995).
4. Empirical research has documented the role of poor father–daughter relationships in the development of eating disorders (Cole-Detke & Kobak, 1996; Evans & Street, 1995; Mueller, Field, Yando, & Harding, 1995). Conversely, there is evidence that a positive father–daughter relationship can buffer the negative effects of other risk factors for eating disorder, such as early pubertal timing (Smolak, Levine, & Gralen, 1993; Swarr & Richards, 1996).
5. See Chapter 2 for a more detailed discussion of White's method.

CHAPTER 5

DEPRESSION
AND SUICIDE

When Peter Brandon called me about his daughter, I could tell from the resignation in his voice that he had just about given up hope. He had been referred to me by a colleague who was seeing Jenny individually but believed that the individual therapy was not getting anywhere and suggested family therapy. Jenny had been to four other therapists, and she was hospitalized for 3 months after she tried to slash her wrists. While hospitalized, Jenny had tried to hang herself. She had been on many different medications, including Prozac, lithium, risperidone, and Klonopin, with little success. Eventually, the staff told the parents that Jenny might be in the early stages of schizophrenia. Although Jenny had apparently exhibited no overt psychotic symptoms such as delusions or hallucinations, the hospital staff could find no other explanation for her erratic behavior.

Peter, Jenny's 52-year-old father and an executive in a major insurance company, was devastated by this news, since his own mother, now deceased, had been diagnosed with paranoid schizophrenia over forty years earlier. Peter and his wife, Clare, a registered nurse, had raised a son who was now married and living away from home. When Jenny told her parents that she had been depressed for many months prior to her suicide attempt, they were stunned. They never even suspected that their happy, outgoing daughter was experiencing such unbearable emotional pain.

The prevalence of depression and suicidality significantly increases at puberty (Compas, Ey, & Grant, 1993; Lewinsohn, Rohde, & Seeley, 1996). Some studies have reported that as many as one-third of adolescents experience periods of depressed mood, and between one-third to one-half of these meet the criteria for a diagnosis of major depressive disorder at some time during their adolescence (Compas et al., 1993; Petersen et al., 1993). Suicidal ideation is also more common among adolescents than among adults or younger children. Between one-third and one-half of adolescents in community samples report having experienced suicidal ideation, and between 6% and 13% of adolescents report that they have attempted suicide at least once in their lives (Dubow, Kausch, Blum, Reed, & Bush, 1989; Garland & Zigler, 1993; Lewinsohn et al, 1996). Suicide is the third leading cause of death among 15- to 24-year-olds, and the suicide rate has increased more dramatically among adolescents than in the population at large (Garland & Zigler, 1993; Lewinsohn et al., 1996). Contrary to what many adults believe, the vast majority of adolescent suicide attempts are premeditated, not impulsive reactions to frustration (Lewinsohn et al., 1996).

Why is depression so common during adolescence? Some authors claim that adolescents are susceptible to depression because of the developmental changes that take place during this phase of life. Hormonal factors might play a role, though it is believed that the effect of hormones on mood is small compared to the much stronger influence of environmental stressors (Buchanan et al., 1992). The physical changes that accompany puberty lead some adolescents, particularly girls, to feel inadequate about their appearance (Allgood-Merten, Lewinsohn, & Hops, 1990; Petersen, Sarigiani, & Kennedy, 1991). The new capacity for formal operational thought makes it possible for adolescents to reflect on themselves in ways that were previously not possible (Elkind, 1967), contributing to brooding and self-denigration. Family conflict, which is a major precipitating factor in adolescent depression (Cole & McPherson, 1993; Lewinsohn et al., 1996), becomes more common during the teenage years. Increased cultural pressures toward independence can push many youngsters into roles for which they are not ready, while also promoting disengagement from parents and other potentially supportive adults.

THE ROLE OF GENDER IN ADOLESCENT DEPRESSION

Among adults, it is widely recognized that depression is more common among women than among men (Culbertson, 1997). It is during adolescence that this gender difference first emerges. Prior to adolescence, depression is more common among boys than among girls, but by age 14, this gender ratio shifts (Petersen et al., 1993).

Many explanations for the gender difference in depression have been proposed, and most experts agree that gender-specific stresses and coping mechanisms play a major, if not decisive, role (Allgood-Merten et al., 1990; Hart & Thompson, 1996; Nolen-Hoeksema, 1987; Petersen et al., 1991). Early adolescence is a more stressful time for girls than for boys. Girls begin developing earlier and are therefore more likely than boys to be experiencing several transitions simultaneously, such as entering junior high school at the same time they are going through the first stages of pubertal development (Simmons et al., 1987). Girls and boys also employ different methods of coping with stress. Girls are more likely to react to stress by internalizing their feelings, while boys are more likely to distract themselves or turn their feelings outward (Cramer, 1979). Even when exposed to the same degree of stress, girls are more likely to react by becoming depressed (Nolen-Hoeksema, 1987).

Alexandra Kaplan (1991) has argued that the socialization pressures on women to inhibit anger and to assume responsibility when relationships fail increase a woman's vulnerability to depression. Girls experience tremendous pressure to silence their own voices in order to preserve relationships that are important to them (Brown & Gilligan, 1992; Jack, 1991). Mary Pipher (1994) has pointed out that many girls miss the open, warm relationship with their parents, which they have felt forced to sacrifice in order to fit in with peers. Girls are discouraged from expressing or even acknowledging anger, and so might have no option but to suppress these feelings and in some cases turn them back against themselves (Miller, 1991). The latter might occur following an incident when the experience of disconnection and isolation is particularly acute, as the following case illustrates.

> Connie had lost everything that was important to her, but her parents, Tom and Ellen, didn't seem to realize it. They had just moved to Philadelphia from a small city in the Midwest because Tom had been offered a promotion. Connie didn't want to move and on the day of the move had to be dragged, sobbing, by both of her parents onto the plane. They were living in a rented apartment while they were waiting for their new house to be finished. Connie spent most of her time in her room, refusing to talk with her parents except to angrily rebuff them when they attempted to engage her. She had begun attending school, but the counselor had already contacted Ellen because Connie seemed so withdrawn and unhappy. The final straw came when Tom and

Ellen told Connie that after 15 years of being an only child, she was going to have a little brother or sister. Upon hearing the news, Connie ran out of the apartment. Three hours later, Tom found her sobbing and wandering aimlessly in an unsavory part of the city.

After a few sessions with the family, I was able to piece together a hypothesis. For one thing, Connie's difficulty with the move helped to distract her parents from their own grief about leaving their friends and family behind. But another dynamic was also operating. Prior to the move, Tom had been despondent about his career prospects. He worked long hours and interacted little with Connie or his wife. As might be expected, Connie and her mother had developed a close bond that typically excluded Tom, who hardly seemed to notice anyway. When Tom got news of his promotion, his mood brightened and, much to Ellen's delight, he became fun to be with again. Meanwhile, Connie was so morose over the move that she had become unpleasant company for her mother.

Neither Tom nor Ellen knew what to do to help Connie. Eventually, they concluded that she'd "get over it" as she became accustomed to their new surroundings, and they decided that the best thing to do was to leave Connie alone. They had long ago given up hope of having another child, and when Ellen learned she was pregnant, she and Tom were thrilled. The news fueled the exhilaration they were feeling for one another. For Connie, however, it was just one more loss—her home, her friends, her special bond with her mother, and now her status as an only child. She had lost everything that mattered to her, while her parents, caught up in the excitement of a new city, new house, and new baby, hardly seemed to notice.

While depression and suicide attempts are more common among girls, boys are more likely to die from a suicide attempt, probably because boys are apt to resort to more lethal methods (Berman & Jobes, 1991; Lewinsohn et al., 1996). Thus, though males are considered to be relatively more privileged than females in our culture, adolescent boys, particularly white adolescent boys, are more likely than girls to die at their own hand. This disturbing finding requires us to examine the possibility that gender-related pressures are implicated in the etiology of depression and suicide in boys as well.

Olga Silverstein and Beth Rashbaum (1994) argue that the expectation in our culture for children, especially males, to leave home at age 18 can put unbearable pressure on a young man. They write, "There's no permission in our culture for them to postpone the leaving-home rite of passage. . . . For a young man who is determined not to leave, the alternatives are covert maneuvers, such as . . . procras-tination . . . sickness . . . or really drastic actions like suicide attempts" (p. 161). The young man who is not ready or willing to accept the culturally prescribed role of a male might begin to view himself as inadequate and unsuited for life (Pleck, 1981, 1995). For some, suicide might seem the only escape from this apparently hopeless situation.

Conflicts related to gender-role expectations are particularly in-tense for gay adolescents, and might be one reason for high rates of attempted suicide among these youngsters (Remafedi, 1994), as the following case illustrates.

> Bart had threatened to kill himself with his father's hunting rifle. Now, he sat sullenly next to his mother, Lois, a frail, depressed-looking woman in her 40s. She was seated next to Bart's father, Ed, a balding, overweight businessman in horn-rimmed black glasses. Next to Ed sat Bart's younger brother, whose baseball hat and athletic build reinforced his self-description as a "jock."
>
> At age 16, Bart had not been to school for the past 3 months because of intractable abdominal pain that had not responded to medical treatment. He had undergone what sounded like a tortur-ing round of tests run by one of the foremost gastroenterologists in the region, and still nothing had shown up. Yet, Bart continued to complain of debilitating pain that kept him confined to his home most of the time. He had lost touch with his friends, except for the few who continued to visit him on weekends.
>
> Patient at first, Ed became increasingly irate at Bart as the medical reports seemed to confirm Ed's suspicions that Bart might be malingering. Because Lois still believed that Bart had an undiagnosed illness and agreed with Bart that he couldn't attend school, Ed felt unsupported in his efforts to get Bart to resume a "normal lifestyle." To underscore his point, Ed would harass Bart daily about his appearance and about minor household chores that Bart had failed to carry out to Ed's satisfaction.
>
> Though Lois sympathized with Bart, she restrained herself from intervening during these arguments, because she didn't want to undermine Ed, as she used to do when Bart was younger. In couples therapy 3 years earlier, she had learned that her marital difficulties were fueled by her siding with Bart against Ed, so she stopped interfering and left Bart and Ed to resolve their problems on their own. She remained steadfast even when Bart pleaded with her for support, though she inwardly ached to comfort her son and intervene with Ed on the boy's behalf.
>
> When Bart's abdominal pain began, there was a brief reprieve in the battles between Bart and Ed, as attention shifted to trying to find out what was wrong and how to treat it. But, as Bart became more and more withdrawn and lethargic, Ed became increasingly

impatient. At times, he couldn't help comparing Bart to his brother, in an attempt to shame Bart into "acting more like a man." It was after one such particularly volatile confrontation that Bart had made his threat to shoot himself.

One of my colleagues suggested that I work to break the "covert coalition" between Bart and Lois by challenging Lois to be more active in her support of Ed's expectations of Bart. Though I understood the rationale behind this suggestion, it didn't sit right with me. How would it help Bart if he were even more overtly abandoned by his mother, the one person in the family who seemed to have sympathy for him? I decided to try a different approach. I noted that Bart never actually said "no" to his father, but instead would plead illness whenever his father made demands on him. Could I help Bart find his voice so that he could verbalize his resistance in words rather than through physical complaints?

I presented the family with the idea that Bart's pain was related to powerful feelings that he apparently was not ready to express in the family sessions. I suggested that I meet alone with Bart to help him "get in touch" with these feelings and to explore the reasons why he held these feelings back. When I met alone with Bart, I told him that he had to stop using pain as an excuse for not doing things his father expected him to do. If he believed that his father's request was reasonable, then he should do what his father asked, and try to ignore his pain. If he didn't believe that his father's request was reasonable, he should simply say so, loud and clear, rather than pleading illness. If he wanted to get over his pain, he would have to take the risk to challenge his father directly.

With my support, Bart did as I suggested. As Bart began to speak up, Lois became more active, sometimes supporting Ed, sometimes mediating, sometimes supporting Bart. I encouraged Lois and Ed to air their disagreements about parenting in private, so that they could present Bart with a unified front. I also encouraged Lois and Bart to have a person-to-person relationship that didn't involve mutual enmity toward Ed. Bart's pain decreased, but it didn't go away. He started to resume some of his activities, and he went back to school.

It was at this point that Bart nervously confessed to me in an individual session that he was being harassed at school by a group of boys who taunted him about being "a faggot." "The problem is," Bart said, "I am. I really am gay. And you're the first person I've ever told."

That session began a lengthy process of helping Bart come to terms with his sexuality, eventually "coming out" to his parents, who were, to my surprise as well as Bart's, supportive. A year later, Bart was back at school, had no abdominal pain, and had begun dating another young man.

FAMILY DYNAMICS AND ADOLESCENT DEPRESSION

Not surprisingly, family discord is linked to both depression and suicidality among adolescents (Asseltine et al., 1994; Brent, Kolko, Allan & Brown, 1990; Forehand et al., 1991). Joseph Richman (1979) pointed to disturbances in the family structure, including role conflicts, blurring of boundaries, coalitions, and secretiveness as contributing factors to adolescent suicide. Susan Harter (1990) proposed that suicide might result if an adolescent feels that he or she has disappointed parents whose support is conditional on meeting their high expectations. Krieder and Motto (1974) noted the association between adolescent suicide and "parent–child role reversal," whereby the adolescent is placed in the position of assuming a caretaking role for a helpless or dependent parent. Charles Fishman (1988) described the suicidal adolescent as "a stranger in paradox," torn between "contradictory directives [that] emanate from a split between the parental figures" (p. 161). Fishman also described the families of suicidal adolescents as "prematurely disengaged," in that the family has misjudged the emotional age of the youngster and has withdrawn the support that the adolescent needs.

Cynthia Pfeffer (1981) noted that conflicts between parents might be displaced onto the child, who might feel that he or she is not doing enough to prevent the parents' unhappiness. Parents might even communicate to adolescents that they are a burden to the family and the family would be better off without them. A suicide threat might be the child's desperate attempt to call attention to a problem that the rest of the family is ignoring. Consider the following case.

I had warned Tony's parents that after he recovered from his depression, they might wish he hadn't. They dismissed this with a laugh. "Don't worry, we can handle it. Just get us our son back."

The family had certainly weathered its share of crises over the years. Tony's older brother, Al, had been paralyzed in an automobile accident, was confined to a wheelchair, and required almost constant care. Accompanied by his full-time companion, Al had recently left home to attend college and seemed to be doing well. Twelve years earlier, Tony's parents, Paul and Lena, lost their infant daughter to crib death. They still commemorated her birthday and Lena still got teary-eyed when the baby's name was mentioned. Their youngest child, now 10, was identified by the family as "learning disabled and having attention-deficit/hyperactivity disorder." The family was in constant financial crisis. Paul ran a small business at home and Lena worked as a recreational aide in a nursing home. Tony had always done well in school and was a star basketball player—until he injured his knee in a game. He had a good relationship with both of his siblings and seemed devoted to his family. The problem was that he had stopped going to school. He sat in his room with the lights dimmed, shuffling around the house, not eating, and refusing to talk.

It seemed almost too obvious to wonder if Tony was mourning his brother, but I decided to explore this possibility anyway. Tony acknowledged that he missed his brother but also pointed out that he was relieved that Al was no longer living at home, because he was getting tired of taking care of him. If anything, Tony said, he was happy that his brother had finally moved out. The rest of the family echoed these sentiments. I decided I'd have to search elsewhere for a hypothesis. Did Al's leaving home reawaken for the parents the grief they felt when they lost their daughter? Was Tony "helping" them by providing them with a distraction for their grief?

Pursuing this direction was a bit more fruitful. Tony challenged Lena on not having let go of the baby. He expressed his frustration at his parents for not putting this tragedy behind them. Tony's mood seemed to brighten a bit when he expressed his anger at his parents. Yet I didn't really believe that talking about this topic was particularly new for this family. If anything, they had the same kind of conversation every year on the deceased baby's birthday.

What I noticed, however, was the process that emerged when Tony began to verbalize his feelings. Tony first attacked his mother for crying every time the baby was mentioned. Lena wept helplessly and Paul reprimanded Tony for hurting his mother's feelings. Tony then lampooned his father, challenging him for "letting" his mother carry on the way she did. This activated Lena, who then angrily began defending herself to Tony. Eventually, Tony gave up, hinting that "Maybe you'd be better off without me." As Tony retreated back into his shell, both parents then rushed to reassure Tony that they loved him and would never want to lose him.

The third time I saw this sequence enacted, it finally hit me. I asked Lena to restrain herself from interfering while Tony confronted his father. Though I had to remind her several times, she eventually got the message. Tony challenged his father, first about his passivity and eventually about the condition of the home, which was in serious disrepair because of years of neglect.

"What kind of man are you anyway?" Tony screamed at his father as Paul sat speechless and tearful.

Trying to activate father, I said provocatively, "Are you going to let your son talk to you that way without answering?"

Lena started to intervene, but she restrained herself after I gestured to her to keep silent. Tears in his eyes, Paul looked at me. "What is there to say? He's right. He's right. What kind of man am I?" Paul sobbed.

Lena spoke up, now angry at me, "This is what we've always been afraid of happening. What are we going to do if Pauly can't work? How are we going to live?"

Unrelenting, Tony now challenged his mother. "That's what you always do. You're always protecting him. You let him get away with everything. No one is ever supposed to upset Dad. Dad is too sensitive. Bullshit! If I've got to pull myself together to get to school, feeling the way I am, then he can pull himself together and start acting like a father."

Paul came to life. "OK, Mr. Know-it-all. You want me to be a father, I'll be a father. Tomorrow you're going to school if I have to drag you out of bed and drop you off there in your underwear."

I wasn't really surprised when Tony only halfheartedly rebuffed his father's threat. The next day, Tony went to school. He began to go out with his friends and push all of his parents' limits. He seemed to be functioning again, but in family sessions, there were many more tears and confrontations as Tony unleashed torrents of resentment at both of his parents that he had been storing up, unexpressed, for years.

Despite the association between dysfunctional family dynamics and depression, it is encouraging to note that positive parent–child relationships can in some cases buffer the youth from the harmful effects of other family stressors (Forehand et al., 1991). Cole and McPherson (1993) reported that the effect of marital conflict on adolescent depression was mediated by the quality of the relationship between the child and parents. Tannenbaum and Forehand (1994) reported that a good father–child relationship buffered the youngster from the negative effects of a mother's depressed mood. Petersen et al. (1991) found that a close relationship with parents moderated the negative effects of early-adolescent stressors and decreased the probability of the youngster becoming depressed later on. Kandel and Davies (1982) found the lowest rates of depression among teenagers who were able to maintain positive relationships with parents and peers.

Next, I present key principles for working with depressed and suicidal adolescents. These principles are based on the idea that depression arises in a family context where the adolescent has felt abandoned and disconnected from the family. Treatment, therefore, focuses on restoring these connections.

TREATING ADOLESCENT DEPRESSION

While many factors contribute to depression, a basic process underlying depression and suicidality among teenagers is isolation and disconnection from supportive and validating relationships. Thus, *a key theme in the treatment of depressed adolescents is to reconnect the youth with the family*. This process involves the following three steps:

1. Ensuring the adolescent's safety by helping the parents to take appropriate measures to prevent a suicide attempt.
2. Offering hope by opening up dialogue between the child and parents, particularly in those areas where dialogue was previously not possible because of topics that were "off limits."
3. Helping the family provide nurturance that does not infantilize, overindulge, or deprive the youngster of age-appropriate autonomy.

Step 1: Ensuring Safety

When an adolescent is potentially suicidal, protection takes precedence over all other goals. Measures must be taken to prevent the youngster from acting on self-destructive impulses. This does not mean, however, that treatment is delayed. To the contrary, the therapist can use the crisis around the prospect of suicide as a way of beginning the process of change in the family.

One way to provide a protective environment for the suicidal child is to organize a family "suicide watch." This means that the family, under the supervision of the parents, arranges for the adolescent to be personally supervised by a responsible party 24 hours per day until the youngster is no longer suicidal. The institution of a suicide watch can be a powerful message to the child that the parents can and will take care of him or her. At the same time, effective implementation of the watch will require the parents to work together collaboratively to make sure that they don't "burn out" before the crisis is over. The therapist must be willing to hold additional sessions and must be available by telephone to coach the family as needed.

Sometimes, a therapist feels that a family is not capable of conducting a suicide watch. Perhaps the parents cannot be relied upon to provide effective supervision because of problems of their own (e.g., severe depression, drug abuse). Perhaps the parents are underreacting to the adolescent's suicidality or do not believe that the youngster is "really" suicidal. In some cases, the parents unconsciously want the adolescent to die.

Even if the family is not capable of carrying out a responsible suicide watch, the therapist must take steps to keep the family as centrally involved as possible. Reinforcements should be recruited first from the extended family or neighborhood. In some communities, specially trained crisis teams can be sent into the home to help the parents supervise the suicidal youth. The key principle is to arrange support that keeps the parents involved and does not supplant the parents as the primary caregivers for the child.

Sometimes hospitalization is necessary and, despite its drawbacks, may be the only alternative. If the therapist has a relationship with a psychiatrist with admitting and attending privileges who supports the therapist's treatment goals, it may be possible for the therapist to arrange to work collaboratively with the hospital staff and keep the parents centrally involved. If the therapist does not have this kind of relationship with the attending physician or hospital staff, the therapist can continue to meet with the parents during the hospitalization as a way of keeping them directly involved in planning how the family will reorganize in preparation for the adolescent's discharge.

Step 2: Opening Up Dialogue

In many cases, following a suicide attempt the adolescent denies an intent to die or claims that he or she no longer wishes to die. In part, this occurs because the suicide attempt has had the effect of eliciting a desired response from the parents—either the parents have demonstrated concern for the child or parents have rallied in response to the crisis and no longer appear so distressed by their own problems. At other times, the adolescent feels enormous shame following a suicide attempt. In still other cases, the suicide attempt did not have the intended effect on the family: Rather than rallying to support the child, the family angrily rejects and criticizes the youngster. In yet other cases, the rigidity of the family structure is such that the factors that precipitated the suicide attempt cannot be discussed. To continue to appear suicidal runs the risk of being ostracized from the family because of the danger of calling attention to these "forbidden" topics.

The following procedure, elaborated from one proposed by John Sargent (1987b), is a useful template for promoting dialogue in families with suicidal adolescents:

Step 1. The therapist connects with the parents by acknowledging their concern for the child, emphasizing the parents' strengths and the positive aspects of their relationship with the child.

Step 2. Using the relationship with the parents as the springboard, the therapist encourages the parents to take a hierarchical position by telling the adolescent that suicide is forbidden. The parents must make it clear that they value the relationship with the child above all else, so suicide is forbidden precisely because it is a decisive threat to this relationship. The parents should be discouraged from communicating that they forbid suicide because it harms the parents or shames the adolescent. The parents must emphasize that preserving the relationship with the child is their top priority.

Step 3. The parents then express in a calm, caring manner a desire to understand why the adolescent attempted suicide. The parents communicate to the child that they acknowledge that the child must have been experiencing tremendous pain and felt that suicide was the only option at the time. The parents express regret that the adolescent chose not to come to them for help and ask the child to explain the reasons why she felt that she could not come to them. It is important that the parents communicate this message in a way that does not accuse or blame the adolescent, but rather recognizes that the child turned to suicide as a last resort. The parents are in effect, saying, "Nothing you could tell me could be so bad that killing yourself is the only answer. Tell me what led you to this point so that I can help you. Our relationship is strong enough to sustain it." In this way, the parents remove the adolescent from the "tell me/don't tell me" bind.

Step 4. After the parents have communicated their sincere desire to listen, then they must give the child a chance to explain why she tried to commit suicide. It is important that this step follow and not precede Step 3, because this step has a very different meaning when it occurs in the context of Step 3 already having taken place. If Step 3 has not taken place, disclosure by the adolescent could mean that the adolescent is trying to distract the parents from the "real" reasons for the suicide attempt. After Step 3 has taken place, the adolescent's disclosure occurs in a context where the parents have already expressed a desire to listen, have acknowledged failures to listen in the past (deliberate or not), and have reassured the child that they are ready to listen now.

Once the adolescent begins the disclosure to the parent, the therapist must see to it that the parents listen. Most of the talking at this stage must be done by the adolescent. The therapist should intervene as little as possible to facilitate the dialogue and to discourage the parents from responding too quickly.

Many parents are quick to defend themselves when they feel criticized by their child. This defense leads either to pointless bickering or to the adolescent shutting down. At other times, parents are too quick to offer reassurance or comfort, thus communicating the message that they have heard enough and can't handle hearing any more. The parents must be helped to listen nondefensively, to restrain themselves from offering comfort prematurely, and to apologize if they cut off the dialogue with self-defense.

Step 5. Finally, after the adolescent has explained why she attempted suicide, the parents must make it clear that they have heard what the youngster has said. Parents who react by saying, "I've heard this before," might confirm the child's hopelessness about the relationship. The parents should be encouraged to respond in a way that indicates that they have heard something they had not heard before, or have heard it in a new way, or have come to a new kind of understanding about what the child needs. The parents must make it clear that what the adolescent has disclosed to them is important and will be taken seriously. As I stated earlier, the therapist should encourage the parents and adolescent to identify a specific, concrete way in which the youngster's concern could be addressed. A behavioral change on the part of the parents communicates clearly that they are committed to improving the relationship with the child.

Step 3: Providing Support

It is important that the therapist not stop at simply encouraging mere words of support from the parents. *It is essential that the parent find specific ways of demonstrating that they are willing and able to take care of the adolescent.* The therapist should encourage the child and the parents to identify specific behaviors that would demonstrate that the parents are seriously committed to helping the youngster.

At the same time, the therapist should ensure that the parents do not infantilize or overindulge the adolescent. Parents should be cautioned against being "too helpful" and not allowing him or her to grow by taking reasonable risks. The goal is not to protect the youngster from failure or disappointment, but to provide an adequate safety net. One of the ways that parents can express their support is to encourage the young person to take on new challenges and reassure him or her that failure is neither inevitable nor catastrophic.

Remove the Child from the Parentified Role

While helping the parents in provide support for the child, the therapist must also encourage the parents to take care of their own needs. The adolescent will notice if the parents are not taking care of themselves. In order to prove that they are indeed seriously committed to their relationship with the child and determined to remove the burden of feeling responsible for them, the parents must acknowledge the adolescent's concern for them and demonstrate that they are taking concrete steps to take care of themselves.

Parents who try to pretend that they are "OK" will only make the problem worse. The adolescent will recognize that the parent is indeed "not OK," and the parent's dishonesty will contribute to the atmosphere of mistrust in the family. In an effort to protect the child from worrying about them, parents might try to hide their own distress. In fact, the child might become even more vigilant if the parents lie about how they feel. The message that is most likely to foster the adolescent's growth is:

> "I'm not feeling very good right now, but I recognize that. I plan to do something to help myself, and there's no reason for you to worry or to feel that you have to take care of me. If you think that I'm not taking good enough care of myself, please tell me as soon as you notice it. But you aren't responsible for taking care of me."

In some cases, either because the adolescent is particularly empathic toward the parent or because the parent is in severe need, it is advisable to identify specific ways in which the child can help the parent (similar to an approach recommended by Madanes, 1984, p. 163ff.). This suggestion does not contradict the idea that the adolescent must be removed from the parentified role. Rather, it facilitates the strengthening of trust in the family because it recognizes that the child indeed has something of value to give to the parent. By identifying a specific way in which the adolescent can help the parent, the child can derive self-esteem from having given something to the parent while being relieved of full responsibility for the parent's welfare.

PITFALLS AND COMPLICATIONS

Therapist Gets Angry at the Parent

When an adolescent attempts suicide, the sympathies of most therapists are with the youngster. Parental flaws emerge in sharp relief, and even the best of therapists are tempted to see the parents as villains and the child as victim. This reaction is even more likely if the parents indeed have done something to betray the relationship with the adolescent and fail to acknowledge this betrayal. The child might be trying to tell the parents how they have hurt him, while the parents simply refuse to own up to it.

Expressing anger at the parents can confirm their belief that they are a noxious influence on their child, leading the parents to distance themselves from the child even more in an effort to protect the youngster from their harmful influence. The therapist's anger at the parents might prompt the adolescent to protect the parents from the therapist. The child simply shuts down again and minimizes the significance of the suicide attempt to shield the parents from the therapist's anger.

Feelings of anger at the parents are a signal that the therapist has missed something, namely, what is making it too painful for the parents to hear what the child is saying. In order to listen to the child, the parents will need to feel more secure in their relationship with the therapist. Anger at the parents hardly contributes to the climate of safety they need. The therapist's anger should be a signal that he or she needs to reach out to them and try to empathize with their position. The therapist must create an experience of "we-ness" (Surrey, 1997) with the parents that can bolster their lack of confidence in themselves.

Parent Underreacts to the Suicidality

In some cases, parents minimize the seriousness of a suicide attempt, or claim that they did not believe that the adolescent "really" wanted to die. Communicating this message can be tantamount to telling the youngster that he is not being taken seriously, and that the parents' offer to listen was bogus.

It is best in these circumstances for the therapist to interpret the parents' underreaction as a defense against the anxiety generated by the suicide attempt, as a sign that the loss of the child is too painful for them even to contemplate. Once again, by acknowledging the parents' love for the child, the therapist can provide enough of a "holding environment" (Winnicott, 1965) to allow the parents to tolerate the idea that their child might actually have succeeded in killing himself.

To generate intensity, the therapist might lead the family through a guided fantasy of imagining the child's funeral, seeing the child in the coffin, hearing the eulogy, then leaving the cemetery (similar to the technique "Contaminating the Suicidal Fantasy" described in Sherman & Fredman, 1986, p. 207ff.). The narrative is drawn out in great detail so that the parents can actually imagine details of the situation and how they would feel. This fantasy will often elicit from the parents an outpouring of emotion and show the child how much they really care.

This exercise is most useful when the therapist suspects that mixed in with their love for the child are unconscious desires to be rid of him. By emphasizing one side of the ambivalence, the parents' defenses against their hostility are activated and the tender feelings might come to the fore, allowing the therapist to connect with this loving aspect of the parents and bring it into the relationship with the child.

Parent Expresses Anger

Sometimes, parents will express anger at the adolescent for having made a suicide attempt. Often, their anger reflects their terror and helplessness. The child, however, might interpret the parents' reaction as confirmation that they don't care about him.

The therapist should reframe the parents' anger as an expression of their concern rather than rejection of the child. The therapist should temporarily block the dialogue between the parents and the child, and speak directly to the parents. The therapist should encourage the parents to verbalize their feelings about the suicide attempt and then listen nonjudgmentally. The child can be asked to leave the room if necessary, but adolescents often benefit from watching the therapist express concern for the parents, since it removes the child from that position.

The therapist should emphasize the parents' concern for the child, even if the primary way this concern is being expressed is through anger. In many cases, the parents are angry at the adolescent because of things the youngster had done long before the suicide attempt. In these cases, it is important to acknowledge the validity of the parents' anger while at the same time exploring with the family how the situation got so bad that the child resorted to a suicide attempt.

Sometimes, the parents are angry because the suicide attempt added one more burden onto an oppressive load of responsibilities. In these cases, the parents' anger is appropriate but it is misdirected at the adolescent. While acknowledging how overwhelmed the parents feel, the therapist must help them recognize that the source of their feeling overwhelmed is not the adolescent, but rather the absence of other supportive adults in the parents' lives. For example, when a single mother expresses anger at a child for suicidality, the anger is more appropriately directed toward the child's absent father, who has victimized both the mother and the youngster by his absence.

The parents might be envious of the attention that the adolescent is receiving as a result of the suicide attempt. The parents might express their envy by declaring that the suicide attempt was merely a way of "getting attention." The therapist should not challenge the parents' perception that the adolescent was seeking attention. Rather, the therapist should invite the parents to consider why the child felt that such an extreme way of getting attention was necessary. Often, what the parents are really saying is that they themselves want more attention. The therapist needs to be the one to provide this attention, so that the child is not in the position of competing with the parents or denying his own needs to make room for the parents' needs.

Adolescent Refuses to Talk

In some cases, despite genuine efforts on the part of the parents to listen, the child refuses to disclose the reasons for the suicide attempt. The appropriate response to this impasse depends on the dynamics that the therapist observes.

Sometimes, the parents ask the child halfheartedly what led to the suicide attempt. The adolescent senses the parents' lack of conviction and accurately identifies this as a "tell me/don't tell me" bind. The parents are communicating to the adolescent that they are not confident that they can help him. The youngster picks up this message, and so remains silent, feeling even more acutely abandoned as a result.

The therapist might ask the child if he is worried that the parents might not understand or might become upset. The therapist should acknowledge that the adolescent might have had valid reasons for coming to this conclusion in the past, but point out that now the parents seem ready and able to provide the needed support. The therapist should first communicate his or her own belief in the parents' competence, and then explore how the parents could convince the adolescent that they are stronger now and ready to hear what the child has to say to them.

If the therapist observes that the parents are showing genuine concern but the adolescent is still not opening up, then a modification of this approach is appropriate. Perhaps the child is attempting to keep the parents engaged, and silence is the only way to do so. The adolescent might have had earlier experiences of being abandoned by the parents once a crisis had passed.

The therapist might offer support to the parents by trying to engage the adolescent him- or herself. It is important that the therapist do so in a way that does not upstage the parents. The therapist should first ask the parents for permission to intercede, and always refer to "we" when talking about him- or herself to the adolescent, indicating that the therapist and the parents are part of the same team.

If the child still refuses to talk in the parents' presence, the therapist might suggest a private meeting with the youngster, but in this case the therapist's goal must be to reintroduce the parents to the dialogue rather than to establish a separate relationship with the adolescent. The therapist might begin the dialogue by talking for the youngster, perhaps relating reasons "other kids" had given for attempting suicide. The therapist could adopt a strategy of passive refusal, for example, saying to the adolescent, "I'm interpreting your silence as a sign that I'm right," or "Speak up and stop me if I say something that isn't true." Needless to say, persistent silence on the part of the child indicates that the suicidal risk has not abated and the protective measures should continue.

Adolescent Minimizes the Problem

As a variation of the aforementioned complication, the adolescent talks but minimizes the problem that led to the suicide attempt. The youngster professes that he "doesn't know" why he did it, or mentions a seemingly trivial disappointment as the cause and declares, "I don't feel like killing myself anymore," without a clear reason why his feelings have changed so abruptly.

The therapist should not too quickly dismiss what the adolescent is saying. The adolescent might actually not know why he attempted to harm himself. In some cases, the suicide attempt occurred in a dissociative state and the adolescent might not recall it. In other cases, the adolescent lacks the vocabulary to express the intensity of despair he was feeling. Perhaps in the past, the child has felt ignored unless the issue raised was of a magnitude deemed significant by the parents. Now the adolescent might be "testing the waters" by raising a seemingly trivial issue. The therapist might explore with the youngster what this seemingly trivial issue represented to him, and thus expand the focus of concern to a more general issue.

If the therapist suspects that the adolescent is minimizing the problem because he does not believe that his parents could handle the "real" problem, the therapist could suggest that the adolescent "test" the parents by making up something that is really terrible but that "might not" be true, simply to see if the parents could handle it. Alternatively, the therapist could ask the parents to close their eyes and imagine the worst thing their child could tell them. The therapist should linger on this moment and request that the parents imagine this disclosure in vivid detail, and also imagine their handling it in a way that is helpful to the adolescent. The next step is very important. After the parents have indicated that they have successfully imagined the "worst possible thing" their child might tell them, the therapist should say,

> "There is a saying that no matter how bad things are, they could always be worse. Now I'd like you to imagine that your child is telling you something that is even worse than what you imagined the first time, [pause] and now I'd like you to imagine that you are handling it."

The results can be quite dramatic. In one case, a girl who had insisted that there was "nothing wrong" burst into tears and threw herself into her father's arms after watching her father struggle through this exercise. She then proceeded to tell her religiously conservative father that she had been sexually active with her boyfriend and was convinced that she was pregnant.

A Caveat

Provoking too much emotion in the family too soon can strengthen the family members' defenses and weaken their confidence in the therapist. I suggest the following guideline: When the intensity is generated by the family, therapists should refrain from decreasing this intensity. Instead, carefully track the way the family handles these conflicts and intervene only to block triangulation, detouring, or other ways of restoring the intensity to manageable levels. If more intensity is necessary, then start with the least anxiety-provoking intervention first and gradually shift to more confrontive and anxiety-provoking interventions as the family members' defenses are relaxed. A direct assault on these defenses is rarely productive. Instead, attend to the security of the therapeutic context as a "holding environment." Work not to dispel anxiety but rather to enhance the ability of the therapeutic system to contain the anxiety. Therapists can achieve this goal by working to strengthen their individual connections with each member of the family.

Let's now return to the case introduced at the beginning of this chapter. This case illustrates many of the principles I have just reviewed. Noteworthy are the ways in which gender issues manifested in this family and how I utilized my relationship with each parent to create a more secure holding environment for the adolescent girl.

CASE EXAMPLE: THE CRYING FATHER

In the first session with Jenny and her parents, I observed a familiar interchange. Clare, who, as mothers are in most families, was in charge of the emotional life of the family, turned toward Jenny and asked, "Don't you want to know about yourself? Don't you want to find out what's making you so depressed?"

Jenny, not surprisingly, answered in the negative: Perhaps the knowledge was too frightening or dangerous to her or to her family, so she elected to remain blind to a part of herself, even if this part of her had to be silenced through suicide.

Clare pressed on: "Don't you like yourself?"

"No, I don't," Jenny replied.

"Why not? So many other people like you," Clare pleaded.

Though Clare was clearly attempting to express support by pointing out to Jenny that she is indeed likable, she was also giving Jenny the message that one's evaluation of oneself comes from outside, not inside, that one is really not competent to assess oneself. Also embedded in her statement is the "tell me/don't tell me" bind—after asking Jenny why she doesn't like herself, Clare doesn't wait for a reply. Rather, she reassures Jenny that other people like her, thus implying that she has no good reason not to like herself, and that the basis for judging oneself is pleasing other people. Meanwhile, Peter sits on the sidelines, commenting briefly but offering little—the familiar pattern of the seemingly overinvolved mother and peripheral father.

Later in the session, Clare remarked to me, "I think Jenny and I are too close." Neither Peter nor Jenny challenged this idea. When I asked Peter what he thought, he answered, "Well, maybe Clare is right. Maybe Jenny is just trying to tell us that she isn't a little girl any more and she doesn't want to be around us all the time."

I asked Jenny for her opinion. "I don't know," she replied. "I just can't talk to my parents."

I asked her why she felt she could not talk with them, and she answered, "I guess I'm afraid of hurting them."

Clare, struggling to understand, asked incredulously, "So you're hurting yourself so that you don't have to hurt us?"

This interchange suggests that Clare has bought into the cultural stereotype that she is hurting her daughter by being too close to her. Attempting to give Jenny the space that she thinks she needs, Clare backs off, but this only intensifies the abandonment the girl is already experiencing. Meanwhile, Jenny and Peter both imply agreement by not challenging Clare's statement. Peter, already peripheral, offers the interpretation that it is Jenny who wants more "space" because she doesn't seem to want to be around them. Presumably, he is referring to "space" from Clare, since he and Jenny apparently don't have much of a relationship.

Jenny offers a different perspective: She points out that the problem is not "too much" relationship, but the absence of one: "I can't talk to my parents." In this respect, Jenny is similar to most adolescent girls, who want to stay close to their parents even as they become more independent and individuated (Kaplan et al., 1991).

Interestingly, though, Jenny does not blame her parents for the absence of dialogue between them. Rather, she blames herself—she is afraid of hurting them. Silence is her only option, because to speak what is on her mind risks hurting her parents, and ultimately herself, because the relationship between them will suffer. Young women often find themselves in this bind. They must suppress their feelings and their own voices in order to prevent the loss of a relationship (Brown & Gilligan, 1992; Jack, 1991). Jenny is in a no-win situation. If she silences herself, she contributes to her own isolation. If she speaks, she risks hurting her parents and damaging her relationship with them, which in turn will intensify her isolation. Therapy must help Jenny and her parents find a way out of this bind. The way out is to help them open up the dialogue without sacrificing their relationships.

Throughout this session, Peter remained aloof. I knew that he cared about Jenny—in fact, it was he who first contacted me for help. But the pattern in the family session underscored his peripheral position. He remained on the sidelines, entering only to contradict Clare or to speak for Jenny when the tension threatened to escalate between Jenny and her mother. Perhaps he was trying to reconnect with Jenny, to communicate that he did indeed want a relationship with her. Unfortunately, he was doing so in a way that robbed Jenny of her own voice and undermined his relationship with his wife.

I also noted that Clare was willing to accept responsibility for part of the problem: "I think Jenny and I are too close," while Peter stated the problem more impersonally, framed in a way that relieved him of blame: "Jenny doesn't want to be around us." Peter was using his peripheral position to exonerate himself: How can I be responsible for this problem if I've really not been around very much?

Later, to explore further the relationship between the parents and to see how I might capitalize on their strengths, I asked Peter and Clare to talk together about how they thought they could be helpful to Jenny.

PETER: (*to Clare*) So what do you think we should do?

CLARE: Well, I think we should keep on what we are doing. We're trying to listen to her, trying to find out how she would like us to change, and . . .

PETER: (*cutting her off*) Yeah, but that doesn't seem to be getting us anywhere. She still won't talk. I think we're back at square one, almost.

CLARE: Well, I don't. I think Jenny is really interested in finding out what's bothering her.

PETER: But what *is* bothering her? We keep asking and asking and she doesn't tell us.

CLARE: I think she is telling us. She's telling us that she's afraid to hurt us.

PETER: And we tell her not to be afraid. So where does that leave us?

CLARE: (*with a sigh*) Peter, I don't have the answers.

PETER: So what are we going to do?

Here, again, we see the familiar pattern of the father attacking Jenny and the mother defending her. Peter has little to offer; he expects Clare to have the answers. But when Clare does propose a solution, Peter criticizes it. Finally, Clare admits, "I don't have the answers." But she doesn't challenge the idea that she *should* have the answers, or that Peter is not offering any himself, or that he should take responsibility to get to know Jenny himself rather than using Clare as an intermediary. As Betty Carter (1988) has pointed out, "Finding direct involvement with his daughter frustrating and upsetting, father turns the job over to mother and then complains about the way she does it" (p. 113).

The pattern was more complicated, as I later learned. Peter's job took him away from home on extended trips several times a year. During his absences, Clare functioned essentially as a single parent. When Peter returned, Clare would step aside to give him an opportunity to be a parent, which reinforced the idea that it was Peter who was really in charge ("Wait until Dad comes home"). Rather than parenting as a team, Peter and Clare took turns acting as single parents. While this may not have been Clare's intention (perhaps she was simply trying to take a break from full-time parenting), the pattern spoke for itself. From Jenny's perspective, it meant that her relationship with each parent was mediated by the other: Her closeness with her mother depended on father's physical presence or absence; her relationship with her father existed only when mother stepped aside. I would need to help Jenny develop a person-to-person relationship with each parent, one that was not mediated by the other parent.

I recommended that Peter and Jenny spend time together, a suggestion they dutifully followed. But the interactions between them remained bland. Though Jenny and her mother argued more, there was more passion in their relationship, more connection, and ultimately more investment by both parties. Peter and Jenny were cordial, but scarcely intimate, and it was clear that simply prescribing time alone together would not stimulate more intimacy between them.

I wondered if Peter's experiences with his schizophrenic mother had frightened him away from Jenny, who had been labeled "preschizophrenic" by the staff at the psychiatric hospital. It would not be the first time that a diagnosis ostensibly given to help an adolescent results in more intense isolation between the child and parents. Peter told me that his father had died when he was only 13, and after his father's death, his mother's male psychiatrist told Peter that it was his responsibility to take care of his mother. I wondered if Peter felt resentment toward his parents for having abandoned him, leaving him essentially orphaned throughout his own adolescence and saddled with the impossible responsibility of taking care of his own mother. However, when I tried to pursue Peter to talk about his inner pain, he pushed me away, dismissing me with reassurance that he had "gotten over" his grief when his father and then, years later, his mother died. Though Peter's mother had died 8 years ago, it was clear that her ghost still haunted him.

We appeared to be at an impasse, but then, as it often does, a crisis arose that provided another opportunity for initiating change. Late one night, I received an urgent message from Clare. Jenny had been rushed to the emergency room after taking 50 acetaminophen tablets. Peter was out of town, couldn't be reached, and wasn't scheduled to return for 3 more days. Jenny had been admitted to the hospital, but the doctors had told Clare that she would be all right and could probably go home the next day. I scheduled an appointment with them late the next afternoon, so that Clare and Jenny could come to my office directly from the hospital.

The story Jenny told was almost unbelievable. She and her mother had just finished eating dinner together. Jenny went up to her room while Clare started the dishes. Hardly 10 minutes later, Jenny came into the kitchen and told her mother that she had taken the pills. Jenny offered no objection as Clare ushered her into the car and drove her to the emergency room.

I began the session by asking Clare to talk with Jenny about the reasons she tried to kill herself.

JENNY: I honestly don't know. I just saw the pills there and I took them.

CLARE: Did it have anything to do with what we were talking about at dinner?

JENNY: I don't even remember what we were talking about at dinner.

CLARE: That's just it, hon, we weren't talking about much of anything, just everyday stuff.

JENNY: I know, Mom. I don't know why it happened.

CLARE: Were you hearing voices?

JENNY: No.

CLARE: Were you planning it all along?

JENNY: (*a bit more annoyed now*) No, Mom. I told you, I don't know why I did it! It just popped into my head.

CLARE: (*getting exasperated*) But I was right in the other room. Why couldn't you come to me?

JENNY: (*sighing*) I told you, I don't know. I just don't know.

I felt sympathy for both Jenny and Clare. I could imagine the guilt Clare felt, since this happened "on her watch," and only minutes after she and Jenny had parted. On the phone the night before, Clare had frantically asked, "Does this mean that I can't leave her alone even for a few minutes?" Though Jenny herself was mystified about her state of mind at the time she took the pills, Clare still felt responsible.

I felt sympathy for Jenny, too. I believed that she really didn't know why she had taken the pills. To her credit, though she knew that she could rescue her mother from her helplessness by fabricating a reason that seemed to satisfy us, Jenny didn't give in to this temptation. But it was poignantly obvious just how much Jenny had lost access to her own voice. Less than 24 hours ago she had taken a near-lethal overdose with no warning and now could offer no explanation.

It crossed my mind that Jenny might have attempted suicide in response to command hallucinations or while in a dissociated state, but I chose to emphasize a different aspect of the problem. It was clear that pleading with Jenny to explain why she took the pills was only pushing her farther away, because our request for a reason presumed that Jenny had knowledge about herself that she really didn't have. The only thing that linked us all was our profound helplessness before a powerful force that none of us understood or could even name. If I was going to be of any help at all, I would have to admit that we were all in the same boat.

I recognized the paradox: By working so hard to save Jenny, we were giving her the message that she was unacceptable as she was. We had been inducted into the cycle of control, as the suicide attempt most poignantly brought to the fore. My relationship with Jenny was predicated on helping her to change (though into what was not entirely clear). Her parents, too, insisted they would "do anything for her," which only underscored how desperately they wanted her to change. Meanwhile, Jenny remained lost. She didn't know herself either, but we were working so hard to help her become who we thought she wanted to be that we inadvertently perpetuated her isolation.

But we were not prepared to allow her to die, even if she believed she wanted to. The bottom line was that we wanted a relationship with Jenny, and that meant she had to stay alive. If living was unbearable for her, then we would do what we could to help share the burden and make it possible for her to go on. But we would never agree that suicide was the only answer. We would keep trying to connect with her even if she wanted to give up.

Stuck as we were in this impasse, I realized the futility of demanding that Jenny tell us why she had attempted to kill herself, an act so extreme that it was really not possible to justify. Jenny knew that she could never adequately explain what she had done, and would not play along. Why should she fabricate a reason only to have it shot down by us as insufficient justification for having attempted to kill herself? She was in a bind: Give us a reason, and we'll contradict it; don't give us a reason, and we will continue to pursue you ever more frantically until you give us one. The only way out was to let go of our need to understand, to remove the requirement that she placate us by satisfying our need for a reason.

To break the cycle of control, I realized that I needed to help Clare focus back on herself rather than on Jenny. This would be difficult, since Clare's heart ached for Jenny. I asked Clare to tell Jenny how she felt about her suicide attempt. Though I was risking the possibility that Clare might express anger, I thought that my relationship with her was strong enough to allow me to reframe anger as an expression of her anxiety over losing Jenny.

I needn't have worried, because upon hearing my question, Clare paused, and then began to weep.

"How do I feel?" she asked, incredulously. "Devastated. Absolutely devastated."

Jenny looked as if she was going to speak up, but I indicated that she should let her mother go on and not interrupt her.

After a tearful few minutes, Clare said, "No matter how big she gets, she's still that little girl I loved. I wish I could take the pain away from her when she feels that way. I've never felt pain like hers. I can only imagine how agonizing it must feel."

Jenny was now listening intently. Clare wept some more, then went on. "If she had died, I think I would cry until the end of time. I just couldn't be consoled. I would go on, I would live my life, but there would always be this big empty space because Jenny wasn't there any more."

Clare sobbed. Jenny, also in tears, put her arm around her. After a few minutes had passed, I asked Jenny if she had any reaction to what her mother had said.

Jenny, drying her eyes with a tissue supplied by Clare, spoke as her eyes watered again, "I never knew she cared so much. 'I'd cry until the end of time.' That's, that's like, all the tears in the world wouldn't be enough." Jenny looked at her mother, "I never meant to hurt you, Mom."

Clare held her as Jenny burst into tears again.

"I know, honey," Clare said, "I know. I just wish I knew what to do when that feeling comes over you, sweetie."

I wanted to build on this moment. Clare didn't know what to do to keep Jenny from trying to hurt herself again, and I didn't know either. But Clare knew a lot about being a mother. I wanted to capitalize on the strength of her relationship with Jenny, using Clare's wisdom as the springboard.

"Clare," I asked, "What did you do when Jenny was little and she was sick, but you couldn't do anything but wait until the fever broke?"

Clare looked at Jenny with loving maternal eyes, then back at me, "I did what any mother would do. I'd sit with her, I'd hold her hand, I'd tell her that it would be all right, that I'd stay with her until she felt better."

I restrained myself from speaking, though I smiled and nodded. I waited for Clare to make the connection for herself. A glimmer of insight appeared in her eyes, "So maybe all I can do now is wait, and hold her hand until the feeling passes."

Out of the mother–daughter relationship, strength had emerged, and a discovery that freed Clare from the responsibility that the need to control brings with it. The answer, like many profound truths, was startlingly simple. In surrendering to her helplessness, Clare realized that she was not responsible for keeping Jenny alive. The feeling that afflicted Jenny, like a childhood fever, was temporarily in control. All Clare could do was to hold Jenny's hand, lending Jenny her own strength to fight the emotional fever that had her in its grip. This Clare knew how to do, and she didn't need me or Peter to tell her how to do it. All she needed to do was to be with Jenny, hold her hand, and stay with her until the feeling passed. Jenny also appeared to relax at this realization. No longer was she caught in the bind of having to help her mother by giving her mother a promise she could not keep—that she would not try to harm herself again. But she could surrender herself to her mother's soothing presence while they waited together for the suicidal feeling to pass.

When a suicidal adolescent like Jenny backs away from her parents, it is almost always out of a misguided sense of love, duty, and responsibility. The adolescent realizes that she hurts her parents when she hurts herself. She knows that they want nothing more than for her to stop harming herself. But the suicidal adolescent is in a bind. If she goes to her parents for help, they go into overdrive trying to reassure her and, in the process, unwittingly discount her feelings. She can't bear to see her parents hurt, so she avoids them, retreating into even more intense isolation, but at least secure in the knowledge that she is not hurting anyone but herself.

If the parents, like Clare, can embrace their own powerlessness, admit that they cannot prevent their child from taking her own life, no matter how much they wish they could, then they can truly be a resource for the adolescent. The child can rest in their arms, secure in the knowledge that she needn't produce anything in order to stay cradled there. All she has to do is ask. And the parents need not find a way to prevent the child from feeling bad. All they need to do is listen, to be there, to hold her hand until the feeling passes. After our therapeutic techniques have failed to produce the changes we seek, all we really have is the healing power of the relationship.

The question now was how to bridge from this pivotal event to the next session, when Peter returned. Sometimes, a mother will display more competence in a father's absence, only to regress to her previous appearance of incompetence when the father is present. Would Clare revert to her old self when Peter returned? Would she be angry at Peter, holding him responsible for Jenny's suicide attempt? Would she clutch more tightly to Jenny, or would she be able to move away enough to allow Peter in, without letting go of Jenny's hand completely?

I knew that Clare would have liked me to bring Peter up to speed, but I believed that it would enhance Clare's sense of her own competence if she could do it herself. I began the session by telling Peter that we had met the day before, and that I believed that Clare had made a very important discovery that I hoped she could share with him now. Clare then took over and explained to Peter what she had discovered the day before. Peter listened, and I could see that he was struggling to understand. For Peter, as for many men in our culture, helping often means doing something concrete, taking a definite action. Simply sitting together and holding hands did not seem to him as if he was doing his duty as a parent.

After listening to Clare, Peter immediately turned to Jenny. "So is that all you need from us, to hold your hand?"

I inwardly winced: Referring to this simple act of connection as "all" that Jenny needed seemed to devalue it. But Jenny had evidently not picked up on this implication. She replied, "Yeah, that's all. If I knew that I didn't have to talk, that I could just tell you that I was feeling bad, and that you'd stay with me, I think I'd feel better."

Peter was not satisfied, "But why can't you talk to us, Jenny? Why can't you tell us what is making you feel so bad?"

I could see a shadow come across Jenny's face again, "I told you Dad, I don't know. Maybe I just don't want to hurt you."

Peter, more agitated now: "But why do you care about hurting me? Don't care how I feel. Just tell me whatever you need to say."

Jenny just sighed this time. Peter went on, "You've got to help me, honey. I need to hear from you what I'm doing to make you feel this way."

Here is the double bind, explicitly stated. Peter has contradicted himself—don't care how I feel, but help me. In addition, the focus was now off Jenny and onto Peter. The issue was no longer what Jenny needed at that moment, but on what Jenny must give Peter so that Peter could feel better, namely, an explanation that Peter could understand.

But I also sympathized with Peter's frustration. I knew he wanted to do what was best for Jenny, and if that meant that he would have to hear very hurtful things about himself, so be it. What he could not tolerate was the feeling of helplessness. Clare could sit and hold Jenny's hand, but Peter, like most men, needed to do something specific in order to feel worthwhile. He needed to call the doctor, go out to buy medicine, heat up chicken soup, carry the portable television up to Jenny's room. He needed to do something concrete, something active, to feel that he was helping.

As a man, I could empathize with Peter's position. How often we men are put in the position of feeling that we must be instrumental if we are to feel good about ourselves. But, in Peter's case, I sensed that something else was also going on. He was frightened of the emotions associated with helplessness and surrender. The seeming irrationality of Jenny's behavior reawakened the ghost of his mother, and offering to share her burden had too much potential to open up his wounds. But these wounds had to be opened if he was going to relate to Jenny person to person and not as a container of his own projected fears. I realized that it was now time to pursue Peter. He must confront his own demons if he was going to understand Jenny. But I knew that I had to proceed gently, lest I become the rejecting parent or his mother's psychiatrist who told him to suppress his feelings for her sake.

MICUCCI: (*to Peter*) I want to know about your sadness.

PETER: (*looking at me as if I had spoken in a language he didn't understand*) What do you mean?

MICUCCI: I can see the sadness in your eyes. I can hear it in your voice. I want to know about it.

PETER: I don't know what you are talking about.

MICUCCI: Just tell me how it feels right now.

PETER: I feel like there's a pounding jackhammer in my chest.

MICUCCI: So you're feeling anxious?

PETER: I guess.

MICUCCI: Do you know what's making you feel anxious?

PETER: I don't know. I guess it started when you asked me about being sad. Like, maybe you see into me and I don't like that.

MICUCCI: See into you?

PETER: Yeah, like maybe you know me better than I want you to.

MICUCCI: And do you know why that would make you feel so scared?

PETER: I guess it scares me to be so close. I just feel better when I can keep a bit of a wall up, I guess.

Like many men, Peter was threatened by intimacy with another man, what Stephen Bergman (1995) has called "male relational dread." I understood that, and I didn't want to push so hard that I scared him away. On the other hand, if I was going to help this family, I was going to have to push Peter farther than he had gone before. I wanted him to get in touch with his emotional side, and learn that he could not only tolerate it, but could also be enriched by it.

MICUCCI: OK, Peter, I understand. Can you let me in just a little? If it gets too bad, you can always put the wall up again.

PETER: (*hesitantly*) Sure, but I don't know what you want.

Many men are so unaccustomed to intimacy with another man that they are not sure what it means. They are a bit suspicious, wondering what they might discover about themselves if they allow another man to get close.

MICUCCI: All I want is to understand that sadness in your voice and in your eyes.

PETER: (*sighing, letting go just a bit*) I don't know. I'm so confused. Clare looks like she knows what to do for Jenny. The two of them look so close together. I guess I just feel out of it, like a third wheel.

Here was Peter's isolation. Clare looked as if she was about to speak, perhaps to reassure Peter, but I gestured to her to remain silent for now.

MICUCCI: So you're feeling left out. Alone?

PETER: Yeah, alone, helpless, like they don't need me.

MICUCCI: You'd like to feel needed.

PETER: Sure, I'd like to. But then, what do they need me for? I don't have any answers for them. I don't know what to do. (*I noticed tears welling in Peter's eyes.*)

MICUCCI: It's OK, Peter. I can imagine how bad that must feel for you.

PETER: It's like when that doctor told me I had to take care of my mom. I didn't know what to do. I was only a kid. What was I supposed to do?

The tears came. Clare looked at me for a sign, and I gestured that it would be all right for her to move over to Peter and put her arm around him. Jenny didn't wait for a sign from me. She went to Peter's other side and put her head on his shoulder.

One theory to explain what had happened in this family is that Peter had projected the threatening and disowned parts of himself onto Jenny. By doing so, it helped Peter feel that this split off part of himself was more controllable because it was someone else—Jenny—who was losing control, not he. The cost, however, was that Peter then lost access to the parts of himself that could feel, that could let go, that could surrender, and as a result, the rational, intellectualized parts of him hypertrophied. If Peter could reclaim even some of these disowned parts of himself, he would have a better opportunity to know Jenny for who she was, and so have a more genuine and intimate relationship with her.

In subsequent sessions, we talked about Peter's loneliness and how Clare and Jenny had misinterpreted it as lack of interest in them. Jenny told her father that she often felt intimidated by him. I could see that Peter winced on hearing this: He didn't want to be seen in this way by his daughter, yet he could understand how it had happened. As the discussion unfolded, the family members both figuratively and literally held each others' hands. They listened to each others' pain, to fragments of thoughts and ideas that came up but didn't necessarily connect in a meaningful sequence, and in so doing, Jenny, Peter, and Clare become both more connected and differentiated. They could see each other as individuals rather than as projections of their disowned feelings.

Eventually, the parents, on their own, solved the dilemma of "what to do when Jenny wants to hurt herself." They decided that they would simply ask her on a regular basis how she was feeling. If she was feeling bad, they would keep her company and hold her hand. She did not have to produce an explanation or even an elaboration. They would just be there for her until the feeling passed, keeping her company, lending her their strength, and, in the process, they all realized that they felt stronger.

SUMMARY

A basic process underlying depression and suicidality in adolescence is isolation and disconnection from supporting and validating relationships. Thus, a key theme in treatment must be reconnecting the adolescent with the family. This process involves the following three steps:

- Ensure the adolescent's safety by helping the parents to take whatever measures are necessary to prevent a suicide attempt.
- Open up dialogue. Often, the "tell me/don't tell me" bind is powerful in these families. Depressed and suicidal youngsters often feel too responsible for their parents' welfare, or fear rejection if they share their true feelings with their parents. Therapists must provide support to the parents to enable them to listen to the child without becoming defensive, angry, or dismissive.
- Help the parents find specific, concrete ways of demonstrating that they have heard the adolescent's concerns and are committed to addressing them.

CHAPTER 6

VIOLENCE, DELINQUENCY, AND OTHER PROBLEM BEHAVIORS

As it so often happens, the boy before me belied the description I had received from his mother on the phone only 4 hours earlier. With wavy brown hair stuffed carelessly beneath a baseball cap and an impish smile, 15-year-old Keith greeted me with a firm handshake that reminded me that he had been a leader in the military boarding school he had attended until he was expelled for his behavior 3 months ago. This was not the angry, bitter boy I had expected to see.

His mother, Pam, had called in desperation on the recommendation of a colleague who suggested they see me. Keith was becoming increasingly disruptive and confrontational in his behavior, culminating recently in an incident in which he threatened his mother with a kitchen knife when she refused to give him $20. Pam was sure that Keith was using drugs, certainly marijuana and possibly hallucinogens, because she had overheard some of Keith's telephone conversations. Keith made no attempt to conceal his drug use, declaring, "Marijuana is not a drug."

Keith respected none of his parents' limits. He defied his 11 P.M. curfew, and several times a week stayed out all night, coming home midafternoon the next day in a disheveled state, falling into bed and then sleeping until 10 P.M., only to repeat the pattern. When his parents challenged him, he'd defiantly retort, "Try to stop me. I'm making my own rules now." After being expelled from military school, he enrolled in the local public school but had stopped attending. On three occasions, Pam had discovered money missing from her purse, and she suspected that Keith was stealing from her. Keith's father, Stu, a shy, soft-spoken man in his mid-40s, had sometimes tried to block the front door to prevent Keith from leaving, but Keith would push his father aside. These confrontations had grown more violent, as both Stu and Keith stood their ground more decisively. A week before our session, Stu and Keith were wrestling on the floor of the living room while Pam looked on in horror. Unable to take it any more, Pam cried out, "Just let him go, Stu. Let him go." Stu stopped struggling, and Keith ran out of the house. The next day, Pam quit her job so she could stay home all day to supervise Keith. It didn't work. Keith continued his rampage, and Pam was even more frightened now, because she was alone in the house most of day.

———•◦•———

"We just don't know her any more," Helen sighed in response to my question about the problem in the family. She and Tammy's father, John, had been divorced for 5 years but had maintained a good relationship "for the sake of the kids," John said. Their older daughter was attending college, and their younger daughter, Tammy, age 14, was, in their words, "running wild." She was a good student until she started ninth grade this year, and then "all hell broke loose." An early maturer, she attracted the attention of older boys, and before long, she was associating with a "bad crowd." Within months, she was pregnant and had an abortion. Now, she was being treated for a sexually transmitted disease.

Tammy didn't deny that she was sexually active, and described herself as "serially monogamous," a rather sophisticated term for a 14-year-old, I noted. When I asked her what she meant, she replied that she never slept with more than one boy at a time, but that she had "hooked up" with "five or six" different boys over the past 6 months. Each relationship burned with intensity for a few weeks, then fizzled, only to be replaced by the next.

Tammy's grades had fallen from A's and B's to C's and D's. She was skipping school but did attend most of the time. She violated curfew regularly but had never stayed out all night. Though verbally disrespectful to her parents, she had never physically assaulted them or anyone else. The worst incident she and her parents could recall was when she threw a book at the wall in a fit of anger.

Tammy admitted that she had tried marijuana and alcohol but

didn't use them on a regular basis because she didn't like them. "I don't know what all the fuss is about," she said, "I don't need that stuff to feel good." She associated with friends who used drugs and alcohol but denied that she was tempted to join them: "It's cool, you know, like they do their thing and I do mine." When I asked her what "her thing" was, she thought for a moment and answered, "Life, man. I just want to enjoy my life. And I am. They [indicating her parents] just need to chill."

———⇒•⇐———

Tyrone had been diagnosed with attention deficit disorder and was taking Ritalin. Seen for his late afternoon appointment when the Ritalin was wearing off, Tyrone fidgeted in his seat. He came to sessions 10 or 15 minutes late, sheepishly apologizing that he had "lost track of time." He didn't wear a watch and seemed surprised when I suggested that he might consider obtaining one, preferably one with an alarm that could go off at preprogrammed times to remind him he had to get somewhere.

Tyrone and Lureen, his mother, agreed that they had a good relationship. They spent time together and talked often about Tyrone's plans for the future. He was involved in sports at school and had a part-time job on the weekends. Tyrone denied using drugs, and his mother believed him, because she trusted Tyrone and knew that he had never lied to her.

"He's a good boy," Lureen said, smiling at Tyrone, "but I'm scared. He's so close, now, and I don't want him to fall."

Tyrone had, indeed, accomplished much compared to the other boys in his neighborhood. He was in his senior year at high school and had won a track scholarship to college. But his grades had slipped, and he wasn't coming home on time. He and his mom were having more and more arguments, and Tyrone was staying away just to avoid the confrontations. Tyrone had been dating a girl for 6 months and was very attached to her.

"When I'm out with Cindy, I just find it so hard to leave," Tyrone said. "I'm having such a good time that I can't break away. I know I should, but I can't."

Lureen snapped back, "Well if you can't now, what will you do when you get to college? You tell me, Tyrone. If you can't walk the walk now, how are you going to make it in college?" Tyrone sighed and didn't answer.

———⇒•⇐———

Illustrating three different faces of adolescent problem behavior, these cases seem so different from one another, it's easy to miss what they have in common. In each case, there is conflict between the parent and the child about what constitutes "appropriate" behavior. The adolescent's misbehavior has seized the attention of the parents, and arguments about the youth's behavior have begun to dominate the family interactions. The parents feel frightened, helpless, angry, and guilty. Their sense of control over their own environment has been shaken, and they cling desperately to what little power they have left.

There are also important differences among these three families. Keith's family is on the brink of chaos, and the possibility of him or someone else getting hurt is imminent. Tyrone, and even Tammy, though crossing the limits, still maintain a relationship with their parents, still see their parents as important figures in their lives, and want to stay connected to them. While Keith seems so self-involved that he can't fathom what his parents might be feeling, Tammy and Tyrone seem to be able to empathize, at least partially, with their parents' predicament. Tyrone, on the verge of leaving home, has already accomplished much, but Tammy is still in the dawn of her adolescence and still has 3 years of high school ahead of her, 3 years in which she could drift farther and farther into trouble.

HOW COMMON IS PROBLEM BEHAVIOR DURING ADOLESCENCE?

It's difficult to obtain accurate estimates of the prevalence of problem behaviors among adolescents. Statistics are based either on self-report or arrest records, and both sources are likely to be biased, the former by the veracity of the reporters, the latter by varying community definitions of what constitutes a delinquent act. Summarizing the literature, McCord (1990) estimated that between 12% and 18% of males had been arrested at least once prior to age 18.

Boys are arrested about five times more often than girls. African American youth are more likely to be arrested than white youth. One factor contributing to this racial difference in prevalence is that police are more likely to arrest a black youth suspected of an offense than a white youth suspected of a similar offense. Another factor is the correlation between poverty and delinquency (Elliott & Ageton, 1980). Furthermore, because of the tendency for problem behaviors to cluster together (Jessor & Jessor, 1977), a small number of adolescents account for a high proportion of serious criminal activity (Yoshikawa, 1994).

National surveys conducted in the early 1990s revealed that over

80% of high school seniors have drunk alcohol, nearly 40% have tried marijuana, about 10% have tried LSD or other hallucinogens, and less than 5% have tried cocaine. Although 28% of seniors and 14% of eighth graders reported having abused alcohol within the past 2 weeks, only 2–3% of seniors report daily use of alcohol or marijuana (Johnston, Bachman, & O'Malley, 1994). Because these statistics are based on self-report, they probably underestimate the actual prevalence of substance use among adolescents. Regional differences in prevalence must also be considered.

McCord (1990) provided a succinct summary of the prevalence of problem behaviors among adolescents:

> Most teenagers have played truant, trespassed, or committed traffic offenses at one time or another. Only a minority, however, have committed serious crimes. Most adolescents have tasted alcohol, and a majority appear to be regular drinkers, but only a minority have become problem drinkers or incipient alcoholics. A majority of adolescents have experimented with marijuana, though only a minority have tried other illicit drugs. (p. 420)

GENDER ISSUES IN ADOLESCENT PROBLEM BEHAVIOR

Delinquent and aggressive behavior is far more common among boys than girls (McCord, 1990). Recent scholarship has argued that cultural gender-role prescriptions encourage the development of aggressive behavior in boys. According to the "gender-role strain paradigm," the contradictory demands of the male gender role place many men in an impossible position (Pleck, 1981, 1995). Boys and men fall prey to feelings of shame because they can't live up to what is defined as necessary behavior for a man in our culture. Sometimes this shame is transformed into other behaviors that feel more empowering, such as aggression. This tendency is reinforced by "alexithymia," an inability to label feelings, common among traditional males (Levant, 1995).

Support for these ideas comes from research that has linked a host of problem behaviors such as school suspension, drinking, use of drugs, being arrested, and forcing sexual activity with highly traditional attitudes toward male roles (Pleck, Sonenstein, & Ku, 1994). These findings imply that male aggression and violence are not the result of undersocialization but rather oversocialization—too much identification with traditional attitudes toward masculinity (Brooks & Silverstein, 1995).

DEVELOPMENTAL PERSPECTIVES

Contrary to what many adults believe, hormonal changes are not a primary cause of erratic behavior during adolescence (Buchanan et al., 1992). Timing of pubertal development appears to be a risk factor for girls but not for boys. Early-developing girls are at higher risk for behavior problems, but only if the girls had problems prior to adolescence, or if they associate with older peers (Caspi & Moffitt, 1991; Magnusson et al., 1985; Silbereisen et al., 1989). For young adolescents (and older adolescents who are delayed in their development), the "personal fable" of invulnerability leads them to underestimate the risks involved in potentially dangerous activities (Elkind, 1967; see also Chapter 3).

Some adolescents have difficulty appreciating the effects of their actions because of delayed development in perspective-taking abilities (see Selman, 1980, and Chapter 3). Most adolescents, by age 14 or 15, can appreciate the perspective of another person, but some teenagers are unable to hold in mind at the same time their own perspective and the perspective of another, a necessary step in arriving at a solution that meets the needs of both parties.

In terms of Kohlberg's stages of moral development, most adolescents are at Stage 3, where earning the approval of others constitutes the basis for making moral decisions. If adolescents associate mainly with deviant peers, then their decisions are likely to be based on what they think will earn the approval of these peers. Youngsters who have not yet reached Stage 3 are motivated primarily by concrete rewards (Stage 2) or avoidance of "getting caught" (Stage 1).

According to Kegan's theory, most adolescents are at the "interpersonal" stage of development (i.e., they have not yet fully differentiated themselves from the reference group of peers). Thus, many adolescents have difficulty distinguishing their own values from those of the peer group. As an additional complication, deviant peers are likely to comprise the primary reference group for adolescents who exhibit problem behavior.

THE ROLE OF THE PEER GROUP

The role of the peer group in inciting problem behavior among adolescents deserves special consideration because of the widespread belief that the reason adolescents engage in problem behavior is association with "bad companions." The research literature does not support this belief.

Peer influence is indeed strong during adolescence, but the relationship between peer-group norms and the behavior of individual group members is bidirectional: Peer-group norms do influence individual behavior, but it is also true that "birds of a feather flock together" (Brown, 1990). Adolescents gravitate toward deviant peers, and they then reinforce each other's deviant behavior. True, there are some adolescents who have such low self-worth and are so famished for approval that they will do almost anything to get accepted. But this case is the exception rather than the rule. Most of the time, troublesome kids find each other and then egg each other on (Dishion, Patterson, Stoolmiller, & Skinner, 1991).

What leads an adolescent to associate with deviant peers? The literature is clear on this issue as well. Adolescents who maintain strong attachment to their parents are least likely to become involved with a deviant peer group (Gottfredson & Hirschi, 1994; Steinberg & Silverberg, 1986). Adolescents from authoritative households are less likely to be swayed by peer influence and give more weight to parental opinion than do adolescents from authoritarian, indulgent, or neglectful homes (Fulgini & Eccles, 1993). The amount of parental supervision and monitoring is also important (Steinberg, Fletcher, & Darling, 1994). Some parents are unable to provide adolescents the supervision they need, either because the parents are impaired in some way (e.g., by their own emotional or medical problems) or because they are distracted by other concerns (e.g., another child with problems, a demanding job, marital problems). Inadequately supervised kids tend to flock together and then mutually reinforce deviant behavior. As the youngster's behavior becomes more disruptive, parents lose even the little influence they had, and eventually many parents just give up monitoring the kid altogether.

A third factor that appears to influence the adolescent's choice of associates is the degree to which the adolescent is attached to societal institutions such as school, home, church, or place of employment (Hirschi, 1969). Adolescents who are involved in a variety of activities are less likely to gravitate toward deviant peers. An adolescent who does reasonably well academically, seems to have decent relationships with teachers, is involved in some extracurricular activities, has a job, or regularly attends religious services is less likely to be attracted to (or attractive to) a deviant peer group. If an adolescent's school experience has been frustrating and humiliating, the adolescent might repudiate the importance of school in his or her life. This can snowball into repudiation of all activities associated with school, such as organized sports or clubs. Once adolescents have earned a reputation of being irresponsible, it is harder to redeem themselves and harder for them to compete with the more successful youngsters for the limited job opportunities for teenagers. These kids will have plenty of time on their hands to find the other disenchanted youth in their community.

THE IMPORTANCE OF RELATIONSHIPS

Aggression, delinquency, and other problem behaviors represent a rupture in the adolescent's relationships with the family. Since attachment to the family varies inversely with attachment to deviant peers, the more the child gravitates to the deviant peer group for the sense of belonging he fails to feel in his family, the more the family is likely to ostracize the child, pushing him even more into close association with deviant peers.

Meanwhile, in the family, an unproductive cycle has emerged. The more the adolescent defies parental rules and restrictions, the more the parents attempt to control the adolescent. These attempts to control the youngster intensify his humiliation and exacerbate the problem, since the kid feels even more mistreated and misunderstood, and more likely to gravitate to deviant peers. The power struggle escalates until there is a precipitous separation and often an irremediable breach in the relationship between the child and the parents—he leaves the family by running away or prematurely separating, the parents withdraw from him in helplessness, or the parents actively extrude him from the family (see Figure 6.1).

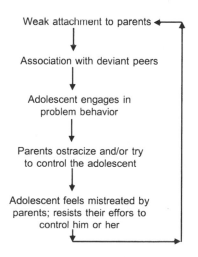

FIGURE 6.1. The symptomatic cycle in adolescent problem behavior.

The key to successful intervention is to break this cycle by working to reestablish relationships within the family. The approach must balance the roles of the parent as authority figure and nurturer for the child. Some approaches to working with families of difficult kids emphasize the importance of shoring up the parental hierarchy (e.g., Price, 1996). However, approaches that err on the side of encouraging parents to impose stringent restrictions and consequences on the child as a way of asserting their authority run the risk of alienating the adolescent by shaming her even more, perhaps driving her into even more serious deviant behavior. Similarly ineffective is an approach that extrudes the parents from the process and works only with the child, either in a confrontational or nurturing role.

One of the biggest challenges in working with families with defiant adolescents is to resist the pull to control the youngster. Without completely ignoring the symptomatic behavior, the therapist must look beyond the symptom—however serious it might be—to the cyclical processes underlying the symptom and work to disrupt these patterns by introducing family members to new ways of interacting with one another. Therapy must balance efforts to establish or restore a failing parental hierarchy with efforts to stimulate the parents to provide age-appropriate nurturance and support for the child. Thus, the therapist must often shift back and forth between supporting the parents and supporting the adolescent, between strengthening the hierarchy and repairing dislocated relationships (Micucci, 1995). How these ingredients are blended, however, depends upon the severity of the problem behavior.

ASSESSING THE SEVERITY OF THE PROBLEM BEHAVIOR

Problem behaviors in adolescence often cluster together, so that involvement in one tends to predict involvement in another (Jessor & Jessor, 1977). However, I find it useful to think of problem behavior as falling on a continuum from mild, to moderate, to severe, depending on the variety and frequency of the behavior and the potential for harm to self or others (see Table 6.1).

When the problem behavior is *mild*, the adolescent might "test limits" by violating rules or showing verbal disrespect to the parents. However, there are also many instances of compliant and prosocial behavior, with no incidents of violence against property or people. A youngster, such as Tyrone, who comes in after his curfew, talks back to his parents, or refuses to clean his room, would be classified as exhibiting "mild" problem behavior.

TABLE 6.1. Assessing the Severity of Adolescent Problem Behavior

<u>Mild problem behavior</u>

- Adolescent tests limits by violating rules or showing
- Many instances of compliant and prosocial behavior
- No violence against property or people

<u>Moderate problem behavior</u>

- More persistent pattern of defiance
- Might be regular users of alcohol or drugs
- Might be engaging in promiscuous sexual activity
- Marginal school performance
- Frequent arguments with family members, involving cursing, threats, fits of temper
- No violence to anyone in the home
- Legal involvement, if any, has been minimal

<u>Severe problem behavior</u>

- Possibility of serious danger either to the adolescent or to other family members
- Pattern of running away or staying out overnight
- Daily use of drugs and/or multiple drug use
- Problems with the law
- Theft from the family
- Physical violence
- Truancy, failure, and/or serious behavior problems at school

When the problem behavior is *moderate*, the adolescent will show a more persistent pattern of defiance in a number of areas. These kids might be regular users of alcohol or drugs, or, like Tammy, might be engaging in promiscuous sexual activity. School performance is often marginal, and there are likely to be frequent arguments with family members, often involving cursing, threats, and fits of temper. However, they have never assaulted anyone in the family, and legal involvement, if any, has been minimal. Adolescents who are failing at school, known to be using marijuana on a regular basis, regularly defy curfews, and curse at their parents would be classified as exhibiting "moderate" problem behavior.

Severe behavior problems includes the possibility of serious danger either to the adolescent or to the family. There might be a pattern of running away, staying out all night, repeated and/or multiple drug use, problems with the law, a pattern of theft from the family, or physical violence. If these kids are attending school at all, they are likely to be truant, failing, and defiant. The case of Keith, which opened this chapter, exemplifies severe problem behavior.

INTERVENTIONS FOR MILD PROBLEM BEHAVIOR

The key to successful intervention in cases of mild problem behavior is to facilitate more effective conflict resolution by the family around the problem behavior. Unlike cases of more serious problem behavior, which will be discussed later in this chapter, the focus should not be on strengthening the parental hierarchy. While it might indeed be the case that parents are not consistent or united in their response to the problem behavior, concentrating exclusively on empowering the parents runs the risk of minimizing the strengths of the adolescent and other family members. Rather, the emphasis should be on strengthening relationships, encouraging dialogue, improving conflict resolution, and helping the parents provide age-appropriate guidance for the youth. Concentrate on what the family is doing right, direct attention away from the problem behavior, and put the kid's behavior in the context of the developmental transitions that the family is facing (Table 6.2).

It is important to expand the dialogue beyond the problem issue. While it is certainly important to help the family negotiate rules and consequences for the household, limiting the discussion to these issues implies that the adolescent's noncompliance is the major problem in the family. In fact, the emergence of mild problem behavior in an adolescent otherwise developing normally often signals that the family is experiencing difficulty making a developmental transition. Limiting the dialogue to the overt behavioral symptom runs the risk of missing an opportunity to help the family over the developmental hump.

Frequently, cases of mild problem behavior reflect an adolescent's attempt to manage anxiety associated with increased demands for independence. By encouraging direct discussion of the adolescent's and parent's worries, the therapist can facilitate the identification of more appropriate solutions. Youngsters can be encouraged to talk with their

TABLE 6.2. Interventions for Mild Problem Behavior

Key = Facilitate more effective conflict resolution by the family around the problem behavior.

- Focus should not be on strengthening parental hierarchy.
- Concentrate on
  Strengthening relationships
  Improving dialogue
  Improving conflict resolution
  Helping parents provide age-appropriate guidance.
- Build on what the family is doing right.
- Put the problem behavior in the context of the developmental transitions the family is facing.
- Expand the dialogue beyond the immediate problem issue.

parents about their feelings about growing up, their plans for the future, and worries about the years ahead.

Often, anxiety about the future consequences of the adolescent's behavior distracts the parents from listening and pushes them to assume a more controlling or abandoning position. At these points, the therapist can intervene to soothe the parents' anxiety by providing a developmental perspective and emphasizing the ways in which the young person is displaying responsible and mature behavior.

In Tyrone's case, for example, I expanded the dialogue beyond the issue of Tyrone's curfew violations. His difficulty saying good-bye to his girlfriend at the end of the evening was framed as a metaphor for the developmental transition that was about to take place in this family: Tyrone was leaving for college, and saying "good-bye" to his mother, his home, and his neighborhood. As we explored the implications of this metaphor, Tyrone began to understand that leaving his girlfriend's house in time to make his curfew would be good practice for the bigger "good-bye" he was to face in a few months. Lureen realized that berating Tyrone for his lateness or imposing more severe consequences didn't really help. While these measures might encourage more compliance from Tyrone around curfew, it would actually undermine what she really wanted, namely, that Tyrone would come to monitor and regulate his own behavior. She realized that the issue was, in fact, "leave taking" in general, not obedience to rules. With my encouragement, she decided to leave the hour of curfew up to Tyrone. However, before leaving the house, he would commit himself to coming home at a specific time. Thus, both goals were served: Tyrone would recognize that leave taking was inevitable, and he would be responsible for regulating himself to meet a commitment he had made rather than simply capitulating to his mother's limits. Meanwhile, I encouraged Tyrone to challenge himself to grow by forcing himself to leave his girlfriend's house on time and then writing down his feelings in a journal after he returned home.

INTERVENTIONS FOR MODERATELY SEVERE PROBLEM BEHAVIOR

When problem behavior has escalated to the point of repeated defiance, open hostility toward the family, or a persistent pattern of potentially dangerous behavior (e.g., frequent drug use), then more decisive interventions are required. At this point, the family interactions more often than not revolve around struggles with each other about the adolescent's behavior. External systems, such as the school or the police, might now be involved, and the parents might be in direct conflict with each other and with the external systems about what to do about the adolescent. The youngster is likely to feel misunderstood and alienated, and may redouble efforts to assert independence in ways that invite only more efforts at control from the adults.

When problem behavior has escalated to this level, it is often the case that attempts to control the adolescent have supplanted efforts to maintain an age-appropriate relationship. In contrast to cases of mild problem behavior, where problem behavior is the exception rather than the rule, where there is little physical danger to anyone, and where family members retain positive relationships with each other, in cases of moderately severe problem behavior, the family interactions are dominated by the problem. Anger and frustration pervade the family. The more ineffective the parents are in reining in the adolescent, the more their authority erodes in a repeating cycle. The involvement of other systems (school, legal authorities) reinforces the parents' feelings of failure. While the therapist cannot discount the degree of frustration experienced by the parents, it is imperative to keep in mind that the adolescent is also experiencing intense feelings of alienation and abandonment.

The central principle of intervention at this level is to redirect the parents' efforts away from control toward rebuilding their relationship with the adolescent (see Table 6.3). This is not an easy task, since the youth's behavior invites controlling responses from the parents. The parents are understandably reluctant to relinquish what they feel is the last vestige of control over a young person who seems determined to self-destruct. They may be convinced that the kid is "out of control" and needs them to impose even firmer controls on him "for his own good."

Often, the parents have tried reasoning with the kid. When this approach failed, perhaps they resorted to more authoritarian methods, such as yelling, humiliating the youngster, or physically restraining him. Sometimes the parents simply give up, abdicate responsibility, and

TABLE 6.3. Interventions for Moderate Problem Behavior

Key = Redirect the parents' efforts away from control toward rebuilding their relationship with the adolescent.

- Discourage control-based methods of influence.
- Emphasize the parents' emotional investment in the adolescent.
- Help the parents distinguish between what they can and can't control.
- Maintain an alliance with the adolescent.
- Recognize stereotypes and social prejudices against young people.

withdraw in defeat. Both strategies are likely to increase the child's alienation from the parents and promote involvement with deviant peers who are in the same boat.

From Control to Relationships

There is a way to reconcile the importance of supporting the parents while also discouraging efforts to dominate the adolescent: Encourage the parents to employ methods of influence that are grounded in their emotional investment in their child rather than methods oriented toward restricting or overpowering the child. A case discussed in Chapter 3 (see pp. 75–76) provides an example. Rather than continuing their futile arguments with their son, these parents began to express honestly and directly to their son their feelings about his behavior. While anger was among these feelings, they had other feelings as well, which were usually eclipsed by the anger. These other feelings–hurt, betrayal, sorrow, anxiety–were rarely, if ever, expressed for fear of implying to their son that they were defeated. Yet they felt defeated, and relying on ineffective control-based methods of influence simply intensified this feeling. When they acknowledged to the boy that they indeed could not control what he did, but that his actions had an emotional impact on them that *he* could not control (because these were *their* feelings), the focus was shifted to their relationship with the boy. Sometimes parents are reluctant to share their feelings of hurt with their children for fear of "laying a guilt trip." But guilt can be a powerful motivator for changing behavior, and many times defiant adolescents experience far too little of this important emotion.

But expressing feelings is not simply another way to manipulate the adolescent. The feelings the parents express must be genuine, and their disclosure of them must be honest. The primary reason for expressing these feelings is to emphasize that the relationship is still important, at least as far as the parents are concerned. The adolescent might choose to disregard the importance of the relationship, but he can't "make" the parents stop caring about him. The youngster, who is striving to assert his own autonomy by claiming that his actions have consequences for him alone, comes face-to-face with the reality that when one is in a relationship, one's actions always have consequences for other people.

Case Example: "Daddy, Don't Worry about Me."

Let's return to the case of Tammy that was introduced at the beginning of this chapter as an example of "moderate" problem behavior.

Tammy's parents had been trying to rein her in by restricting her, ineffectively grounding her when she violated curfew, only to find out that she had sneaked out of the house later that night. In the family session, Tammy glared at her parents, as if daring them to start an argument that was almost sure to end in her leaving my office in a fit of high dudgeon. I had seen this pattern in the second family session and didn't want to risk letting it happen again.

John began the third family session by telling me with a mixture of fury and resignation in his voice that the weekend before our session Tammy came home at 2 A.M., 2 hours later than their negotiated curfew. When he confronted her, she blithely told him that she was "hanging out" with her most recent boyfriend, a 22-year-old, unemployed high school dropout, whom her parents had expressly forbidden her to see. Interrupting her parents' account of the events of that night, Tammy interjected with a provocative tone, "Don't worry, we're using condoms. I won't get pregnant again."

John was fuming, but I caught a glimpse of great sorrow on Helen's face. I turned to her and asked if she would share her feelings about what Tammy has been doing. She burst into tears.

"It's breaking my heart," she sobbed. "I can't bear it any more. Every day I wonder if today might be the last time I see her."

Tammy looked incredulous. "Oh, Mom, don't be so dramatic," she sighed.

"No, it's true, honey." Helen continued, "I can't sleep at night for worrying about you. I know there's nothing else I can do to convince you to change. And it hurts me so much I can't think of anything else."

Helen burst into sobs again. I noticed that John, like most men when they feel powerless, was about to shift into anger, and I wanted to prevent what was sure to be another unproductive outburst that would overshadow Helen's poignant self-disclosure.

"John, I can see that you're angry at Tammy for putting you and her mother through this," I said, "but I also sense that you may be having some of the same feelings that Helen just talked about."

"Of course I do," he said. "How couldn't I? Tammy is my daughter. Sure I get angry, but it's just to keep me from crying my eyes out over what this girl is doing to herself."

"Daddy, don't worry about me," Tammy feebly interjected. "I can take care of myself."

"Honey, I do worry about you," John said. "And no matter how many times you tell me not to, I will. I love you and I don't want to lose you."

"You won't lose me," Tammy replied unconvincingly.

"I'm not so sure, honey," John continued. "Just the other day, I read in the paper about that girl they found in the river. They said she was probably raped. I couldn't even finish the article, because all I could think of was that it could have been you."

Tammy tried to bait her parents with remarks that seemed designed to pull from them an angry or controlling response against which she could react. But I was able to help the parents stay with their own feelings of helplessness, frustration, and anxiety, and to communicate these feelings to Tammy. Eventually, Tammy shifted from defending herself to trying to soothe her parents, claiming that her parents really had no reason to worry and that she didn't want them to feel bad. All she wanted was to be left alone. I encouraged John and Helen to continue to state their position and to let Tammy know in every way they could that they were committed to a relationship with her.

I helped the parents distinguish between what they could and could not control. Short of monitoring Tammy around the clock, they could not control what she did. They could not control what she said about her sexuality, and they could not control what gave her pleasure. They had more control over what they permitted in their home, but even in this arena, their control was limited because they were not prepared to ask Tammy to leave if she violated their prohibitions. They had some control over their own feelings, more control over their actions, and thus some control over the kind of relationship they would have with Tammy. The latter depended on at least three considerations: what they wanted, what Tammy wanted, and what they thought would be best for Tammy. Both parents claimed that they wanted a close relationship with Tammy. Tammy said that she wanted a relationship with her parents, but she did not want them to "force" her to do anything. After some discussion, both parents agreed that it would be best for Tammy if they were available and supportive to her, and that little would be gained from giving her an ultimatum that could lead to her leaving the house and living on the streets.

The parents struggled with the question of what to do when Tammy was late and they did not know where she was. They concluded that all they could do was call the police. Tammy bristled at this idea: "How could you call the police on me? I thought you just said that you loved me?" Her parents explained that they were calling the police not to get her into trouble (though it might) but because they were worried about her and they didn't know what else to do.

This distinction was an important one. If the parents were calling the police in yet another ploy to control or reform Tammy, then they were playing into the symptomatic cycle. However, if the purpose of calling the police was not to punish Tammy, but rather to allay their worries about her and to carry out what they saw as their duty as parents, then the pattern of mutual reactivity would be broken.

Maintaining an Alliance with the Adolescent

When the severity of problem behavior is moderate (rather than severe), building an alliance with the adolescent must take precedence over encouraging the parents to exercise more authority. The therapist might offer a few individual sessions with the youngster at the start of treatment in order to build a relationship with her and to attempt to engage her in treatment.

One purpose of these sessions, besides communicating empathy for the youth's predicament, is to identify a specific goal the youth wants to work on that the therapist can support. To secure the family's cooperation, the therapist might frame these individual sessions as a period of extended evaluation that is necessary before he or she can give appropriate recommendations to the parents about how they should respond to the child's behavior.

Acknowledge Prejudice against Adolescents

Adolescents may be subject to prejudice resulting from stereotypes about teenagers. The boy who is accosted by the police simply because he looks suspicious is experiencing the effects of this prejudice. When parents use the argument, "You are not old enough to do that," they are in fact responding to their teenager not as an individual, but as a member of a class. Responses such as these are likely to frustrate young people and reinforce the view that they are not being respected for their individuality but rather are being stereotyped as members of a group. Of course, by acting in rebellious ways to challenge these prejudicial beliefs, the kids are reinforcing them.

The therapist must empathize with the adolescent's position as a subordinate in society and try to appreciate how the youth's behavior might be an adaptive response to the power structures of the systems in which she is embedded (see Brody, 1975; Denborough, 1996; Miller, 1991). The therapist must, of course, do so in a way that does not imply that the therapist is entering into a coalition with the child against the parents. The therapist should neither criticize nor defend the parents' position, but should strive to communicate that he or she understands how kids feel when they are stereotyped.

In Tammy's case, I acknowledged the "double standard" of acceptable sexual behavior for boys and girls, and how boys and men sometimes encourage promiscuous sexual activity in girls. We explored how Tammy viewed her sexuality and came to the conclusion that, like many boys and unlike many girls, Tammy was able to dissociate intimacy from sexuality. Without implying that this capacity was pathological, I suggested that Tammy might also explore ways to link sexuality and intimacy. We talked about the differences between physical and emotional intimacy. She realized that she sometimes used sex as a substitute for emotional closeness. Though she didn't really see anything wrong with this, she was interested in developing other ways to experience emotional intimacy. I suggested that she could utilize her relationship with her father as a laboratory for expanding her capacity for nonsexual intimacy with a man. Tammy also decided that she'd like to experiment with postponing sexual relations with her new boyfriend until she felt their relationship had grown more emotionally intimate.

Words, Not Actions

When adolescents are defiant and rebellious, parents focus on the behavior, and the feelings behind the behavior are not addressed. In individual meetings, the therapist can help the adolescent articulate feelings in a way that can lead to productive dialogue in the family.

Many teenagers, especially boys, have great difficulty expressing their feelings in words (Levant, 1995). With the therapist's help, adolescents can begin building a vocabulary that will allow them to enter into productive dialogue with their parents about these feelings. Meanwhile, the therapist helps parents to relinquish the position that they are the "experts" on their children, and instead allow the children to teach them who they are and what they need from them.

INTERVENTIONS FOR SEVERE PROBLEM BEHAVIOR

At this level, the adolescent is engaging in a pattern of disruptive and potentially dangerous behaviors. Examples include running away, repeated drug use, serious thefts, or physical violence against other family members. The youngster appears unconcerned about the potential consequences of his actions either to himself or to others. If he comes to therapy, he does so only under duress and, when there, participates halfheartedly, if at all. Parents feel helpless and defeated. Often, they are so preoccupied with the adolescent's behavior that they have little energy for anything else. Their lives have become so constricted that they are completely isolated from friends and extended family. They might be fearful of the child and go to great lengths to avoid provoking a conflict, even if it means abdicating their parental authority.

Families with adolescents who exhibit severe problem behavior exemplify what Cloé Madanes (1981) has termed a "hierarchical reversal"; that is, the child has more power than the parents, who are terrified of what the child could do to them or to himself if they attempt to wrest authority back. While in the case of mild or moderate problem behavior, the parents still retain some authority, in the case of severe problem behavior the parents feel almost completely powerless. Thus, the first step in helping these families is to restore some power to the parents. The challenge is to do so without alienating the adolescent and thus losing any hope of engaging him in treatment (see Table 6.4).

Engaging Reluctant Adolescents

It's difficult to find an optimal balance between supporting the parents and supporting the adolescent, so therapists should not berate themselves if they can't find a way to engage the youngster in therapy. By helping the parents restore a sense of order to their household, the therapist has stopped the hemorrhaging and has opened up the possibility that therapeutic work with the family or with the child alone might be done. The therapist might refer the adolescent to a colleague for a few individual sessions while continuing to work with the parents, and then, after a while, conduct a few conjoint sessions with the other therapist present as cotherapist and advocate for the adolescent's position. If cotherapy is not possible for financial or other reasons, then the following ideas might be useful.

TABLE 6.4. Interventions for Severe Problem Behavior

Key = Find a balance between supporting the parents and supporting the adolescent.

- Restore power to the parents without alienating the adolescent.
- Attempt to engage the adolescent in therapy.
    Show genuine interest in the kid's side of the story.
    Find a concrete way to benefit the kid.
    Join with the resistance.
    Request a consultation from the kid.
    Invite collaboration.
    Let go.
- Help parents restore order to the household.
    Wiping the slate clean
    Reclaiming control over their own lives
    Reducing isolation from extended family and community
- Shift the emphasis to nurturance.
    Engaging a peripheral father
    Reengage son with mother
- Strengthen ties between the adolescent and social institutions.

Two Sides to Every Story

If the adolescent expresses reluctance to participate in the sessions, the therapist might tell her in the presence of the parents that he understands that there are many sides to every story, and that he sees his role as taking no one's side consistently but rather helping the family members to resolve their disagreements with each other. The therapist points out that at times he might agree with the parents' position and at other times agree with the child's position. The reason the therapist wants everyone at the sessions is to afford him the opportunity to hear all sides of the story before he gives his recommendations. If the adolescent chooses not to participate, then the therapist is left with no choice but to meet only with the parents, but then (the kid is told) it is possible that the therapist will wind up agreeing with the parents.

The therapist then explains that he would like to meet first with the youngster alone and then with the parents. The therapist asks each member of the family to agree that whatever is discussed in the individual session with the child is to remain strictly confidential. Usually, parents will readily agree to this stipulation, but even if they do not, their assent is not essential, because the point of the meeting is to establish a relationship with the youngster, not to explore personal issues in depth. The therapist meets with the adolescent alone and attempts to establish an alliance, perhaps using some of the following suggestions (similar to techniques described by Selekman, 1993; see also Liddle, 1993).

Find a Concrete Way to Benefit the Adolescent

Forging an alliance with adolescents who are engaging in problem behavior can be difficult because, from the kid's perspective, a therapist is another adult authority figure to mistrust. One way a therapist might establish an alliance is to offer a concrete way to benefit the youngster. For example, the therapist might offer to try to convince the court to be lenient with the youth, saying, for example,

> "I'm prepared to write a recommendation to the court that says they should give you another chance. Most of the time they'll go along with my recommendations. But I need to be convinced that if I stick my neck out for you, I'm not going to get it cut off. Before I write this recommendation, you'll need to convince me that if you're given a second chance, you won't prove me wrong."

Join with the Resistance

The therapist can join with the adolescent around his unwillingness to be in treatment. The therapist might say,

> "Your parents seem resolved that you will be in therapy, but what we do here is up to us. How can I help you get something you want? I can be very useful to you because I think your parents trust me. I can be your advocate to try to get some of the things that you want. But I can't lose your parents' trust. If I do, then you're back to square one."

Another possibility is to offer to work with the kid toward convincing the parents he no longer needs therapy. The therapist then explores with the youngster the ways that the kid might successfully convince his parents that therapy is no longer necessary, emphasizing behavior change rather than words alone.

Request a Consultation

The therapist might approach the adolescent as a consultant on the family dynamics. The therapist tells the youngster that she senses that there is a good reason why the kid is so angry at his parents and she'd like to hear the adolescent's side of the story. The therapist might point out something she observed about the parents and ask the adolescent (with genuine curiosity) what this behavior means, or how the family had evolved to this point. In effect, the therapist is joining with the adolescent's refusal to take responsibility for the problem by appearing to shift the responsibility back onto the family system. The art of carrying out this intervention is to do so without engaging the child in a coalition against the parents.

Invite Collaboration

The therapist might inform the adolescent that he is being asked to make a recommendation regarding something that affects the youngster's life. The therapist tells the kid that he will be required to make this recommendation whether or not the adolescent decides to work with him. The therapist invites the adolescent to collaborate in formulating the recommendation. The therapist might say,

> "I want to recommend something that I know you will like. But I can't do this unless you and I talk and come to an agreement. I'm prepared to recommend whatever you want as long as I'm also

convinced that it is reasonable. If you decide not to talk with me, then I'll just have to tell them whatever I think is best, and that decision will probably be based mostly upon what your parents tell me. I'd rather not do it this way, but if you decide not to participate, I guess that's what I'll have to do."

Let Go

Sometimes, the adolescent rebuffs all of the therapist's offers and simply refuses to participate. Rather than engaging in a power struggle, the therapist should communicate respect for the youth's decision but explain that he will nevertheless try to engage the adolescent periodically while continuing to work with the parents. The therapist, from time to time, telephones the kid, sends unsolicited letters and birthday cards, perhaps even visits the youngster at home. In meetings with the family, the therapist invites the parents to consider the child's perspective, representing it himself if necessary. Just as the parents are being coached to manage their side of their relationship with their child, so the therapist can continue to make overtures to the adolescent, even if the kid rebuffs them all.

Meeting with the Parents

Whether or not the therapist is successful in engaging the adolescent in an alliance, he or she then proceeds to meet with the parents and tells them in private that he or she has ideas for handling the defiant behavior. However, before sharing these ideas, *the therapist obtains the parents' assurance that they will carry out the therapist's suggestions in such a way as to make the youngster think that the parents (not the therapist) had come up with these ideas.*

The therapist explains that this "deception" is necessary if there is going to be any hope of ever engaging the adolescent in treatment. While this intervention might strike some as devious, in fact it strengthens the parental hierarchy by restraining the parents from carrying out any of the therapist's suggestions until they are convinced they could do so in a way that does not implicate the therapist in the adolescent's eyes. Thus, the parents assume more ownership of the interventions, and more responsibility for the outcome.

First Step: Restore Order

The treatment then proceeds with the first step of restoring order to the household by returning power to the parents. The goal here is to decrease parental reactivity and to increase planfulness in the way in which the parents respond to the kid. The therapist meets alone with the parents and expresses empathy for their position of helplessness. The therapist acknowledges their powerlessness as well as their caring for the child. The therapist carefully reviews, in detail, all of the failed solutions they had tried in the past. The therapist then suggests that drastic situations often require drastic responses and asks the parents if they are prepared to carry out these measures. If the parents express doubt, it is best for the therapist to continue talking with them about their previous failed attempts to solve the problem, from time to time asking if they are ready to consider a drastic solution. Once the parents agree, then the therapy can proceed.

Wiping the Slate Clean

The therapist suggests that the parents tell the child that they are willing to wipe the slate clean and start all over. Past infractions are forgiven, and they are prepared to begin again. They admit to the adolescent that they have made mistakes in the way they have treated him in the past and they apologize. They invite the child to come to therapy so he can tell them how they have failed him as parents. They then offer to do something small and concrete for the kid, such as buying him a new pair of jeans or preparing his favorite meal. The parents do not push or beg, but instead simply invite the youngster to consider returning to therapy.

In preparation for this intervention, it is important for the therapist to talk with the parents about what it means to wipe the slate clean. The parents should be cautioned against carrying out this intervention until they are committed to it and prepared to see it through. They should be warned that doing so incompletely would probably make matters worse, so they should refrain from acting until they have dispelled any doubts about the decision. The therapist then explores in detail how their relationship with their child would be different if they were seriously committed to wiping the slate clean. How would they act toward him if they had in fact forgiven and forgotten past offenses?

The point here is that by changing the parents' response and, in some cases, even their perception of the adolescent, the symptomatic cycle is broken. The parents are no longer responding in their predictable way, but are instead treating the child as if he were not "the problem." This change opens up space for other new responses to emerge as well.

Reclaiming Control Over Their Lives

The parents must be redirected away from controlling or "reforming" the adolescent and toward a focus on themselves and their own needs—what they need to do to reclaim some control over their *own* lives. The therapist might discuss with the parents how they have suffered from the problem and how their lives have become more and more constricted as a result. The therapist acknowledges that they have lost the feeling of comfort in their own home. The therapist encourages them to think about what they need in order to feel secure again. This discussion shifts the emphasis away from controlling or changing the child and onto what the parents can do to restore their own sense of security.

The therapist helps the parents focus on what *they* can do to restore a sense of order, even without the adolescent's cooperation, thus enabling the parents to see that they can set reasonable limits and stand by them regardless of what the youngster does. Perhaps they need to know that they are safe from violence, so they decide to tell the adolescent (as did Keith's parents) that if he threatens violence, they will call the police and press charges. Perhaps they need to know that their property will not be damaged or stolen. After making reasonable precautions to secure their belongings, they tell the child that if they discover anything missing, they will assume he stole the item, and they will either report him to the police or confiscate one of his possessions equal in value to the missing item. Perhaps the parents have neglected their relationship with each other and need to arrange to spend some time together. Perhaps they have been neglecting another child while they have been preoccupied with the "problem" adolescent. In any event, the therapist should help the parents define what is *essential* for them to reclaim a sense of order and sanity in their own lives.

Exploring Beliefs

The therapist needs to explore the family's beliefs about the problem, with an eye to discerning how these beliefs have interfered with solving the problem. Sometimes parents see the adolescent as a *troubled* youth, and so believe that their responsibility is to give her plenty of leeway and to provide a sense of security and unconditional love. In these cases, the therapist might encounter resistance from the parents when he or she suggests that they set firmer limits. In other families, the parents are so angry at the adolescent that they see her only as a *troublesome* youth. They want to punish her for her actions and be rid of her as quickly as possible. In these cases, the therapist encounters resistance when he or she suggests that behind the adolescent's troublesome behavior hides a troubled teen who needs more understanding and nurturance.

The parents need to expand their views to include other aspects of the kid, to see her as a more complex individual. The adolescent is *both* a troubled *and* a troublesome youth. She needs *both* firmer controls *and* more understanding. The therapist must first assess where the parent falls on the continuum of seeing the adolescent as troubled or troublesome, and then work to move the parents closer to the middle of the continuum.

If the parents are loath to set limits or seem willing to take most of the blame for the problem, the therapist might suggest that the parents talk to other parents in similar situations, might share stories of other families he or she has worked with, or might ignite the parents' indignation and outrage at the way the child has been treating them.

If the parents emphasize the other side of the coin and are so angry at the kid that they are unable to see her as a troubled youth, the therapist might point out some of the adolescent's positive qualities, help them recall ways in which the child had demonstrated loyalty to them in the past, recollect earlier times when they felt some connection to the youngster, or emphasize that the adolescent still needs them and that they have much to offer her. The therapist might consider externalizing the problem so that the parents can separate the adolescent from "the problem" and differentiate their feelings about the child from their feelings about the child's actions. For example, the therapist might explore with the family how the "problem behavior pattern" has victimized them all, including the adolescent (see Dickerson & Zimmerman, 1992).

Sometimes one parent sees their child as "troubled" and the other sees her as "troublesome." Not only does this difference of opinion lead to mutual undermining between the parents, but it can escalate into ugly conflicts between the parents regarding the "right" approach. Some therapists believe that problem behavior in a child is symptomatic of detoured marital conflict between the parents, and so they welcome the surfacing of these conflicts as an opportunity to work on the "real" problem in the family. The problem with this view is that it is linear: It fails to acknowledge that the adolescent's problem behavior is also fueling the conflict between the parents, or may be helping to transform a minor problem in marital conflict resolution into a major impasse.

I recommend an approach that utilizes the crisis created by the adolescent's problem behavior as a way to improve parental collaboration. The parents are advised that the top priority is to reduce the level of danger in the household, and that in order to do so they will have to put aside any other differences between them and join forces. The parents are told that both of them are right, that the child is both troubled and troublesome, and that each needs to consider the merits of the other's position in order to reduce the polarization between them. A useful metaphor is to compare each parent's view with the view from a single eye, and to compare the integration of both views to "binocular vision." Thus, the parents are encouraged to help each other see the "blind spots" in the view that each favors.

Reducing Isolation

Families with aggressive or delinquent adolescents are often isolated from the extended family or their communities. Perhaps the parents have been so preoccupied with the child's outrageous behavior that they have neglected other relationships in their lives. Perhaps the parents are so embarrassed that they have distanced themselves from family and friends, whom they expect will criticize their competence as parents. Perhaps the family was always isolated and cut off from extended family and community, and this lifestyle served them well until the adolescent's behavior began to frighten them, so that now they feel intensely alone and disconnected from other sources of support.

Whatever the reason for the family's isolation, the therapist should strive to help the family reconnect with members of the extended family and the community. For example, the therapist might suggest that the parents contact the parents of the adolescent's peers, to talk with them about what they might do together to solve the problem they mutually share. The therapist might encourage the parents to attend (or start) a parent support group in their community. The therapist might brainstorm with the parents about people they could call to serve as reinforcements if a conflict were to escalate between them and the kid.

Shifting the Emphasis to Nurturance

So far, I have emphasized the therapist's work with the parents to restore order to the household, and I have done so because in cases of severe problem behavior this is the first and most crucial step. But what about the adolescent? Once order has been restored to the household, then the therapist must shift the emphasis to rebuilding relationships in the family.

The therapist helps the parents reconstruct the process by which their relationship with their child deteriorated, and helps them to identify ways in which they might rebuild the lost positive feelings for the child. At this phase, the therapist gradually shifts his primary alliance from the parents to the child. Once the parents' authority is more firmly established, then the therapist begins to explore with the parents the ways in which they might have (deliberately or unwittingly) abandoned the child in the past, thus evoking feelings of rage and entitlement that may have erupted in a pattern of destructive behavior.

The goal at this stage is for the therapist to facilitate the open and direct expression of emotion on the part of each family member, and to give each family member the experience of being heard by the therapist and by each other. The therapist strives to empathize with each family member and to see the problem from each person's unique point of view. The therapist helps family members acknowledge how they have failed each other in the past and helps the parents recall previously unappreciated ways that the child might have tried to help them.[1]

For example, once Keith's parents had begun to feel more control over their own lives, we shifted the emphasis to exploring the reasons Keith seemed so angry at his parents. The revelation came during the ride home after a particularly emotional session in which the family had recounted a crisis the previous night that the parents had handled successfully.

On the way home, Keith revealed to his parents that he "couldn't forgive them" for having sent him to military school. He tearfully related the brutal hazings he had experienced there, and the rage he felt at the upperclassmen who victimized the younger students.

In our next session, Pam asked Keith why he had never told them about the abuse he had experienced at school. Laughing sardonically, Keith told about another boy who had reported the hazing to his parents, who then came to the school to confront the administration. The offenders were punished, but the boy who reported them was victimized even more brutally by other students and literally ostracized by his peers, who feared being associated with him. Eventually, the boy had "a breakdown" and left the school in shame.

Almost in tears, Keith told of the rampant drug use on the campus and the hypocrisy of the administration and faculty, who denied that there was a drug problem at the school. He talked about his initiation into smoking marijuana, and how it helped him to feel a sense of calm he couldn't get any other way. "I begged you to take me home," Keith cried, "but you wouldn't listen. You wouldn't even talk with me about it. Now I'm living by my own rules and you can't stop me!"

Boys like Keith may act out aggressively as a way of asserting their image of a masculine ideal, or as a way of engaging a peripheral father (Osherson & Krugman, 1990). The therapist must challenge the father to help the boy develop a more inclusive image of what it means to be a man. The therapist fosters a relationship between father and son in which they can engage in an activity that bonds them together as men. The therapist encourages the boy's father to find ways to validate his son's masculinity in nonaggressive areas, and to develop those positive qualities of masculinity such as loyalty and commitment to others. Toward this end, I suggested that Keith and Stu plan a weekend camping trip together, something they had done (and enjoyed) before but had not done for years.

Some have argued that problem behavior among boys stems from the mother's precipitous disengagement in an attempt to promote the boy's independence and masculinity (Silverstein & Rashbaum, 1994). The relationship between a son and his mother is difficult to balance. The therapist must help the son and mother to reconnect and to remain connected, while encouraging the mother to acknowledge and prize her son's masculine qualities. The mother needs to be comfortable with giving nurturance, and the boy needs to be comfortable receiving it. If a father is present in the home, he must model appropriate behavior toward the mother and insist that his son respect his mother.

Toward this end, we explored ways in which Pam could remain an important person in Keith's life. We started with simple things, such as buying him a small article of clothing, or cooking him a meal he liked. Keith started coming home at night for dinner with his parents. As many mothers do, Pam was careful to give Keith "plenty of space." She would allow him to decide how much contact they would have. As Silverstein and Rashbaum (1994) point out, while this strategy might appear respectful of the boy's boundaries, it runs the risk of allowing distance to grow in the mother–son relationship: The boy might feel that it is "not manly" to want to be with his mother, and so may not approach her. He reads her reticence to approach him as evidence that she's not interested either.

In family sessions, we talked explicitly about this pattern and explored ways in which Pam might play a more active role in Keith's life. At first, Keith was willing to accept only traditional "mothering" activities such as cooking meals and doing laundry. Pam, a remarkably astute and sensitive woman, was patient. She made him dinner and neatly folded his T-shirts. Eventually, Keith began to help his mother in the garden, and by midsummer, they were redecorating Keith's room together. Stu supported this activity by giving Keith the money to buy the wall paint. And, of course, as Pam and Keith worked, they talked, and their relationship blossomed.

Strengthening Ties to Society

Some theories maintain that a primary cause of delinquency is weak ties to societal institutions (see above, p. 172). The therapist must help the adolescent connect with the institutions from which he has become alienated, perhaps by encouraging the youngster to join a sports team, to do volunteer work, or to return to church. Rather than trying to pull him away from his deviant peers, the therapist strives to engage the adolescent in a process of developing more diversity in his relationships.

Although the family relationships were improving, Keith's parents were still nervous about his friends. Yet, they realized the futility of forbidding Keith to associate with them. Early in treatment, they complained that Keith would receive telephone calls from people they did not know. As one of the strategies for restoring a feeling of comfort in their own home, Pam and Stu decided they would invest in a "caller ID" service offered by their local telephone company. This service allowed them not only to monitor incoming calls, but also to block calls from certain numbers. Though Keith was furious when he heard of this decision, he accepted his parents' explanation that they had a right to have the "caller ID" service because it was their home and their phone. The mysterious phone calls decreased, but they did not stop entirely.

Rather than concentrating on pulling Keith away from his "bad" friends, we tried to think of ways to help Keith strengthen ties with more mainstream youths. Keith wanted to earn money, so he was encouraged to find a job. He wasn't successful. His parents were willing to pay Keith an hourly wage for doing volunteer work at a soup kitchen. Keith accepted their offer. He began spending more and more time at the soup kitchen, and even started attending a youth group at the church that sponsored the kitchen.

A Clarification

In talking about working with these families in stages, I do not intend to imply that one finishes one stage before beginning another. As has been emphasized in other chapters, these phases overlap. In cases of severe aggression, the first order of business is to restore the parents to a position of authority. But the therapist shouldn't postpone working to restore family relationships until the parents are firmly in control. In fact, by addressing both processes simultaneously, the therapist has a greater chance of engaging the adolescent in treatment. On the other hand, to focus exclusively on strengthening the parents' connection with the kid, without helping the parents restore some order in the household, puts the relationships on quicksand. If the parents fear the adolescent, they will not allow themselves to get close enough to him or her to engage meaningfully in the process of mutual understanding.

PITFALLS, CAUTIONS, AND OTHER CONSIDERATIONS

Failing to Assess the Adolescent's Cognitive Functioning

Some adolescents exhibit a pattern of poor judgment not for emotional reasons but because of limited intellectual ability (i.e., low IQ). Others exhibit compromised impulse control because of the presence of a pervasive learning disability or attention-deficit/hyperactivity disorder (ADHD). If the therapist suspects any of these conditions, a comprehensive psychological evaluation could be helpful.

1. ADHD. ADHD is a lifelong developmental disorder, so there must be evidence that it was present since early childhood. Adolescents who present with symptoms of ADHD but do not have a history of at least some symptoms of hyperactivity, impulsivity, or inattention since early childhood probably do not have the disorder. For youngsters with ADHD, medications may improve attention span and may even help to moderate impulsivity, but these are often not the only factors contributing to problem behavior. While the presence of ADHD might increase the chance that the youngster will exhibit problem behavior, there are many kids with ADHD who do not exhibit problem behavior, and many kids with problem behavior who do not exhibit ADHD. Thus, even if ADHD is present, the therapist should not assume that the "cause" of the problem behavior has been isolated.

2. Nonverbal learning disability. Recently, a subtype of learning disability known as nonverbal learning disability (NVLD) has been identified (Rourke, Young, & Leenaars, 1989). NVLD manifests in weak nonverbal reasoning abilities, including difficulty interpreting social cues and appreciating the relationship between cause and effect, particularly with respect to social behavior. NVLD has been associated with depression, and some adolescents with NVLD exhibit problem behavior because of their difficulty relating cause and effect. They drift toward deviant peer groups because of a history of social rejection resulting from their inability to process social cues.

3. Verbal learning disability. Adolescents who have a language-based learning disability might also be prone to exhibit impulsive and/or aggressive behavior because they are unable to use language to resolve conflicts. These youngsters strike out because they can't hold their own in a verbal argument. Often, these kids earn a reputation for starting physical fights because they are the first to throw a punch in an escalating battle of insults. These kids are not necessarily more aggressive, but they appear to be because their aggression is expressed physically rather than verbally.

Overlooking Serious Psychiatric Disorder

Among the serious disorders that might contribute to problem behavior are psychoses, mood disorders, and psychoactive-substance-related disorders. Adolescents who are psychotic may experience hallucinations that command them to engage in aggressive acts. They might harbor delusional ideas that contribute to distrust, withdrawal, alignment with deviant peers, and rebellious behavior. Adolescents with bipolar disorder might engage in seemingly uncontrolled sprees of antisocial behavior during a manic episode.

Sometimes teenagers engage in risky and defiant behavior as a way of distracting themselves from feelings of despair. This pattern has been termed "masked depression" because the problem behavior obscures other symptoms of depression, such as sleep or appetite disturbance. For example, the boy who doesn't get up for school might be experiencing a sleep disturbance, obscured by the fact that he also violated curfew and comes in late. The kid who does not have meals with the family or who has lost weight might be suspected of abusing drugs, but in fact the weight loss could be a symptom of depression. Complicating matters further, many adolescents medicate themselves with drugs as a way of relieving symptoms of depression. In addition, the substances themselves might promote episodes of dyscontrol or the emergence of substance-induced psychotic symptoms. If any of these conditions are suspected, a psychiatric consultation should be sought. If medications are indicated, their use should always be framed as adjunctive to the family work, not a substitute for it.

Intrusion of the Therapist's Values

It is virtually impossible to deal with adolescent problem behavior without venturing into the arena of values, an area that most therapists have been trained to avoid. Yet, many of the clashes between adolescents and parents involve the appropriate values by which to conduct one's life.

Some writers find a way out of this dilemma by pointing out that therapy, by its very nature, deals in values (e.g., Efran, Lukens, & Lukens, 1990). Therapists can never be completely objective, because their own views of what is right or wrong, healthy or unhealthy, progress or regress, inform the way that they conduct therapy. In fact, when therapists claim to be "objective," they are more apt to be naive regarding the impact of values on their work, and therefore more likely to impose these values on clients.

Some have challenged therapeutic "objectivity" from another vantage point. Feminist therapists, for example, claim that a therapist who does not directly challenge traditional gender-role expectations contributes to maintaining the unjust power differential between men and women (Goldner, 1988; Hare-Mustin, 1987; Walters, Carter, Papp, & Silverstein, 1988). These writers exhort therapists to challenge overt attempts by men to wield power over women and to expose covert manifestations of gender hierarchies by calling attention to them in therapy. From this perspective, maintaining objectivity or therapeutic "neutrality" is not only impossible but undesirable. As Walters et al. (1988) write, "Therapy is a political act and cannot be separated from the social issues in which the family is embedded" (p. 29).

In my work, I avoid disclosing my own values to the family. While I do not claim to be objective or neutral, and I strive to be aware of ways in which my own values might influence what I choose to do or say in therapy, I generally believe that my particular values on an issue are irrelevant to the job of doing therapy. I am more interested in process than content, in *how* the family members deal with their differences rather than *what* decisions they eventually make. To put it bluntly, I don't consider it my business to tell family members what they should and shouldn't do. Instead, I see my job as helping family members persist in the struggle to listen to each other and resolve their differences without resorting to bullying one another, pretending their conflicts don't exist, or triangling a hired expert (i.e., therapist) to take responsibility for decisions that are rightfully theirs.

Most of the time, values are but one of many considerations parents are weighing in order to make a decision. For example, parents might have moral objections to premarital sex but their primary concern is not the immorality of their daughter's behavior but rather the potential consequences of this behavior for the girl's future. The therapist can be helpful here by presenting to the parents the results of the available research on the issue under consideration. For example, a recent study by Bingham and Crockett (1996) found no adverse psychosocial outcomes for either male or female adolescents who engage in early sexual intercourse. Parents who are worried about the effects of minor experimentation with drugs might be informed of the findings of Shedler and Block (1990) that adolescents who experimented with marijuana were actually better adjusted than those who completely abstained.

After presenting the relevant research findings (after a trip to the library if necessary!), the therapist should simply monitor the process among the family members as they discuss the issue under consideration, intervening not to defend or refute a point of content, but to identify and remove the obstacles that are preventing the family members from arriving at a decision about this issue on their own.

Expecting Too Much of the Parents

It is important for therapists to consider other stressors in the family's context that might limit the parents' ability to participate fully in treatment.

1. How available are the parents? Adolescents from single-parent households are at higher risk for problem behavior (Dornbusch et al., 1985; Steinberg, 1987a). Often, these single parents are isolated from extended family and their community. Sometimes the noncustodial parent actively undermines the parent with primary custody. One of the top priorities for intervention is to find a way to support an overwhelmed single parent. If at all possible, the noncustodial parent should be involved in treatment, along with stepparents and other adults who live in the home. If the single parent is isolated, steps must be taken to build bridges to the extended family and the community. In some cases, if the extended family resides too far away or the parent is adamantly opposed to their involvement, the therapist might temporarily need to accept the role of coparent, though the therapist should at all times be on the lookout for others in the parent's community to assume that role.

Parents might be unavailable for other reasons, such as their own emotional or physical symptoms, marital discord, another child with problems, or a demanding job. Very early in treatment, the therapist must assess to what extent these factors might undermine efforts to support the parent's involvement with the troublesome adolescent. For parents with emotional or physical problems of their own, it will probably be necessary to recruit support from outside the family. The therapist should always first strive to find support for the parent, and only if all options have been exhausted should the therapist consider finding extrafamilial support directly for the adolescent. The goal should be to shore up the parental subsystem first before declaring the parental subsystem inadequate to the task and bringing in substitutes from outside the family to work directly with the youngster, such as an individual therapist, residential placement, or a foster home.

2. Are there other problems in the family that are as serious or more serious than the adolescent's behavior? In these cases, the adolescent's behavior is simply one of a host of problems in the family. When the therapist tries to focus on the adolescent's problem behavior, other problems distract the family's attention. No single problem is able to hold center stage long enough for a solution to be found. In these cases, when the adolescent's behavior is a symptom of general family chaos, the suggestions in Chapter 10 for working with multiproblem families might be helpful. In short, the goal with such families is not to address the adolescent's problem behavior per se, but rather to help the family as a whole to function more successfully by facilitating the development of more efficient problem-solving strategies.

3. *Know the family's community.* In low-income urban areas where there are high rates of delinquency, kids might conclude that the only way to earn respect and to avoid being victimized is to join the group of victimizers. On the other hand, there might be resources in the community that are not readily apparent to outsiders. Once the therapist has identified these resources, then the task becomes helping the family access them. This might require inviting the community representatives into the therapy sessions or, if necessary, going into the community to meet them.

Expecting Too Little of the Parents

Another pitfall is concluding too quickly that the parents are incapable of change. Madanes (1981) has outlined a number of ways that parents try to avoid the therapist's efforts to help them take charge. These maneuvers include the following:

1. Disqualifying themselves by denying that they have no expertise for dealing with the problem adolescent, or professing ignorance about what expectations and consequences are appropriate.

2. Turning over authority to the problem child by allowing the child too loud a voice in deciding how to handle the problem and how to structure the household.

3. Disqualifying each other by telling the therapist secrets about the other parent, threatening to break up the parental unit, or refusing to collaborate with the other parent.

4. Disqualifying the therapist by directly or indirectly challenging the therapist's suggestions, or simply refusing to comply with the therapeutic contract.

The result is that the therapist is likely to take on an inappropriately central position in the therapy. Signs that this has occurred include the following: The therapist begins to feel responsible for the adolescent's behavior, the therapist begins to feel hopeless or inadequate to the task of working with the family, the therapist begins challenging the youngster directly about the problem behavior, the therapist begins to feel angry at the kid, or the therapist gets caught up in micromanaging the family's decisions.

One way to circumvent this pitfall is to avoid giving the parents specific suggestions on how to handle a problem. Rather than directing the parents on what to do, the therapist should help them identify at least two alternative ways they could respond to the situation. The positive and negative consequences of each alternative can be explored, but the parents make the final decision about which alternative to choose. In some cases, the parents protest that they are unable to choose, and insist that the therapist tell them what is the "best" way to handle the problem. The therapist must respectfully decline these invitations, and instead reiterate his or her confidence in the parents' competence to make the decision that is best for them and for their household.

Another way a therapist might get inducted into taking over for the parents is to get bogged down in the details of carrying out a particular decision. Discussions may devolve into lengthy debates over the specific time of curfew, or the exact words the parents should use in presenting a decision to the adolescent. When therapy begins focusing on the details, it is likely that the parents have failed to grasp that the goal is not to control the adolescent, but rather for them to feel that they are doing the best they can to manage a difficult situation. While therapy can involve some coaching, it is best for the therapist to focus on the broad strokes and leave the parents to work out the details.

SUMMARY

The main point of this chapter is that aggression, delinquency, and other problem behaviors represent a rupture in the adolescent's relationships with the family. The more the parents try to control the kid, the more the kid resists their control and gravitates toward deviant peers who reinforce problem behavior. The key to successful intervention is to break this cycle by working to reestablish relationships in the family.

I suggest that problem behavior be viewed along a continuum from mild to moderate to severe.

- When the problem behavior is *mild*, the adolescent tests limits but generally has maintained positive relationships with the family. At this level, I recommend that therapy should focus not on strategies to eliminate the problem behavior but rather on the developmental transitions that the family is facing. Build on existing family strengths to encourage conflict resolution and to expand dialogue among the family members.

- When the problem behavior is *moderate*, there is a more persistent pattern of defiance. The adolescent might be abusing drugs or alcohol, might be sexually promiscuous, or might be chronically truant. Despite frequent arguments with parents, the adolescent has never been violent at home. At this level, the key principle is to redirect the parents' efforts away from trying to control the youth. Discourage control-based methods of influence and emphasize the parents' emotional investment in the youngster.
- *Severe* problem behavior presents a threat of harm to self or others. In addition to engaging in potentially dangerous behavior, the adolescent might also have been violent toward family members. At this level, the main principle is to find a balance between supporting the parents and supporting the adolescent. Restore power to the parents without alienating the kid. Help the parents to regain some control over their own lives, and then shift the emphasis to helping the parents provide age-appropriate nurturance to the youngster.
- Finally, I discussed a number of pitfalls that could be encountered in treating problem behavior, including failing to assess the role of low IQ or learning disability, overlooking serious psychiatric disorder, pushing one's values on the family, or overestimating or underestimating the parents' ability to handle the youngster with behavior problems.

NOTE

1. These suggestions are derived from the concepts of "acknowledgment" and "multidirected partiality" in contextual family therapy (see Boszormenyi-Nagy & Spark, 1973).

CHAPTER 7

PSYCHOSIS

W*ho was the patient here?* I wondered, as I watched the family behind the one-way mirror. In the room on the other side of the mirror, a woman was sobbing, flanked by her 13-year-old son and an elderly woman who was the crying woman's mother. I later learned that the crying woman's name was Jessie, her mother was Sarah, and the boy was Jamal.

JESSIE: (*frantically*) Momma, I'm losing my mind! I'm losing my mind!

SARAH: No you're not honey, you'll be all right. Tell her she'll be all right, Jamal.

JAMAL: Mom, you'll be all right.

JESSIE: (*sobbing*) No I won't! You don't know what I'm going through. I'm losing my mind.

SARAH: (*to Jamal*) Give her this, hon. (*Hands Jamal a tissue.*)

JAMAL: (*Gives Jessie the tissue.*) Take this, Mom. You'll be all right.

JESSIE: Yeah, I'll be all right. Don't worry about me.

JAMAL: I don't, I won't worry. (*to Sarah*) She shouldn't cry like that.

SARAH: She can't help it, honey.

JESSIE: I can't help it. But I'll be all right. You'll be all right.

JAMAL: I know. I'll be all right.

Jamal was supposed to be the patient. At 13, he had already been hospitalized twice within the past 4 months for psychotic symptoms, which included hallucinations and catatonic episodes. His outpatient therapist, Dr. Steve Simms, was presenting the case to me for a consultation because Jamal appeared to be decompensating again. Jamal lived most of the time with Jessie, a 35-year-old single mother, but both Jamal and Jessie spent time at the home of Sarah, Jessie's mother, who had recently retired after working 30 years as a medical records clerk. Jessie had not seen Jamal's father since Jamal was a baby, and she had no idea of his whereabouts. Jessie was unemployed and had just been discharged from a one-week stay in an inpatient psychiatric unit where she was receiving treatment for depression and anxiety. Jamal carried diagnoses of psychotic disorder NOS (not otherwise specified), learning disorder NOS, attention-deficit/hyperactivity disorder, and mild mental retardation. The family lived on the brink of poverty in the inner city of Philadelphia.

Throughout this book, I have emphasized that interpersonal isolation, overt and covert, contributes to and results from the development of symptoms in adolescence. Every syndrome we have considered—eating disorders, depression, aggressive and defiant behavior—has been related to a cycle of interactions that has at its core the experience of isolation for both the symptomatic adolescent and the other family members. We now consider psychosis, admittedly a rare symptom among adolescents but one with far-reaching consequences.

Psychosis is almost synonymous with profound isolation. Individuals experiencing psychotic symptoms have retreated into a private world populated by terrifying voices and frightening images. They are wracked with uncertainty about what is real—the world around them or the world inside of them. Delusional beliefs about other people contribute to the feeling that they are completely alone in a dangerous world. Their speech is unintelligible, and their loose associations make it impossible for them to communicate about their experiences with others. Their bizarre behavior frightens other people and drives them away.

THEORETICAL PERSPECTIVES

Family Dynamics

In post-Freudian psychoanalytic theory, psychosis was thought to result from severe disturbances in the relationship between the infant and his or her "schizophrenogenic" mother (Fromm-Reichman, 1948). The pioneers of family therapy sought to break from this tradition by emphasizing more complex interactions that involved both parents and the child. For example, Theodore Lidz and his colleagues identified the patterns of *marital schism* and *marital skew* in families with schizophrenic children (Lidz, Cornelison, Fleck, & Terry, 1957). Martial schism involved mutual undermining by the parents and competition for the child's loyalty. In marital skew, one spouse was weaker and dependent on the other spouse, who covertly bullied the weaker spouse into submission. Murray Bowen (1978, p. 107) described families with schizophrenic children as an *undifferentiated ego mass*, characterized by intense emotional reactivity and triangulation. Lyman Wynne and his colleagues (Wynne, Ryckoff, Day, & Hirsch, 1958) emphasized the dynamic of *pseudomutuality* in psychotic families, whereby all family members were invested in maintaining rigid interactional patterns at the expense of developing an individual identity.

Other early family models of psychosis emphasized the disturbed patterns of communication in these families. Gregory Bateson, Don Jackson, Jay Haley, and John Weakland (1956) proposed the well-known *double-bind theory*, according to which the presence of irreconcilable contradictory messages ultimately led to a retreat from reality on the part of the psychotic individual. Margaret Singer and Lyman Wynne asserted that a disordered style of communication, known as *communication deviance*, was the defining characteristic of families with young adult schizophrenics (Singer, Wynne, & Toohey, 1978).

More recently, Mara Selvini-Palazzoli (1986) described a step-by-step process by which psychosis evolves in families, termed the *family game*. According to this model, the child becomes embroiled in a long-standing battle between the parents, each of whom uses the child's symptoms as a way of gaining advantage over the other parent. Selvini-Palazzoli has advocated use of the *invariant prescription*, by which parents are given the instruction to go out alone without telling the children where they are going, meanwhile recording scrupulous observations on any events in the family that seem to be related to this prescription.

Biology

In reaction to perceived efforts on the part of the professional community to blame parents (especially mothers) for psychotic symptoms, the pendulum has swung in the other direction, so that many families now militantly rebel against the idea that parents play a role in the development of psychotic symptoms among their offspring. The growing body of literature linking psychosis to genetic and other biological causes has reinforced this position. There has been a movement to medicalize psychosis and treat it as an illness that can be managed, but not cured.

As in most polarized debates, there is danger in becoming too closely aligned with one side of the issue. Those who view psychosis as a strictly biological disorder run the risk of ignoring important interpersonal interactional patterns that contribute to the emergence or exacerbation of symptoms. Those who minimize the importance of biological factors may misattribute the adolescent's behavior to other factors (e.g., drugs) and fail to acknowledge the adolescent's exquisite vulnerability to family stress. There is also speculation that the symptoms of psychosis may interact with the biology of the nervous system in a cyclical manner, such that the symptoms alter the biology of the brain, which then produces more symptoms (Harrop, Trower, & Mitchell, 1996). Failure to treat the symptoms, therefore, could exacerbate the biological vulnerability, even though the symptoms might not have a purely biological etiology.

A middle ground between a strictly biological and strictly psychological model for psychosis is one that integrates the effects of biology and environment. According to this model, termed the *diathesis–stress model*, genetic factors determine the degree to which a person is predisposed or vulnerable to developing psychosis (Gottesman, 1991). Whether psychotic symptoms actually emerge depends on the amount of environmental stress that the individual experiences. Symptoms appear once the combination of genetic vulnerability and stress exceeds a theoretical threshold. Those with minimal biological vulnerability require a substantial amount of environmental stress before showing psychotic symptoms, while those with a higher vulnerability require less stress. In other words, individuals with a high genetic predisposition to psychosis are more likely to show psychotic symptoms under relatively lower degrees of stress.

Integrated Approaches

One of the consequences of the diathesis–stress model has been a deemphasis on single modes of treatment and a greater emphasis on integrating biological and psychosocial treatments. There has been a shift from identifying the family patterns that cause schizophrenia to identifying factors that influence the course and prognosis of the disorder. For example, relapse rates in schizophrenia have been linked to a family pattern known as *high expressed emotion* (Leff & Vaughn, 1981). These families are emotionally overinvolved with one another, overtly critical of the patient, and express hostility in a rejecting manner.

One example of an integrated approach to treating psychosis is the *psychoeducational* model, such as that advocated by Carol Anderson (1983) and Michael Goldstein and his colleagues (Kopeikin, Marshall, & Goldstein, 1983). According to this model, family members are helped to identify and change the interactional patterns that are presumed to exacerbate the psychotic symptoms, even though these patterns are not necessarily seen as etiological. Family members are encouraged to view the psychosis as an illness in order to promote feelings of sympathy and helpfulness rather than anger or resentment toward the patient. They are coached in ways of relating to one another that minimize levels of conflict and negative affect in the family.

I also advocate an integrated approach to treating psychosis that includes both medication to relieve the psychotic symptoms and family therapy to help the family members change the way they interact with one another. As I have argued in previous chapters, members of families in which there are severe symptoms are often profoundly isolated from one another. As family members become increasingly focused on the symptoms, they neglect other aspects of their relationships with one another, breeding more isolation and more symptomatic behavior in a mutually reinforcing process known as the "symptomatic cycle." Psychosis represents the most extreme form of this isolation, where the presence of delusions, hallucinations, and bizarre behavior constitutes a private world to which others have no access. Thus, the treatment of psychosis must include not only amelioration of the psychotic symptoms but also work with the family to reduce their isolation from one another and from their community. My approach is illustrated in the case of Jamal, which is discussed in detail later. First, however, I identify several key challenges therapists face when they treat psychotic adolescents and their families.

TREATING PSYCHOTIC ADOLESCENTS: CHALLENGES TO THE THERAPIST

Some of the challenges posed in the treatment of psychotic adolescents include the following:

Building a Relationship with the Adolescent

Psychotic adolescents might be paranoid or so self-involved that they cannot enter into a relationship in the usual sense of the term. The challenge is to remain engaged in spite of the absence of the usual kinds of emotional reciprocity one experiences in a relationship.

Relationships with psychotic individuals will have a different "feel"; thus, therapists should not base their assessment of the quality of the relationship on their subjective experience of it. Therapists should instead look at the youth's behavior to evaluate how invested he or she is in the relationship with the therapist. Some questions to consider include the following: Does the adolescent come to sessions? Does the adolescent seem interested in what the therapist says? Does the adolescent follow the therapist's suggestions? How does the adolescent's relationship with the therapist compare to other relationships in the adolescent's life?

Engaging the Family in Treatment

The family members are likely to be so troubled by the adolescent's psychotic symptoms that at first glance they appear highly motivated to participate in therapy. On the other hand, it is also easier for them and the therapist to become so focused on eliminating the symptoms that family dynamics are overlooked. The challenge is to engage the family in the process of change without alienating them by implying that they are to blame for the adolescent's condition.

Therapy should focus on alleviating the adolescent's symptoms, preventing recurrences, and improving functioning, not on uncovering family dynamics that presumably caused the psychotic episode. The therapist serves as a consultant to the family to help them identify ways in which they might facilitate the adolescent's progress. The therapist focuses on interactional patterns, but not with the goal of discovering "why" the psychosis occurred, but rather with the goal of promoting better family functioning as a way to reduce stress on the adolescent.

Respecting the Vulnerability of the System

As noted in Chapter 2, symptomatic cycles retard the individual development of family members. Once the cycle has been disrupted, development is free to proceed. However, in many families, developmental transitions are so threatening that the transitions themselves reactivate the cycle. The therapist must always remain alert to signs that the cycle is reemerging whenever any one in the family takes a developmental step toward autonomy or individuation. The therapist must move back and forth between supporting development and disrupting the symptomatic cycle. As will be illustrated in the case of Jamal, the therapist encourages developmental progress on the part of each family member while ensuring that the connections among the members of the family remain strong.

Coordinating Multiple Helpers

In treating psychosis, it is likely that many professionals will be involved with the family. The problem of coordination then comes to the fore. In some cases, the therapist might be in the role of case manager and head of the treatment team. Ideally, all members of the team share a common view of the treatment goals, decisions are made collaboratively, and periodic meetings with the family and the team are arranged. As team leader, the therapist must attend not only to his or her relationship with the family but also to the relationships among the members of the team. Conflicts among team members can undermine effective treatment and must be resolved. Sometimes, members of the team unwittingly become inducted into the symptomatic cycle, as in the case of Jamal, and a top priority must be realigning the relationship between the professional and the family.

In most cases, the family therapist is not head of the treatment team and might feel out of the loop when major decisions are being made. Complaining about a model that puts a higher priority on medical management than on systemic change will not help. The therapist must find a way to work with the other professionals for the benefit of the patient and the family. Cultivating relationships based on mutual respect rather than competition is essential. The therapist might conceptualize his or her role as that of consultant to the team in matters pertaining to family dynamics and effective team coordination. As with any consultant, the other team members are free to accept or reject the therapist's suggestions, and the therapist should not take this personally. The therapist who has a conflict with another team member must be careful not to triangulate the family by attempting to win the family over to his or her side. The therapist should also watch out for attempts by the family members to triangulate him or her into conflicts between the family and another team member. Rather than becoming involved in these conflicts, even if it is in the apparently helpful role of mediator, the therapist should help the family deal more directly and effectively with the member of the team with whom the family is in conflict.

Resisting the Pull to Underestimate the Family's Capacity

As Haley (1980) and Madanes (1981) have pointed out, family members who are dealing with severe symptoms sometimes attempt to abdicate their parental role by declaring themselves incompetent to deal with the problem. They might try to shift responsibility to the professionals, who are then faced with the paradoxical task of "curing" the symptomatic member without authorization to meddle in family dynamics. If the professionals make a decision that the family does not like, the family asserts its authority by refusing to comply or threatening to seek help elsewhere. What can result is a pattern of mutual blame and abdication of responsibility by the family and the professional team, with the patient caught in the middle.

The therapist must avoid the pitfall of assuming that the problem is too big for the family to handle and instead ask what the family needs in order to handle the problem more effectively. This perspective keeps the family in an appropriately central role and affirms its competence, while also recognizing that the family will need the help of extended family, friends, and professionals. This principle is illustrated in the case of Jamal, where the family was encouraged to mobilize their resources to simulate a hospital at home rather than immediately seeking hospitalization when the symptoms reemerged.

Selecting an Appropriate Treatment Focus

Though amelioration of the patient's suffering is an important goal, therapy should not focus only on removing psychotic symptoms. Symptom removal is a negative goal, while helping the family members reduce tension and cope better is a positive goal. Symptoms can be treated without demonstrable family change, for example, by administering medications. Also, by focusing exclusively or even primarily on removal of symptoms, the therapist is apt to neglect the important interrelationships among the family members that can enable or retard the adolescent's progress.

Therapy should focus on helping the adolescent function better. This goal is accomplished by taking a careful inventory of what the adolescent is currently able to do, and then helping the adolescent to take small steps in the direction of more independence.

For example, after one session, when Jamal met with the therapist alone, Jamal expressed anxiety about taking the subway home and wanted to call his mother to pick him up. The therapist instead suggested that he walk with Jamal to the subway station and wait with him until his train arrived. Over the next few sessions, the therapist gradually expanded Jamal's sphere of independence, first walking him to the station and not waiting for the train, then eventually walking him halfway, until eventually Jamal was traveling to sessions on his own.

Sometimes the emergence of symptoms is an indirect request for help. For example, Jamal expressed his fear of taking the train alone by becoming disorganized and bizarre in his speech. The therapist considered it progress when Jamal could verbalize his fear and no longer relied on symptoms as a way of expressing a need.

Developing Appropriate Expectations for the Adolescent

The therapist must help the family navigate between the poles of underestimating and overestimating the psychotic youngster's competence. If family members underestimate the youth's competence, they might encourage too much dependency that thwarts her development. If family members overestimate the youth's competence, they might fail to provide the support she needs when faced with a developmental demand that appears minor but that may be a substantial stressor for an adolescent vulnerable to psychosis. In other cases, the family members may misattribute the adolescent's behavior to willful defiance and therefore respond in a way that exacerbates the problem.

For example, 16 year-old Gabe Flynn, who carried a diagnosis of bipolar disorder, was belligerent and disrespectful to the other family members. The boy's father had always remained peripheral, aligned in a covert coalition with the boy against his mother, who had taken most of the responsibility for parenting and did so in a rather heavy-handed manner. Initially, family sessions focused on helping Mr. Flynn become more involved in parenting. Mr. Flynn, however, took the opposite extreme: In order to avoid the breakup of his marriage when his wife gave him an ultimatum that he either take a stronger position with Gabe or face losing her, Mr. Flynn flipped over to supporting his wife, which left the boy feeling abandoned and encouraged an intensification of his symptoms. The boy's hostility toward his mother increased, and as Mr. Flynn persisted in supporting his wife, Gabe began directing hostility toward his father. Gabe became more disorganized in his behavior and speech, and claimed to be hearing voices. Nevertheless, Mr. and Mrs. Flynn continued to view Gabe's behavior as "bad," rather than "crazy," and kept punishing him. Eventually, the boy became so symptomatic that he needed to be hospitalized.

This boy was still triangled in the conflict between his parents, albeit in a different way. Previously, the triangle involved a covert coalition between father and son against mother, but now the triangle shifted to a detouring–attacking one (Minuchin, 1974), whereby the parents maintained an illusory sense of affiliation by taking a hard line with the boy. The solution involved shifting the parents' attention from setting limits to developing ways to manage conflict without escalating it.

I encouraged Mr. and Mrs. Flynn to see Gabe as temporarily under the influence of "bipolar disorder" that would pass with appropriate treatment and management. The parental coalition was solidified not by exhorting them to remain firm against the boy, but by prompting them to talk with each other about ways that they could be more helpful to Gabe and more supportive of each other when Gabe's behavior got out of control. Toward this end, I suggested ways to deescalate family conflicts, using techniques such as distraction, focusing on points of agreement, and avoiding unproductive arguing.

The reader might note that Gabe was still, in a sense, triangled in the relationship between his parents. Before, they joined together in attacking him; now, they aligned with each other in an effort to help him. This is often a necessary stage when long-standing parental conflict renders parents ineffective in helping a psychotic youngster. The escalating conflict between the parents poses more of an immediate threat to the youngster than sustaining the triangle by encouraging the parents to put their differences aside in order to help their child. But therapy cannot stop here. After convincing the parents to join forces to help their child, the therapist must help the parents sustain their alliance by learning more productive ways of addressing the unresolved conflicts between them.

CASE EXAMPLE: REDUCING ISOLATION IN PSYCHOTIC SYSTEMS

I now return to the case introduced at the beginning of this chapter. This case chronicles a 2-year effort to help a family deal with recurring psychotic symptoms in an adolescent boy. It is presented in some detail because it depicts the long and often frustrating process of working with psychotic adolescents and their families, where all of the challenges discussed earlier are addressed. The case also illustrates a number of other challenges and principles that will be highlighted at appropriate points in the case discussion:

- How the therapists conceptualized work with a family on the brink of poverty, who had few resources and therefore could easily be dismissed as incompetent or unable to handle the adolescent.
- How the therapists met the challenge of working with a parent who also has serious psychiatric symptoms leading to recurrent hospitalizations.
- How a therapist working alone can get caught up in a symptomatic cycle, and how a brief hospitalization was used to disrupt the cycle.

- How the symptomatic cycle was repeatedly activated whenever a family member took a step toward greater autonomy or individuation.
- How the therapists facilitated the construction of a team that included the family, consultants from the hospital, and members of the family's community.

This case represented a successful effort to prevent hospitalization. After three hospitalizations in a period of 4 months, future hospitalizations were averted, psychotic symptoms were reduced in intensity, and family relationships were improved.

Some Background

Prior to our first session, Dr. Simms had filled me in on the history. Jamal had struggled in school through the first few grades until a psychological evaluation revealed that his IQ was 72, in the borderline mentally retarded range. He was placed in a special education class but didn't seem to be learning much. Over the past year, he had begun to wander aimlessly about the house late at night and seemed to be listening to voices. Finally, he was hospitalized on an emergency basis after he "went berserk" and started screaming and threatening to hurt himself. He was hospitalized for 2 weeks, during which time the team worked with his mother, Jessie, to help her feel more in control of the situation.

They returned home, and Jamal seemed to be better, but within a month they were back in the emergency room, with Jamal actively hallucinating and spending hours unresponsively staring into space. This time, a neurological consultation was requested but showed nothing wrong. Jamal was put on a low dose of risperidone, an antipsychotic medication, and improved.

The inpatient team again worked with Jessie to help her feel more competent to manage Jamal on her own. The team believed that Jessie's parental authority was being threatened by Sarah, who would criticize her in Jamal's presence and overtly undermine Jessie's attempts to take charge. To support Jessie, the team tried to block Sarah's intrusions and focused their efforts on shoring up Jessie's parenting role.

At the end of the second hospitalization, the family was referred to Dr. Simms, who met with Jessie and Jamal twice a week. Initially, they were doing fine, but then Jamal's symptoms returned. Trying to avoid a third hospitalization, Dr. Simms was spending several hours a week struggling to help the family manage Jamal at home. Finally, exhausted, he decided that Jamal had to be readmitted to the hospital.

Because the unit where Jamal had previously been hospitalized didn't have any beds available, Dr. Simms asked me if I would consider accepting Jamal into the unit I was directing at the time. I agreed that I would try to help in any way I could, and asked that we schedule a session the next morning to be attended by Jessie, Sarah, Jamal, and Dr. Simms.

The Assessment Session

At the beginning of this chapter, I recounted the scene I was witnessing through the one-way mirror while Dr. Simms and I met briefly to plan the session. Jessie, weeping uncontrollably, was so overwhelmed by her own problems that she was unable to help her son. Jamal was trying unsuccessfully to comfort his mother, despite the fact that he was about to be admitted to a psychiatric unit. Sarah, faced with two family members apparently in psychiatric crisis, had little more to offer than words of reassurance, which unwittingly distanced Jessie even more because Sarah's calm reassurance contrasted so dramatically with Jessie's sense of herself as out of control.

Therapists involved with a family such as this might find themselves caught up in the symptomatic cycle, which can vitiate their efforts to help the family. Sometimes, the therapist can experience the same sense of isolation experienced by the family members, and might respond to this isolation by calling in a consultant or requesting hospitalization. For this reason, I wanted Dr. Simms to be present at my initial interview with the family. I wanted to assess his role in the symptomatic cycle and help him extricate himself from it. I also wanted to communicate to Dr. Simms and to the family that I respected his role as the primary therapist for the family, and so I began the session by addressing him first. I asked Dr. Simms how he thought we could be helpful to him.

He replied, "Well, until now, I have been unsuccessful in helping this family cope. We've made several plans to deal with Jamal's behavior, but they just don't work. I think we're all stuck." Sarah and Jessie nodded in unison.

Dr. Simms stated nondefensively that he was "stuck," thus situating the impasse in his relationship with the family rather than inside the family. I saw this as a good sign. It told me that Dr. Simms was involved with the family, and that (like a good family therapist) he looked first at the relationships within the therapeutic system for the source of the problem before stepping out of the system and scapegoating the family. The way he described the problem gave a clue to how he might have become inducted. He talked about plans that he and the family had developed, but that didn't work because the family didn't follow through. I suspected that conflict around these plans might be contributing to the symptomatic cycle, so I asked him to elaborate.

MICUCCI: Can you tell me more about these plans?

SIMMS: Well, the most recent plan involved having Sarah and Jessie decide who would be in charge. Sometimes Jessie seems to be in charge, and sometimes Sarah seems to be in charge. It's confusing. So, we agreed, because Jessie seemed to be having so many problems of her own, that Sarah would be in charge, but every time Sarah tried to take care of Jamal, Jessie would step in and take him home with her. Then, Sarah and Jessie would fight about what to do.

MICUCCI: And how do you see the failure of this plan being related to Jamal's symptoms?

SIMMS: The more Sarah and Jessie fought, the worse Jamal got.

I noted that Dr. Simms linked the failure of the plan to conflict between Jessie and Sarah about who should be in charge, but that now he was focusing on the relationships *within* the family, rather than on the relationship between himself and the family. I wondered if his well-intentioned efforts to help might have reinforced the patterns among the family members that he was describing as part of the problem.

One of the ways to increase the understanding of the symptomatic cycle is to request a detailed exposition of the events leading up to the current crisis, so I asked Dr. Simms to fill me in on the the events of the past few days. In response, Dr. Simms presented the following sequence of events:

- Jamal became symptomatic at school, which brought him to the attention of the school psychologist.
- The school psychologist contacted not the family, but Dr. Simms.
- Since Dr. Simms knew that Jessie was in the hospital, he bypassed her, called Sarah, and urged her to take Jamal to the emergency room to arrange hospitalization.

I concluded from this chronology that Dr. Simms had been identified both by the family and by the larger system—in this case, the school—as the person in charge of Jamal. Meanwhile, Sarah quietly accepted the responsibility for arranging hospitalization for Jamal, bypassing Jessie, not out of malice but to protect her.

It appeared that the therapist's willingness to accept responsibility for Jamal undermined the plan that called for either Jessie or Sarah to be in charge. I asked what Dr. Simms proposed as a solution. He said he thought it would help if full custody of Jamal were transferred from Jessie to Sarah. Coming alive, as if for the first time, Jessie balked at this suggestion.

"No way," Jessie said, with conviction. "I want to have custody of my own son. Right now, I'm in a bad way and I need to get help myself by going back into the hospital. But when I come out, I want Jamal to live with me, and I want full custody of him in my own house."

The Symptomatic Cycle

Jessie's response helped to flesh out the details of the symptomatic cycle in this family.

- *Step 1.* As long as Jessie is capable, she parents Jamal alone, with Sarah concerned, but on the periphery.
- *Step 2.* Gradually, Jessie becomes overwhelmed by the responsibility of parenting Jamal alone and responds by distancing herself from him.
- *Step 3.* Cut off from a relationship with his mother, Jamal's symptoms intensify, leading to his first hospitalization.
- *Step 4.* The hospital supports Jessie in her role as parent, blocking Sarah's involvement, which is seen as intrusive and undermining of Jessie's authority.
- *Step 5.* Jamal thereby becomes reconnected with Jessie, and his symptoms decrease. He is sent home with Jessie.
- *Step 6.* Since the hospital has excluded Sarah from the treatment, Jessie now is isolated and cut off from Sarah.
- *Step 7.* Jessie now becomes symptomatic, which leads her to withdraw from Jamal.
- *Step 8.* Seeing Jamal neglected by Jessie, Sarah volunteers to help. She comes back in to take over for Jessie in caring for Jamal.
- *Step 9.* Relieved of the responsibility of caring for Jamal by herself and now reconnected with Sarah, Jessie recovers, which leads back to Step 1 in the cycle.

The symptomatic cycle is summarized in Figure 7.1.

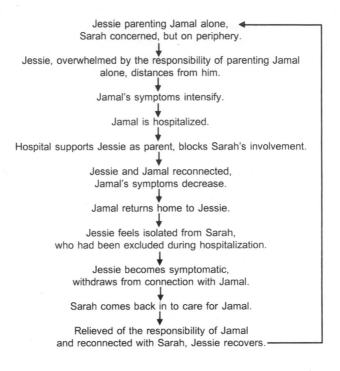

FIGURE 7.1. The symptomatic cycle of Jamal's family.

The Treatment Contract

Based on this understanding of the symptomatic cycle, I proposed that Jamal be readmitted to the hospital. This time, however, the hospitalization would be used to help the family members develop different relationships with each other and to help the outpatient therapist develop a different relationship with the family. Rather than excluding either Sarah or Jessie and insisting that only one of them be consistently in charge, we would urge collaboration between Sarah and Jessie and we would help them work together as a team to help Jamal. We would also help the outpatient therapist adopt a different role with the family. Rather than taking responsibility for Jamal himself, the outpatient therapist would work on helping Sarah and Jessie collaborate more effectively in caring for Jamal.

The Hospitalization

The day after Jamal was admitted to our unit, Jessie readmitted herself to the psychiatric hospital from which she had been discharged only

48 hours earlier, in apparent violation of our agreement that the goal of Jamal's hospitalization would be to help Jessie and Sarah work more effectively as a team. However, in an effort to remain connected with Jessie, our team chose to frame her decision as an effort to make herself better equipped to help Jamal after he was discharged.

We negotiated several hospital passes for Jessie so that she could attend family sessions during Jamal's hospitalization. Sarah was included in all sessions. From the first, our family sessions focused on discharge planning. We intended to discharge Jamal as soon as it was clear that Jessie and Sarah were working collaboratively, and that the outpatient therapist had developed a different relationship with the family. During the hospitalization, in addition to family sessions, Jamal participated in group activities with his peers. Jamal was placed on a low dose of risperidone, monitored by the team psychiatrist.

The Discharge Plan

After a 2-week hospitalization, Jamal's symptoms had improved, Jessie and Sarah were working more effectively as a team, and Dr. Simms reported feeling more comfortable with his new role. The discharge plan included monthly follow-up sessions with me so that we could intervene quickly should the symptomatic cycle reemerge.

At discharge, the inpatient team made two recommendations: First, since Jessie was to be discharged from the hospital shortly after Jamal's discharge, the team recommended that both Jessie and Jamal live for a few weeks with Sarah to allow a smooth transition to Jessie and Jamal returning home together; second, to forestall future hospitalizations and to help the family to deal with crises on its own, the team suggested an alternative to hospitalization. Should Jamal show symptoms again, Jessie should immediately contact Sarah, and they should discuss together what should be done. If they thought that hospitalization might be necessary, before coming to the hospital, Jessie and Jamal should go to Sarah's house, and the family should simulate an emergency room there, contacting the outpatient therapist by phone to receive advice and support. If, after 24 hours of being in this "emergency room" at Sarah's home, the family still wanted hospitalization, then they would meet for a crisis session with Dr. Simms to discuss the next step, with me and other members of the inpatient team available to Dr. Simms for emergency consultation, if need be. The family agreed to this plan and implemented it on one occasion following Jamal's subsequent discharge from the hospital. After a few hours at Sarah's house, Jamal seemed better and hospitalization was averted.

During the hospitalization, we addressed some important goals with this family. First, we deliberately avoided the mistake of excluding Sarah from the process, and instead actively included her in a way that allowed us to cast a more effective role for her. Second, we accepted the reality that Jessie herself had emotional problems, but we refused to allow these problems to disqualify her from her parenting role. Instead, we worked around these problems and insisted that she be involved in Jamal's care to whatever extent possible, with Sarah supporting her as necessary. Third, we acknowledged that a traditional family structure was not working for this family. A traditional structure would have Jessie, as parent, in charge, with Sarah involved, but in the role of supporting Jessie. The fact that Jessie periodically became unable to function because of her own emotional difficulties led us to consider an alternative to this structure.

We decided that a coparenting structure might work better for this family. Rather than having Jessie in charge and Sarah secondary, we wondered if having Jessie and Sarah act as coparents for Jamal might better address the problem of confused hierarchy. If it were made clear that Jessie and Sarah were equally involved in Jamal's care and therefore should negotiate together any major decisions about what to do, it would eliminate the confusion that Dr. Simms had pointed to in the first session: "Sometimes Jessie is in charge, and sometimes Sarah is in charge."

We decided that both women should be in charge, following the model of a two-parent family with father and mother as coparents. In this case, rather than a heterosexual married couple, Jamal's two parents would be his mother and grandmother. We realized that this structure would create problems of its own—for example, Jessie and Sarah had a long history of conflict with one another as mother and daughter—but we decided that these problems would be outweighed by the potential benefits.

First Reemergence of the Cycle

The next crisis occurred 6 months following Jamal's discharge. All had been going well until this point. Instead of three hospitalizations in 4 months, Jamal had been symptom-free for 6 months. Now, however, it looked as if another hospitalization might be imminent. The first sign was Sarah's absence from the session. Jessie reported that Sarah couldn't attend because she hadn't been feeling well. Jessie appeared exasperated and overwhelmed, and was asking us to readmit Jamal, who sat at her side, silent and nearly immobile.

"I can't take it any more," Jessie said. "He's doing it again, walking around the house, talking to himself, staring at the walls. I have to call his name four or five times before he answers me. And he won't do anything I say. I tell him to turn off the TV and do his homework, and he won't do it. I ask him to take out the trash, and he tells me he'll do it later. He's getting sick again and he needs to come back in."

"You must be feeling very stuck," I said.

"Yeah!" Jessie almost shouted. "And my mother, she's at her last wits, she's been ill, she doesn't want us around anymore. I been trying to help her, too, but I just can't do it. I feel like I'm going to fall apart myself."

"And what is it about Jamal that you find most difficult to deal with?" I asked.

"His complete disrespect," Jessie answered, without a beat. "He's totally disrespectful, not doing anything I tell him. The other stuff, the wandering, the staring, I can deal with that, I've dealt with it before, but the disrespect, I can't take that. It's like he'll just do whatever he wants regardless of what I say."

We noted with interest that Jessie was requesting hospitalization for a different reason than before. She acknowledged that she could handle the symptoms that had led to Jamal's three previous hospitalizations. What she couldn't handle was his disrespectful attitude. Previously, Jamal was an unusually compliant adolescent. He did whatever his mother and grandmother asked. Now, Jessie was chagrined by Jamal's defiance and felt unable to cope with it.

We hypothesized that the symptomatic cycle was being reactivated by Jamal taking his first tentative developmental steps into adolescence. Like most adolescents, he was testing his mother's rules. Clearly, the family was not prepared for this transition.

It seemed that Jessie felt isolated and alone, particularly since Sarah was ill. We heard her request that Jamal be rehospitalized as a plea for more support. Though we sympathized with Jessie's plight, we believed that rehospitalizing Jamal could risk reinstating the symptomatic cycle.

We proposed an alternative: Rather than bringing Jamal into the hospital, we would bring the hospital to Jessie. We would allow Jessie to attend support-group meetings for parents whose children were hospitalized, the therapy team would make ourselves available by phone, and we would arrange for Jamal to visit the unit for a few hours and talk with some of the staff. Jessie responded positively to our suggestions and seemed relieved. We also wanted to include Jamal in the plan in a way that communicated our support for his foray into adolescence, so toward the end of the session Dr. Simms addressed Jamal directly:

SIMMS: And the stuff with school, and the other kids making fun of you, how are you doing with that?

JAMAL: OK.

SIMMS: You're dealing with that stuff?

JAMAL: Yeah, I'm dealing with it.

SIMMS: And how's your basketball shot?

JAMAL: (*smiling*) It's good.

SIMMS: You ready to take me on the next time I see you?

JAMAL: Yeah, I'll take you on.

SIMMS: OK, so I'm going to give you two things to do between now and when I see you again, OK?

JAMAL: OK.

SIMMS: First, you listen to your mom. You respect her and do what she says, OK?

JAMAL: OK.

SIMMS: OK, and then, second, you work on your shot. You practice, you hear? Work on that shot. Get ready for our game.

JAMAL: OK, I will.

SIMMS: So let's seal our agreement with a handshake, OK?

JAMAL: OK.

SIMMS: (*Gets up and extends his hand to Jamal.*) Agreed?

JAMAL: (*Takes Dr. Simms's hand.*) Agreed.

Here, Dr. Simms communicated support for Jamal's development by giving him a task that is appropriate for a young adolescent: Obey your mom, and work on your basketball shot. Our goal was to disrupt the symptomatic cycle but at the same time support the developmental transition that apparently had reactivated the cycle. We wanted to encourage Jamal's development as an adolescent while we also supported Jessie's struggle to adjust to the transition.

We did not want to forget Sarah, since, in the past, whenever Jessie demonstrated more competence as a parent, Sarah would fade into the background. We wanted to proceed with our original plan of coparenting, and we didn't want Sarah's absence in this session to lead to her disengaging from the therapy process. To stay connected to her, we decided that Dr. Simms should send Sarah a "get well" card, with a note summarizing the session and reminding her that we looked forward to seeing her next month.

Second Reemergence of the Cycle

Jessie and Sarah returned the following month. Jessie expressed her gratitude for the team's support in the previous session. The family left the session appearing more competent and comfortable with one another.

We anticipated that this conviviality might not last, and our suspicions were confirmed when we met with the family for the next session, now 8 months after Jamal's discharge. In the interval since the preceding session, Sarah had taken a brief trip out of state to visit a relative. During Sarah's absence, Jessie had resumed a relationship with Teddie, a former boyfriend who had been abusive to both Jessie and Jamal in the past. When Sarah returned and found out that Jessie was seeing this man again, she was furious. The ensuing conflict between Sarah and Jessie threatened to tear them apart.

JESSIE: (*addressing Dr. Simms*) I feel as though she should just cut the strings, and let me do what I want.

SARAH: Oh, I will, I will. This is it. You can do whatever you want, I'm out of it.

SIMMS: (*to Sarah*) Now, Sarah, you know we need you here.

SARAH: Well, I'm out. I'm going to say it one last time, and then that's it. (*Now to Jessie.*) You went through hell with this man before, and now you're taking him back. If you didn't learn the first time, then I can't help you. I'm washing my hands of the whole damn situation.

SIMMS: And what does this mean for Jamal?

SARAH: Jamal can come to my house any time he wants. He's always welcome; he's my grandson. But I don't want anything to do with her.

JESSIE: That's fine with me. It's about time that you butted out of my life.

When families are caught in a symptomatic cycle, energies are channeled away from normal developmental tasks. After the cycle has been disrupted, family members are free to proceed on the previously aborted developmental course. Two sessions ago, Jamal's tentative steps into adolescence, made possible by the disruption of the cycle during the hospitalization, triggered the return of the cycle, manifested in Jessie's request for Jamal's rehospitalization. Here we see a similar process in Jessie: We had intercepted the cycle by creating a supportive circle around Jessie. With this disruption of the cycle, Jessie's development resumed, and she began to pursue a relationship with an available adult male. However, Jessie's involvement with this man endangered her relationship with Sarah and so threatened to reactivate the symptomatic cycle.

We had to intervene in a way that supported Jessie's development while helping her stay connected to Sarah and Jamal. If we were to support Jessie against Sarah, thinking, perhaps, that Jessie's move toward autonomy should be encouraged, we could risk alienating Sarah, who, in turn, might abandon Jessie. Instead, we needed to support Jessie in a way that could strengthen her connection with Sarah. This was accomplished by helping Jessie talk openly about her isolation and loneliness.

SIMMS: (*to Jessie*) Who in the family is lonelier, you or your mom?

JESSIE: Me.

SIMMS: Do you think your mom knows how lonely you feel?

JESSIE: No, she doesn't. She thinks that I've just gone back with Teddie, but I haven't. I know what I'm doing. I know he's not good for me or for Jamal. I was just lonely when she was away and when Teddie came around, I felt better.

Rather than attempting to mediate the conflict between Sarah and Jessie, we asked Jessie to talk about the loneliness and isolation that led her to rekindle the relationship with Teddie. In so doing, we hoped to keep Sarah engaged by exposing a side of Jessie that was not often apparent to her. The session ended on this note, without a final resolution of the conflict between the two women. However, we were encouraged, because Sarah appeared to have calmed down, and the fighting had subsided.

The next session, 1 month later, was attended by Sarah and Jessie, and their presence together signaled to us that the relationship between them had been preserved. Meanwhile, Jessie had decided, on her own, to terminate the relationship with Teddie.

Jessie talked about having had a panic attack a week earlier, and as she related the circumstances, it was clear to us that a different relationship was evolving between Sarah and Jessie, one that respected Jessie's competence as an adult. When Jessie had the panic attack, she called Sarah, as she typically would when experiencing these symptoms. Previously, Sarah would immediately take over for Jessie, accepting responsibility for Jamal, intending to support Jessie, but actually encouraging Jessie's dependence on her and unwittingly reinforcing symptom expression as a way to ask for help. This time, however, Sarah responded differently. She supported Jessie over the telephone, encouraged her to weather the panic attack on her own, and reminded her of the progress she had made over the past months. Jessie, supported but not engulfed by her mother's help, successfully handled the panic attack on her own.

Expanding the Team

Though the connections within the family and the therapy team were growing stronger, we wanted to begin the process of helping the family reconnect with its community. Just as the isolation within the family had driven the symptomatic cycle, the isolation of the family from the community could replicate the same pattern. Sarah was planning a 2-week trip to North Carolina to visit her sister, and we thought that her absence could provide an incentive for Jessie to find a "backup" person on whom she could rely for support while Sarah was away. After brainstorming with Jessie about possible candidates for this role, she decided to invite a close friend, LaTanya, to the next session. LaTanya turned out to be an ideal choice. Younger than Jessie, she represented a bridge between Jamal's generation and Jessie's generation. LaTanya's mother was also a friend of Sarah, which provided a link to Sarah. LaTanya began to attend sessions regularly, and over the next few months, we worked to strengthen the connections among Sarah, Jessie, LaTanya, and Jamal.

Challenging Grandmother's Isolation

The next impasse occurred at a session 16 months after Jamal's discharge. Jessie did not attend the session, claiming illness. Sarah attended with Jamal and LaTanya. Jamal had grown remarkably in the past months. He was attending school regularly, played basketball with his friends, and even held a part-time job. In this session, Jamal began to address directly some of his concerns with Sarah.

JAMAL: Grandma, can I tell you something?

SARAH: Of course, Jamal, I'm listening.

JAMAL: Well, I wish you and my mom wouldn't fight so much.

SARAH: Yes, that would be nice.

JAMAL: Yeah, and I wish you wouldn't yell. Couldn't the two of you just talk it out?

SARAH: Yes, that would be a better way.

JAMAL: 'Cause it really upsets me when you yell.

SARAH: Well, that would be a better way. (*pause*) Or, better yet, I can leave the house when the two of you come over. I don't have to be there. I can just let the two of you run me out of my own house.

Again, the threat of abandonment loomed. We resisted the pull to challenge Sarah, recognizing that confronting her could risk pushing her farther away. Instead, we decided to encourage Sarah to talk openly about her concerns. We decided to trust in the principle of isomorphism: that if we listened to Sarah, then Sarah might be able to listen to Jamal.

Not surprisingly, Sarah launched into a diatribe about Jessie. She complained that Jessie would come to visit on weekends and then not help out around the house. Sarah was angry because she felt used, but she was also afraid. "If she can't help me now when I can help myself," Sarah cried, "how can I expect her to help me when I'm older and I really need it?"

Here was Sarah's isolation. She was afraid that she would be abandoned when she was too old and dependent to do anything about it. She was afraid that she couldn't count on Jessie. Nevertheless, like many people who are afraid of their own dependency, Sarah reinforced her own isolation by threatening to cut off her relationship with Jessie when she felt frustrated and anxious. She never reached out to others, never asked for help, and even refused to be on the receiving end when someone offered help. We decided that listening to Sarah ventilate her frustrations would not be enough. We needed to challenge her to reach out when she felt alone and frustrated.

SIMMS: Sarah, I'm hearing what you're saying, but there's something I don't understand.

SARAH: What don't you understand?

SIMMS: I don't understand why you don't reach out to the people who care about you when you are feeling bad.

SARAH: But I do, I do.

SIMMS: No, you don't. You've never asked me for anything. You've never asked Dr. M for anything.

MICUCCI: That's right.

SIMMS: You've never asked LaTanya for anything, has she, LaTanya?

LATANYA: Nope.

SARAH: Oh, yes I have. I ask when I really need something.

SIMMS: Sarah, you don't ask us to help you. And we want to. We want to be there for you.

SARAH: I know, I know.

SIMMS: But you don't do it. When we asked you to be part of the team to help Jamal, you came through for us, didn't you?

SARAH: Yes, I did, and I'm so happy Jamal is doing so well.

SIMMS: But you don't lean on us when you feel bad.

SARAH: But I'm OK. We're here for Jamal. This is for Jamal, not for me.

SIMMS: Sarah, this is for everyone. We're all in this together. You and me and Jessie, and Dr. M, and Jamal, and now LaTanya. We're a team.

SARAH: Yes, that's right, we're a team.

SIMMS: And I'm interested in you for you. Not just as Jamal's grandmother. Not just as Jessie's mother. But as a person. Someone I care about just for who she is.

SARAH: (*a bit sheepishly*) Oh, I know that.

SIMMS: But I never hear from you! You never call me with news. You never tell me when something important has happened to *you*. I want to know. I want to know how you liked your trip. I want to know about the good movie you saw last weekend. I want to know what the doctor told you about your ulcer. I want to be part of your life.

SARAH: You are, you and you (*pointing to Micucci*) are very important parts of my life.

SIMMS: But I don't feel it. Because you never lean on me, and you let me get only so close.

SARAH: It's not you. It's just the way I am.

SIMMS: But that's the problem, Sarah. It's the way you are, not just with me but with everyone. And I worry about you.

SARAH: Don't worry about me.

SIMMS: But I do. I worry about you because you don't let yourself lean on anyone.

SARAH: But I don't need anyone.

SIMMS: Everyone does. And maybe not now, but there will come a time . . .

SARAH: Oh, yes, there will come a time.

SIMMS: So when will you start doing it?

SARAH: But no one will be there when I need them.

SIMMS: How do you know? Have you asked?

SARAH: No, I haven't asked.

SIMMS: Ask LaTanya right now. Ask her right now if you can count on her.

SARAH: (*reluctantly*) LaTanya, can I count on you?

LATANYA: You know you can. You're like a mother to me. I'd do anything for you.

SIMMS: Do you believe her, Sarah?

SARAH: Yes, I do. Thank you, honey. I know you'll be there for me.

SIMMS: So now ask me. Ask me if I'll be there for you.

SARAH: Oh, I know you will.

SIMMS: Well, I will. And so will Dr. M, right? (*I nod.*) We care about you, Sarah.

SARAH: I guess I didn't realize how much.

It was a struggle, but we finally got through to Sarah. We felt confident that she was now connected with us, and from this connection we hoped that she could listen to Jamal.

SIMMS: I know that things are not great between you and Jessie. I know that some of what she does pisses you off. But right now, your grandson is asking you for something. He's asking you to listen to him, and to do something for him. This doesn't really have to do with you and Jessie. This has to do with you and Jamal.

SARAH: OK, I see that now.

SIMMS: So, Jamal, will you tell your grandma again what you started to tell her before?

JAMAL: OK. Grandma, I just wish that you wouldn't yell at my mom. Couldn't you just try to talk it out?

SARAH: OK, Jamal. I'll do it for you. For you, I'll do it. I'll try, no, I'll go one better, I *will* do it. I will stop myself from yelling at your mom and talk things over calmly with her. This I will do for you. I promise.

To reinforce this theme, following the session we contacted Jessie and suggested that she give a surprise birthday party for Sarah at the next session, thereby giving Jessie an opportunity to provide the nurturance for which Sarah longed. The entire inpatient team was invited to the party, and Jamal was given the job to take pictures.

Therapy Ends

In future sessions, we kept playing the same themes: that we were a team that could depend on one another, that together we could handle crises, that relationships were important, and that relationships meant asking for help and giving it when it was needed. We felt that this family had successfully developed new relationships with each other and with their community. They were relating in a more flexible, relaxed manner, showing more acceptance and understanding of each other. Jamal was doing well on the low dose of antipsychotic medication that he had started to take during his last hospitalization. He was attending school and showed no psychotic symptoms.

We continued to meet monthly with the family, but there were no more crises. The complaints revolved around Jamal's minor limit testing, and we encouraged Jessie's newfound ability to stand firm on consequences. We noted that Jamal challenged his mother in typical adolescent style, but always respectfully. In one memorable session, 26 months after Jamal's discharge, Sarah voiced her unqualified support for Jessie: "I agree with her completely. He's still a boy, and he must listen to his mother. When he's older, he can do what he wants, but now, Jessie is the mother and he is the son. I agree with her 100%."

Our team persevered with this family for several months, helping them weather crises and disentangle from the symptomatic cycle whenever it reemerged. The key to our work was countering the isolation that characterizes psychotic systems by building connections with the family, encouraging family members to remain connected with each other, and strengthening ties to resources in their community.

SUMMARY

Patience and persistence are the keys to working with psychotic adolescents and their families. As this case illustrates, the therapist must be alert to signs that the symptomatic cycle is reemerging and act quickly to prevent regression or symptom relapse. Important principles to keep in mind are the following:

- Focus on improving the adolescent's functioning rather than simply removing symptoms.
- Do not imply that family dynamics caused the psychosis. Focus on altering family patterns, with the goal of helping the psychotic youngster to function better and avoid relapse.
- Improve family members' capacity to cope with the psychosis by strengthening relationships with each other and with members of their community.
- Coach the family on handling crises on their own rather than immediately turning the psychotic adolescent over to professionals.
- Develop relationships with each member of the family. See them as individuals, not simply as relatives of the psychotic person. Help them cope better with stress in their own lives, and encourage them to have a life outside of the family.
- Avoid professional isolation by maintaining connections with colleagues. Ask for consultations when you feel stuck, but keep in mind the pitfall of triangulation (see pp. 46–47).

CHAPTER 8

UNDERACHIEVEMENT AND OTHER SCHOOL-RELATED PROBLEMS

The parents of 13-year-old Todd Drucker were distraught because they had recently received notice that Todd was failing three courses. Todd had assured them that he was doing well, despite the fact that they never observed him doing any homework. When they approached Todd to talk about the failure notice, Todd protested that the teachers were being "unfair." He insisted that he was doing his work, and that he did not deserve the failure notice. He also assured his parents that he had improved, and that his most recent test grades in all three courses were A's. Mr. and Mrs. Drucker were not convinced. They phoned the teachers and heard a different story. Not only was Todd getting failing grades on tests and quizzes, but he was also not turning in assignments, and he appeared uninterested in class.

⟫⟪

The parents of 15-year-old Mike Cohen were getting almost daily phone calls from school complaining about Mike's disruptive behavior and poor academic performance. When Mr. and Mrs. Cohen tried to talk with Mike about the school's concerns, within a few minutes they'd be shouting at one another. The argument would escalate, and Mike would storm out of the house, only to return hours later after his exhausted parents had gone to bed.

———◆•◆———

It was only the fourth week of the school year and Dave Coletti, age 13, had been suspended for the second time because he had been fighting on school grounds. It was Dave's father who contacted me and requested "help for our family." Dave was in danger of being placed in a special school program for disruptive students, and his father believed that "it would kill Dave if he had to go to that program."

Both parents, Dave, and Dave's quiet, studious younger brother attended the first session. Mr. Coletti, a sincere, gentle man, opened the session by recounting a long list of school problems starting in the third grade. Dave interjected at several points to clarify details of time, place, or sequence. Mrs. Coletti remained silent, but her expression betrayed her frustration.

After listening to the father for a while, I invited the mother to comment. She burst out, "I've had it! This kid doesn't respect anyone— least of all me. He's headed to reform school, and there's nothing I can do about it."

Mr. Coletti jumped in. "Well, honey, that's why we're here. We're here to find out what we are doing that's making Dave act this way." Mrs. Coletti sighed and looked away, defeated.

It seemed likely that this scene had played out before: The father, the reasonable, supportive parent, wanting to help his son so much that he was willing to accept the blame for the boy's actions, and the mother, the tired, frustrated parent who was reluctantly cast in the role of reminding father how out of control Dave was.

I learned that the dynamics were even more complicated when I contacted the school. The school counselor "confided" in me that she believed that Mrs. Coletti was "the problem." She thought "something was up" with the mother, and that Dave was acting out at school because he was displacing onto teachers and other students his aggression against his mother. At school conferences, just as in our family session, Mrs. Coletti remained silent, allowed the father to do the talking, and, when she did speak, expressed herself in a way that seemed critical of the school. The father, the school counselor believed, was the more reasonable parent, since he was able to be calm at the school conferences and agreed with the school that Dave's fighting was a reflection of "underlying issues."

———◆•◆———

Many families come to therapy with a school problem as the presenting complaint. Usually, the concern is the child's "underachievement" (i.e., the youngster's academic performance is falling short of his or her capabilities). Behavioral problems, such as truancy or noncompliance with school rules, might or might not accompany underachievement.

Harry Aponte (1976a) was one of the first family therapists to recognize that effective family therapy must also include work with the larger system or *ecosystem* of which the family is a subsystem. For school-related problems, Aponte advocated working with the family and school together rather than with the family alone. Evan Imber-Black (1991) has also extended traditional family therapy concepts to the larger system or *macrosystem*. She makes two observations that are particularly relevant to the relationship between the family and the school:

1. Neither system (i.e., family or school) need be inherently dysfunctional in order for problems to arise in their interaction. This point extends to larger systems the principle that relationships within the family may be dysfunctional even in the absence of individual psychopathology.

2. Patterns of relationship between the family and larger systems may replicate existing patterns within the family. This is known as *isomorphism*. For example, in a case reported by Power and Bartholomew (1985), detouring of conflict between the parents through the symptomatic child was isomorphic to the pattern of detouring conflict between the parents and the school through the child.

I believe that academic underachievement is usually the result of multiple factors that interact with one another. Rather than attempting to isolate a single "cause" of the school problem, I recommend that the therapist evaluate the relative importance of all of the following common contributors to academic difficulties in order to arrive at the appropriate intervention strategy.

FACTORS CONTRIBUTING TO ADOLESCENT UNDERACHIEVEMENT

Why do students fail to meet academic expectations? Some of the more common reasons are discussed here and summarized in Table 8.1.

TABLE 8.1. Factors Contributing to School-Related Problems

- Learning disability
- Attention-deficit/hyperactivity disorder (ADHD)
- Motivational factors
- The school environment
- Peer relationships
- Problematic family relationships
    Passive–aggressive underachievement
    Autonomy struggles
    Overprotectiveness
- Problematic relationship between the family and school
    Family disqualifies the school
    School disqualifies the family
    Family and school disqualify the student

Learning Disability

Learning disability may be broadly defined as failure to master academic skills despite adequate intellectual ability (Chalfant, 1989). In most cases, learning disability will be identified during the early years at school, though in some cases it will not be detected until adolescence (Kline, 1972). Adolescents with undiagnosed learning disability often compensate for their deficits during the early school years but falter when work demands increase. Because of their previous success at school, these adolescents are frequently not considered learning disabled but are rather viewed as inadequately motivated—which they might also be, since learning disabled students are at higher risk for a variety of other problems at school (Brier, 1989; Cohen, 1985; Cook, 1979).

Learning disability can accompany any of the other problems discussed in this chapter. Since learning disability in adolescence is often misdiagnosed but can have substantial importance for academic planning, the therapist should consider consulting with a qualified psychologist to determine if a complete psychoeducational evaluation is indicated.

Attention-Deficit/Hyperactivity Disorder

Attention-deficit/hyperactivity disorder (ADHD) is a syndrome of presumed but unknown neurological etiology that affects the capacity to direct and sustain attention to tasks (Pennington, 1991). In some cases, learning disability may also be present. In many cases, the child will also exhibit problematic behavior associated with the impulsivity and hyperactivity that are part of this syndrome (Wender, 1995). Follow-up studies of adolescents with ADHD have shown that they are at higher risk for antisocial behavior and other forms of marginal adjustment in adulthood (Gittelman, Mannuzza, Shenker, & Bonagura, 1985; Mannuzza & Gittelman, 1984; Mannuzza, Klein, Bonagura, & Malloy, 1991).

Three subtypes of ADHD are identified in the fourth edition of the *Diagnostic and Statistical Manual of Mental Disorders* (DSM-IV; American Psychiatric Association, 1994): the predominantly inattentive type, the predominantly impulsive type, and the combined type. Although most adolescents with ADHD will exhibit signs of impulsivity and hyperactivity, it is important to note the possibility that an adolescent might have an attentional problem even though signs of hyperactivity are absent. This subtype of ADHD might be mistaken for depression and can be differentiated from it by the absence of other symptoms characteristic of a depressive syndrome and the presence of attentional deficits on psychological testing.

In many cases, treatment with stimulant medication such as methylphenidate (Ritalin) can improve the student's attention span, though it is important to evaluate the potential for abuse of the medication. Antidepressants are sometimes prescribed as an alternative (Faigel, Sznajderman, Tishby, & Turel, 1995). Cognitive-behavioral methods to train youngsters to modulate their impulsivity have also been effective (Kendall, 1991) as well as psychoeducational interventions (Barkley, Guevremont, Anastopoulos, & Fletcher, 1992).

The procedure for diagnosing ADHD includes psychological testing, behavioral ratings of the student by parents and teachers, and, in some cases, direct observation (Pennington, 1991). Even with comprehensive testing, ADHD can be difficult to detect, particularly when it occurs comorbidly with other disorders, or when it is embedded in a context of other social or interpersonal problems. When the diagnosis is uncertain, a trial on medication may be undertaken, though some experts caution against this practice, pointing out that stimulants will often improve performance even in cases where true ADHD is not present.

Motivational Factors

Although motivation and academic performance typically decline when kids enter high school (Elmen, 1991), students who are more oriented toward intrinsic goals and more confident in their abilities are more likely to demonstrate persistence and eventual success on academic tasks (Ames & Archer, 1988; Ginsburg & Bronstein, 1993).

Academically successful students tend to attribute their success to internal factors ("I studied hard"), while underachieving students are more likely to attribute their success to external factors ("The test was easy"; Carr, Borkowski, & Maxwell, 1991). Some students, especially girls, believe that their achievement is not under their control and so feel helpless in response to failure (Dweck & Licht, 1980). Underachieving students may not benefit from feedback regarding their academic performance because they don't usually see a connection between success and anything over which they have control, such as effort or study strategies.

Many students have never learned how to study, lack basic academic skills, and spend insufficient time on their studies (Mullis et al., 1994). In particular, those adolescents who are above average in intelligence may have been able to succeed in elementary school without exerting much effort. When they get to junior high school, where more independent work is required, their grades plummet. The shock of encountering failure for the first time can begin a downward spiral of underachievement beginning in middle school and continuing into high school.

It is important to differentiate low motivation in school from low motivation in general. Students who are not academically oriented might nevertheless be highly motivated in another area, such as sports or the arts. Students who appear unmotivated in general (what Erikson, 1968, might consider an example of "identity diffusion") are more likely to experience other individual and interpersonal problems in addition to academic difficulties.

The School Environment

After reviewing the literature, Jacquelynne Eccles and her colleagues (1993) concluded that the typical middle school is often unsuited to the needs of the developing adolescent. Compared to elementary school teachers, middle school teachers are less likely to trust their students and more likely to emphasize control and discipline in the classroom. They are also likely to be perceived by their students as less friendly, less supportive, and less caring than elementary school teachers. Eccles et al. argued that a poor fit between the adolescent's needs and the school environment is a major factor contributing to academic underachievement.

Just as a family can be termed "dysfunctional," a school can be dysfunctional because of conflicts within the faculty or between the faculty and the administration (Fisher, 1986). Teachers who feel overworked or unappreciated might displace some of their frustration onto students, who, in turn, might personalize the teacher's attitude toward them and respond in ways that only serve to intensify the teacher's frustration.

One obviously bright girl told me that she deliberately failed a course because she "hated" the teacher and refused to do any work "for her." For this girl and many other adolescents, achievement is strongly influenced by the quality of their relationships with teachers. Erratic performance at school, with a wide range of grades and no consistency in patterns of high and low grades, often suggests that the personal relationship with a teacher is an important factor in an adolescent's academic performance.

Peer Relationships

Students who associate with high achievers arc likely to value high achievement, while students whose friends are underachievers are likely to underachieve as well (Epstein, 1983). Undermining of academic competence by peers is particularly intense for African American students, whose peers might accuse them of "acting white" when they get high grades (Fordham & Ogbu, 1986).

Students who are strongly oriented toward peers tend to perform more poorly in school, but the strength of an adolescent's peer orientation depends on the quality of his or her relationship with parents (Fulgini & Eccles, 1993). According to these authors, adolescents who are most strongly oriented toward peers are those who come from authoritarian homes in which they are afforded few opportunities for decision making. Other studies have shown that authoritative parenting (warm but firm) is associated with school success (Steinberg et al., 1992), while strict and punitive parenting is associated with diminished school achievement (DeBaryshe, Patterson, & Capaldi, 1993).[1]

Another, less obvious feature of the adolescent peer context is the socialization pressures experienced by girls and boys in the school. Pipher (1994) has called attention to the prevalence of sexual harassment of girls by boys in middle school, a practice that can poison girls' entire school experience. Boys are also subject to gender-specific socialization pressures at school, such as intimidation and violence among the male peer group (Denborough, 1996). Boys who deviate from culturally prescribed standards of masculinity as represented in the peer culture face ostracism or victimization by other boys, male coaches, and male teachers (McLean, 1996). The myth that boys must be independent has led to the emotional abandonment of boys by parents, especially mothers, intensifying boys' alienation from the family and amplifying the dynamics of the male peer culture (Silverstein & Rashbaum, 1994).

Problems in the Relationship between the Adolescent and the Family

Passive–Aggressive Underachievement

Weiner (1971) identified a family pattern that can be associated with underachievement in adolescence. This pattern, which he terms "passive–aggressive underachievement" includes (1) underlying hostility toward parents that cannot be directly expressed, (2) concerns about rivalry with parents and siblings leading to intensified fears of failure, and (3) a preference for passive–aggressive means of coping with difficult situations.

This pattern may be particularly salient in families where achievement is highly valued. In these families, the adolescent often gets a clear message of conditional acceptance, whereby one's worth is measured by how much one achieves in the academic arena. These adolescents find it difficult to differentiate parental disappointment about their achievement from global disapproval by the parents.

Autonomy Struggles

School performance can become the battleground on which autonomy struggles between the adolescent and parents are fought. The more parents try to force the child to conform to school expectations, the more the youngster stands his ground or rebels, perhaps recruiting deviant peers into a coalition to strengthen his position in the family struggle. The parents might respond to this move by attempting to recruit a therapist into a coalition to help them regain their power over the adolescent, thus intensifying the struggle, unless the therapist recognizes the systemic dynamics.

Overprotectiveness

Many parents unwittingly reinforce irresponsibility on the part of the adolescent by working too hard to ensure the student's success at school. Typically, these are families in which achievement is highly valued and parents are overidentified with the child's academic performance. Whenever the child is in danger of failing, the parents go into overdrive to prevent the failure. While, at times, this parental response might be helpful in that ultimate failure is averted, in the long run this pattern discourages the adolescent from assuming responsibility for his or her own academic performance.

Advising parents to "back off" and allow the student to take more responsibility in the academic arena is often not enough. The simple behavioral act of backing off, if not correlated with a shift in parental attitudes and beliefs about the importance of achievement and the implications of failure, can simply move the battle from the overt to the covert. The therapist needs to work on helping the parents emotionally differentiate themselves from the adolescent in order for the backing off to be more than a simple move in a game for more control.

Problems Involving the Adolescent, the Family, and the School

At times, the relationship among the adolescent, the family, and the school contributes to the academic problem. Several patterns are common, and more than one may be present. These patterns involve the dynamic that has been termed "disqualification" (Madanes, 1981), that is, the undermining of one member of a system by another. With respect to the adolescent-family-school system, three patterns of disqualification may be observed: (1) Family disqualifies the school, (2) school disqualifies the family, (3) family and school disqualify the student.

Family Disqualifies the School

Once, many will lament, authority was respected. Parents supported teachers, and vice versa, and the student had no quarter for appeal. It was assumed that the student and even the parents should defer to the judgment of the teacher as the expert on the student's educational needs. In our (so-called) enlightened times, such naive submission to authority and expertise is no longer commonplace. In the 1960s, we were paradoxically admonished to "question authority," and we have been dutifully following this dictum ever since. Needless to say, children often follow this rule in dealing with parents and other authority figures. What is not so obvious to many parents, however, is that they themselves might follow this practice in their relationship with other authority figures (e.g., teachers) in their child's life.

One family presented with a 14-year-old boy who was receiving poor grades in his social studies class and was quick to point out that the teacher was widely regarded by students as "a fag." This label was applied because the teacher apparently behaved at times in an effeminate manner. The parents passionately denounced the rumored sexual practices of the teacher, of which there was no hard evidence, and beamed proudly at their son when he reassured them that he "hated fags" and would poke out the teacher's eye with a pencil if he even so much as touched him on the shoulder. The student was in danger of failing the class, not only because he was not completing assignments, but also because he was a ringleader in the class's disruptive behavior.

These parents saw no inconsistency in their admonitions to their son to "just do as he was told" so he could pass the course, while at the same time joining him in disparaging the teacher. In fact, for the parents, there may have been no inconsistency. As adults, they have achieved a more sophisticated level of cognitive awareness that allowed them to differentiate the teacher's authority qua teacher from his alleged homosexual behavior. Perhaps the parents simply intended to communicate to their son that they understood his contempt for the teacher's effeminate mannerisms, while nevertheless insisting that these feelings were not excuses for poor performance in the classroom. A 14-year-old, however, could not be expected to appreciate this distinction, given his minimal experience with formal operational thinking. The boy heard his parents' support for his disapproval of the teacher's presumed sexual practices as vindication for his refusal to participate in class.

Other parents might not be so overt in their criticism of a teacher's competence, but communicate their disapproval of the teacher's methods indirectly. For example, the parents might not criticize the teacher openly in the adolescent's presence, but repeatedly complain to the school administration about the teacher. Or the parents might not challenge the youngster when she argues that she is failing in school because the teacher does not "like" her, thereby giving tacit approval to the idea that the student is not responsible for her own academic success or failure. While, indeed, it is possible that a teacher is treating a particular student unfairly, this issue needs to be dealt with in a way that does not undermine the authority of the teacher or school in the eyes of the adolescent.

Overinvolvement of the parents in the student's academic projects can also be construed by the adolescent as lack of support for the school. One parent whose son had a long history of underachievement despite above-average intellectual abilities would "help" her son with his homework by agreeing to do half of it for him if he would agree to do the other half. She would plead with the school to give her son extensions on assignments that he had left to the last minute. Routinely, on the eve of the renegotiated due date, she would sit with her son at the word processor, liberally "editing" what he dictated to her to help the paper "flow better." Not only did this practice undermine the school's expectation that the boy accept responsibility for his own assignments, but it also gave the message to the boy that he was incapable of doing his work without his mother's help.

School Disqualifies the Family

In recent years, the heightened awareness of child abuse has led to the practice of requiring professionals who work with young people to report parents to the authorities if there is evidence that the child has been abused by the parents. While this practice certainly has its merits, one of its disadvantages is the possibility that it might undermine the parents in the eyes of the youngster.

In one case, a teacher had become so overly involved in a student's personal life that she would routinely allow the girl to visit her on weekends, go on trips with her, and join her for meals. The well-intentioned teacher felt genuine compassion for the child, who lived in an impoverished household where her needs and those of her seven siblings were often neglected. The teacher, believing that the student's academic success depended on her being safe and appropriately nourished, attempted to compensate for the neglect in her family. Unfortunately, the more the girl confided in the teacher about the conditions at home, the more disrespectful the child became to her own parents, to the point that whenever they tried to discipline her, she threatened to run to the teacher's house and report them for abusing her.

In a less dramatic case, at a school conference attended by the teacher, principal, school counselor, parents, and the therapist, it was evident that the school staff viewed the poor, uneducated, immigrant parents as incompetent. Though the parents, perhaps naively, trusted the school's judgment regarding what would be best for their son, the message came across that the school did not respect their ideas about their son's education.

Schools might also disqualify families by failing to keep them informed about the student's progress. In some cases, particularly with older adolescents, it might be appropriate for the school to deal directly with the student rather than involve the parents. However, if the student is in serious academic trouble, some communication with the parents is warranted. By failing to contact the family, the school maintains a rigid boundary between itself and the parents that can be exploited by the adolescent, who can "split" the two systems to his own advantage.

More subtly, a school can disqualify parents by disregarding their priorities for their own children. One school counselor confided in me that she believed that a parent's expectations of one of her students exceeded the student's ability. She did not consider the student to be "college material," though the parents were encouraging her to pursue an academic track. The counselor believed that the student would fare better in a track that prepared her for a technical trade, and in private conversations with the student she discouraged her from attending college. During these meetings, it was not uncommon for the girl to complain to the counselor about the "pressure" her family was putting on her, while the counselor listened supportively. When I suggested to the counselor that she invite the parents to a meeting at school to discuss the girl's academic plans, the counselor dismissed this idea: "You don't know these parents. There's no reasoning with them. They'll never agree to let Janie attend technical school." Clearly, the battle lines were drawn and the possibilities for dialogue were remote.

Perhaps the most common way that families feel disqualified by the school is when the school refers the family to therapy, with the implication that the student's problems at school are a result of family problems. These families come to therapy under duress and react defensively whenever the therapist attempts to explore family dynamics. These cases require special handling by the therapist and will be discussed later in this chapter.

Family and School Disqualify the Student

Attempting to present a unified front, the parents and school sometimes fail to acknowledge the student's responsibility for setting his own academic goals. While this practice might be defensible for younger children, it is inappropriate for adolescents, who should be encouraged to assume more autonomy in setting goals. If the parents and school act as if the student is incompetent to take responsibility for his academic career, they may create a "self-fulfilling prophecy" (Rosenthal & Jacobson, 1968).

School conferences sometimes involve the parents and exclude the adolescent. While this practice communicates to the student that the adults in her life are working together on her behalf, excluding her can also give the message that the adults will assume responsibility and she need not. It is small wonder that many students in this position fail to apply themselves to their schoolwork. Having been giving the message that their opinions regarding their education are not important, they comply by abdicating responsibility for their academic career. Unfortunately, a symptomatic cycle quickly arises, whereby the adolescent fails to perform in school, which elicits only more concern from the parents and school, who redouble their efforts to close ranks to "help" the student.

Often, the parents and school have a benevolent attitude toward the student, who is viewed as a "nice kid," though incompetent to meet the expectations of the school. The parents and teachers see themselves as working well together to help the student, and a therapist might be enlisted to support these efforts. In these situations, the therapist's adopting a competency-oriented approach should help the parents and teachers see the student's unrecognized strengths and find opportunities for the student to take more responsibility for his own academic performance (Fishman, 1993).

Timmy was almost 18 and in his senior year in a Catholic boys' high school. A thin, pimply youth with wispy blonde hair, he shuffled into the first session with eyes downcast and his windbreaker zipped to the collar, flanked by both of his parents. As is typical in my first sessions with adolescents, I addressed Timmy first, but his mother immediately launched into the concerns she had about Timmy because he was doing poorly in school and was in danger of not graduating. His father nodded in assent, while Timmy remained mute, staring at his hands that lay clenched in his lap.

Quickly reading the family structure as one where mother was in charge of representing Timmy's interests to the world on his behalf, I decided to join with this family by supporting this structure for the present. As a side benefit of this decision, I learned much about Timmy's academic career. He had always been a "quiet, good boy," who was viewed by parents and teachers alike as not particularly academically talented. His mother beamed proudly as she related the efforts Timmy had put forth to succeed in previous school years, though it was clear that these efforts were very much amplified by her own participation. Whenever Timmy had a problem with a teacher, his mother was there to intercede on his behalf. Timmy was shy, his mother pointed out, and tears welled in her eyes as she described the paroxysms of anxiety Timmy experienced when he so much as had to call for a pizza to be delivered. Eager to spare Timmy the anguish that would debilitate him for days, his mother would simply take over. Whenever a phone call needed to be made, his mother would be there, whenever a problem arose with anyone at school, his mother would intercede.

After listening to this story for several minutes, I decided to risk challenging the structure by asking Timmy if he felt that his mother's efforts had been truly helpful to him. He nodded his head in reply, and again his mother jumped in, simply demonstrating *in vivo* the pattern she had just been describing. This time, she added that the school "liked Timmy a lot" and always "went the extra mile" to help him. She and the school administration hand picked Timmy's classes every year, careful to select teachers who would understand his problem and not expect too much of him in the classroom.

Unfortunately, this year, Timmy had to take a required mathematics course in order to graduate, and there was only one section of the course available. This section was taught by a teacher who had a reputation for being one of the toughest in the school. When Timmy did not complete an assignment, rather than phoning his mother as previous teachers had done, the teacher challenged Timmy directly. He would call on Timmy in class and rather than accept Timmy's silence as an appropriate reply, would remind him that his grade would be diminished by poor class participation. Though he was stern and structured, the teacher was nevertheless dedicated to his students and made himself available every day after school for extra help. He even reached out to Timmy by extending a personal invitation to help him prepare for the next exam.

Unaccustomed to dealing with teachers directly, Timmy rebuffed the teacher's overtures, did not appear for the extra help, and failed the examination. When his mother contacted the teacher to explain "Timmy's situation" the teacher replied that he would be happy to help Timmy if he saw evidence that Timmy was willing to help himself. To prove his support, he guaranteed that he would give Timmy a passing grade in the course as long as he came for extra help three times per week for the next 3 weeks. Timmy, however, remained intransigent. He never appeared after school, failed the exam, and seemed unconcerned and unsurprised when he received an "F" for the marking period.

Until then, the school and his parents had defined Timmy as incompetent and, in the guise of supporting him, had actually infantilized him to the point that he was essentially incapacitated. Meanwhile, his fears, as they are wont to do, intensified through avoidance. The more Timmy avoided facing other people, the more fearful he became of doing so. At the same time, taking a "hard line" with Timmy would not be fruitful, since it was clear that he would collapse under even the slightest pressure or adopt a rigid posture, which his family interpreted not as stubbornness, but as being frozen with fear.

In cases like this one, an approach that gradually expands the student's degree of responsibility is indicated. Though it was clear that Timmy would not (or could not) deal directly with the math teacher on his own, it was also clear that some steps in this direction were imperative. His mother's role was redefined as supportive rather than intercessory. Every small movement Timmy made toward autonomy was emphasized and encouraged, and framed as evidence that he "was ready" to start assuming more responsibility for himself. At first, even microscopic moves in the direction of independence were magnified, such as Timmy "thinking about" calling for a pizza or being willing to unzip his windbreaker during a therapy session.

While accepting Timmy's fears, I consistently addressed Timmy as a 17-year-old, inquiring about his interests and plans for the future. I steadfastly refused to accept his incompetence and framed his difficulties as resulting from a long imprisonment by "fears" that had oppressed him as well as the rest of the family. By "externalizing the problem" in this way (White & Epston, 1990), Timmy could be separated from the problem, which could be seen as something outside of him rather than part of him. I encouraged him to "starve the fears" by refusing to "feed them" through his avoidance. In this way, the math teacher ceased to be the enemy, but rather became another potential ally against the fears, which were Timmy's real nemesis.

Implicit in this case, though not in the foreground, is another pattern that might emerge when parents and the school collude to disqualify the student. Sometimes the parents and school are in intense conflict over what is best for the student. Each disqualifies the other, but they remain engaged in an attempt to win the struggle through one-upmanship. Whatever the content of the conflict, the process remains the same: The student's failure and the family-school conflict elicit one another. Rather than working collaboratively to help the student succeed, the family and school battle with one another over whose approach is right. To the extent that the parents and school are distracted by their conflict with one another, they are less available to support the student. Consequently, the student is more likely to fail, which only elicits more parent–school conflict in an unending cycle— though the cycle often does end with the student being removed from the school, only to repeat itself in the next school the student attends.

Kelli Chase was about to enter her third school since starting ninth grade 2 years earlier. In her first school, her father related, she was in danger of failing English and Math because the teachers at the school were "incompetent." Kelli's parents decided to remove her from the public school and place her in an exclusive private school that had a reputation for outstanding teachers.

During the admission process, Mr. Chase claimed, they were promised by the headmistress that Kelli would be permitted to take electives in Drama and Music, two areas in which Kelli admittedly excelled. Apparently, it was not clear to her parents that these electives were open only to students who had already completed a number of required English and Math courses.

Consequently, Kelli would be ineligible for the Drama and Music electives until the next school year. To compound the problem, the parents averred, they were unable to convince the headmistress to place Kelli in a creative writing class, one that was open only to students who had completed a course in Basic Writing, which Kelli had not.

Kelli was doing poorly in her English class, at least partially because she was not completing the assignments, which her parents described as "busywork" that did not elicit Kelli's "creativity." Phone calls to the headmistress had increased in frequency, which only served to intensify the conflict between the two systems. To make matters worse, the family had come to me for "documentation" that Kelli had special learning needs that necessitated her being placed in the Creative Writing class, though the only evidence that could be obtained that Kelli had such special needs was in the eyes of her parents.

Interestingly, I was spared from having to provide the requested documentation when the school, probably out of fatigue, decided to relent and moved Kelli into the Creative Writing class. Not unexpectedly, her performance continued to be marginal. Now, however, Mr. and Mrs. Chase were furious at the school for having moved Kelli into the Creative Writing class "too late," so that she was behind the other students and unable to keep up. They were already looking for another school for Kelli. When Kelli was accepted into a high school that emphasized the performing arts, the family decided that their problem was solved, thanked me for my help (what help?), and vanished into the throng of satisfied but unchanged therapy visitors.

In cases like Timmy's and Kelli's, the student's needs dissolve into the agendas of the adults in the student's lives. In Timmy's case, the benevolence of parents and school had deprived him of the opportunity to learn how to negotiate on his own behalf. In Kelli's case, academic weaknesses that set her up for failure were submerged in the torrent of conflict between the family and the school. Now, I discuss strategies for intervening in conflicts involving the family and the school, highlighting common pitfalls in this work and how they can be avoided.

STRATEGIES FOR INTERVENTION

The first step in developing an appropriate intervention strategy is to *assess whether a learning disability or ADHD is contributing to the underachievement.* As I have already pointed out, many adolescents who present with underachievement have one or both of these disorders.

Since the presence of a learning disability or ADHD can have a major influence on academic performance, it is important to evaluate whether these disorders are present. In some cases, the student might already carry one of these diagnoses, in which case the therapist should determine whether the school is providing the necessary remedial education. In other cases, the learning disability or ADHD has not been diagnosed before, and it will be important to refer the student for a comprehensive psychoeducational evaluation. As I pointed out earlier, the presence of learning disability or ADHD does not mean that systemic dynamics do not also contribute to the adolescent's under-achievement. However, neglecting to consider the possibility of learn-ing disability or ADHD can create unnecessary frustration and vitiate other interventions.

The second step is to *assess the relationship patterns among the adolescent, the family, and the school* so as to identify the appropriate points of intervention and the level of involvement the therapist should assume with each system. I shall describe three strategies that represent different degrees of involvement by the therapist in the family–school macrosystem. Each of these strategies has advantages and pitfalls. In *coaching*, the therapist refrains from direct contact with the school and directs all interventions through the adolescent or family. In *mediation*, the therapist has contact with both the family and the school but does not attempt to intervene directly in the relationship between the two systems. In *direct intervention*, the therapist convenes the family and school personnel together in order to intervene directly to change the problematic relationship patterns between the two systems. These strategies are depicted in Figure 8.1.

In general, it is wise to select the least intrusive method of intervention that is appropriate to the problem at hand; that is, the therapist should first evaluate whether the problem can be resolved from the position of coaching and consider moving to a more intensive level of involvement only if coaching has not been effective.

Coaching

Coaching the Adolescent

The therapist can coach the student in ways of handling problems at school more effectively. If the parents are involved, they remain in a supportive role, allowing the youngster to take the lead in solving the problem. The following case illustrates this approach.

Beth, a 17-year-old senior, was struggling in her math class. She was typically a mediocre student in math, but had never before been in danger of failing. To make matters worse, she had been poorly

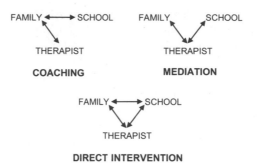

FIGURE 8.1. Three models of intervention for school-related problems.

motivated at the beginning of the school year, hadn't turned in several assignments, and had lost favor with the teacher. Beth had tried on her own to approach the teacher, but she felt the teacher was unresponsive to her. Now, Beth was convinced that she would fail the course because the teacher didn't like her. Beth's parents were prepared to intercede for her, but I believed that it would be more appropriate if Beth handled the problem on her own.

I listened sympathetically as Beth explained in detail her frustration with the class and her anger at her teacher. At first, the two feelings were merged in her experience, but, as we talked, she began to differentiate them. Beth was a bright, intuitive girl, and it did not take her long to recognize that her feelings toward the teacher were fueling her frustration with the subject matter. We then explored several options. She decided that she would write the teacher a note, apologizing for not working at the beginning of the year, and ask if she could meet with him after class to try to convince him that she was now serious about passing the course. I wondered aloud how Beth might feel if the teacher did not respond to her note. Beth replied that she would feel hurt, but that she would try to put her feelings aside and approach the teacher in person a few days later to ask what he thought about her note. As a last resort, if the teacher still seemed unwilling to help, then Beth would ask her school counselor to intercede.

Coaching the adolescent is most appropriate when the school problem is relatively circumscribed and has not expanded to include dysfunctional interactions between the family and school. It is likely to be most suitable for older adolescents who are able to take some distance from the conflict and not personalize the teacher's behavior. This approach is almost essential for adolescents with learning disability or ADHD who are preparing to enter college, and who will need to advocate for themselves in order to receive the appropriate academic supports.

Coaching the Parents

If the adolescent is not motivated to handle the problem independently, or if the problem is so severe that parental involvement is necessary, coaching the parents might be the appropriate strategy. Coaching is a strategy advocated by Mary Eno (1985):

> Parents can be coached to work with schools, that is, to learn how to get the kind of information they need, how to evaluate that information, and how to negotiate with school staff members for specific changes. This therapeutic approach is in line with the guidelines of minimal intervention—the parents are nudged to do as much of the work as possible themselves. (p. 166)

I used the strategy of coaching to help the family of Todd, the 13-year-old boy introduced at the beginning of this chapter. I first considered the possibility of a previously undiagnosed learning disability or ADHD. However, Todd did not fulfill the criteria for ADHD, and his previous academic performance was exemplary. The therapeutic issue appeared to be helping the parents and school close ranks so that Todd would not be able to split them.

I encouraged Mr. and Mrs. Drucker to make contact with Todd's school counselor, who could be a resource to them and a liaison to the faculty. I suggested that the parents discuss with the counselor the possibility of instituting a procedure by which Todd would write down his assignments in a special notebook and at the end of class check them with the teacher for accuracy. Todd would then show his assignment book to his parents every night. They would supervise his completing his homework and sign the assignment book after the work was completed.

The counselor readily agreed with the plan and the teachers welcomed the parents' involvement. Todd balked at being treated "like a little kid," but his parents reminded him that as soon as he could demonstrate that he was capable of monitoring his school performance on his own, they would consider discontinuing the plan. Todd was also told that he would not be permitted to watch television or talk on the telephone until his assignments for the night were completed satisfactorily. If Todd "forgot" to bring his assignment book home, then he would not be allowed to watch television or talk on the telephone at all that night, and he would still need to spend 2 hours in his room studying. Over the next few weeks, the family and school worked out the "glitches" in the plan, and by the end of the marking period, Todd's grades had improved enough that he was passing all of his courses.

Pitfalls of Coaching

When the therapist does not have direct contact with the school, he or she must rely on the family's report as an accurate account of the transactions taking place between the family and school. Reports from a single perspective are always biased to some degree. Family therapists have long recognized that a complete understanding of a relationship can be obtained only by superimposing the perspectives of each participant, a process Bateson (1972) called "double description." By relying strictly on the family's account of its interactions with the school, the therapist runs the risk of accepting the family's biased perceptions of the school. For this reason, coaching is not an appropriate method in cases of intense conflict between the family and school. This pitfall can be minimized by obtaining indirect information from the school, for example, report cards and written evaluations.

While it might seem that relying on the family's account of the interaction with the school will put the family in the most favorable light and cast the school in the role of culprit, it is also possible that the school might be contributing to the problem in ways not apparent to the family. For example, there might be a conflict between the student's teachers about how best to handle the student. The school might be failing to intervene in harassment of the adolescent by peers or by a teacher. If the therapist suspects that one of these situations applies, then more direct involvement with the school (e.g., mediation or direct intervention) might be appropriate. Alternatively, the therapist could coach the parents how to obtain information that could help determine whether an internal dysfunction in the school is contributing to the adolescent's problem.

A second pitfall of coaching derives from the principle that triangulation can occur even when there is no direct contact between parties involved in the triangle. In coaching, the family and school have direct contact, the therapist and family have direct contact, but the therapist avoids direct contact with the school. Families can avoid conflict with the school by citing the therapist as the source of the advice. The school, attempting to respect the alliance between the therapist and the family, might refrain from contacting the therapist, either accepting the family's account as veridical, or, more dangerously, detouring the problem by blaming the therapist rather than dealing directly with the family. If therapists sense that triangulation is occurring, they have several options:

1. The therapist can request a (single) meeting with the family and school to clear up the "miscommunication." In this case, the therapist must be prepared to move to a more intensive level of involvement if it appears difficult to return to the less involved position of coaching.

2. The therapist can confront the parents (tactfully) on their role in the triangulation. Generally, this approach will be effective only with those families that have already demonstrated the capacity to reflect on their relationship patterns.

3. In some cases, the therapist might want to encourage the triangling. This strategy is, of course, fraught with risks. Therapists might choose to pursue this course if it appears that triangling the therapist substitutes for the more destructive pattern of triangling the adolescent. Therapists, presumably, can take care of themselves while in the triangled position, and eventually work toward de-triangling themselves.

Mediation

Mediation represents a step up in the level of involvement between a therapist and the school. In coaching, the therapist avoids direct contact with the school. In mediation, the therapist engages directly with the school in the role of liaison or go-between.

Mediation is similar to the approach advocated by Don-David Lusterman (1985) for "situations in which negative contact between the school and the family has increased pressure on the parents to produce change in the child's school behavior, but has in fact produced more negative behavior, and exacerbated existing problems in the home" (p. 24). Lusterman proposed a five-step process:

1. The family therapist advocates complete disengagement between the family and the school.
2. The therapist contracts with the family and school that, for a period of time, the school will not contact the family if the student has difficulties in school, but rather will contact the therapist who will then work with the school to develop appropriate school-based interventions for the problem.
3. The therapist works with the family on problems not related to school.
4. When the home situation has improved, the therapist gradually

reintroduces contact between the parents and school, adopting
the position of coach for the family.
5. The therapist withdraws when it is clear that family and school
are working together more productively.

My work with the family of Mike Cohen, introduced at the beginning
of this chapter, represents an example of mediation. It appeared that
the parents and school had developed a dysfunctional cycle of interactions: The parents' efforts to solve the school problem were only
increasing the tension at home and making it even less likely that
Mike would change his behavior at school. Mike himself agreed that
he was very upset about the tension in the house, and he wished that
he and his parents could get along better. He claimed that he was
often so upset by the arguments of the night before that he had a
"bad attitude" in class the next day and displaced his frustration onto
the teachers.

I decided that I might be able to disrupt this pattern by inserting
myself between the parents and the school. Adopting Lusterman's
strategy, I contracted with the parents and the school that they would
have no contact with each other for 6 weeks. Instead, the school would
contact me if Mike misbehaved, and I would provide consultation to
the school on how to handle the problem without contacting the
parents.

Meanwhile, I encouraged Mr. and Mrs. Cohen to "back off" and
allow Mike to decide how he would manage his school responsibilities.
I worked with Mike and his parents to draft a contract specifying that
by the end of the 6-week period, Mike would be expected to bring
home passing grades in all of his subjects and not have been suspended
from school for any reason. Any discussion about school would be "off
limits." If Mike needed advice on how to handle a problem at school,
he was to contact me. I would work with the family on other issues,
such as balancing supervision and autonomy for Mike in other areas
of his life, helping Mr. and Mrs. Cohen work more collaboratively as a
team, and encouraging the parents to resume some of the outside
activities that they had been neglecting because they had been so
consumed by Mike's school problems.

Privately, I challenged Mike to prove to his parents that he was
"right all along" in claiming that he didn't need them to monitor his
schoolwork. At the beginning of each session, I spent a few minutes
alone with Mike, checking in with him about his progress and coaching
him on how to handle problems at school. The remainder of the session
was focused on other family issues. Twice a week, I contacted Mike's
school counselor for a report on Mike's behavior and to offer sugges-

tions on how the school might respond when Mike was uncooperative. I met with Mike's teachers and helped them to develop a consistent strategy for working with him.

Gradually, the relationships between Mike and his parents improved. At the end of the 6-week period, Mike had brought up his grades, though he was still failing one subject. I decided to use this as an opportunity to reinvolve the parents with the school.

I suggested that the Cohens contact Mike's teacher to find out why he was failing the course. After gathering this information, we would discuss how Mr. and Mrs. Cohen could help Mike if he was interested in passing the course. I emphasized, however, that whether Mike passed or failed the course was his responsibility, and that his parents would take neither the credit if he passed nor the blame if he failed. They would not, however, sign permission for him to take a part-time job after school unless he passed all of his subjects. Essentially, I was encouraging the parents to detriangle themselves, following Kerr and Bowen's (1988) advice that rather than telling their child what the child should do, parents should simply state clearly what they would do in response to the child's behavior.

When to Use Mediation

In many cases, poor boundaries between the family and school can underlie family–school conflict. Mediation is an appropriate strategy to consider when the parents are either too involved with the school or not involved enough. As Lusterman points out and Mike's case illustrates, by serving as mediator the therapist can reduce the tension and associated reactivity between the parents and school. The therapist can draw a clearer distinction between "home" problems and "school" problems, restoring the former to center stage in the family sessions and moving the adolescent to a more central role in dealing with the latter.

When the family is disengaged from the school, the therapist can decrease the gap by serving as a bridge. Mediation has an advantage over coaching in that the mediating therapist has direct contact with both family and school and is thus able to see the problem from both perspectives rather than relying exclusively on the family's account. From the position of mediator, the therapist can positively reframe the actions of the family and school to each other, thus countering biased perceptions that can contribute to heightened conflict. The therapist can selectively underscore points of agreement between the family and school to build a stronger coalition between them, while ensuring that the student is not scapegoated.

Pitfalls of Mediation

A pitfall of mediation is the possibility that either family or school could cede all authority to the therapist. Either or both systems could refuse to engage in the process of negotiation and instead appeal to the therapist's "expertise," while abdicating responsibility for the consequences of the decisions.

To avoid this pitfall, therapists should clearly negotiate their role with both the family and the school at the outset of the mediation process. Therapists should adopt the position of advocate for "what is best for the student" and use this position as leverage to effect a structural change in the family's relationship to the school. For example, if the parents are protecting the student from appropriate consequences at school, the therapist can support the school's position by blocking messages from the school to the family.

Direct Intervention

Of the models discussed in this chapter, direct intervention requires the greatest involvement of a therapist in the family's relationship with the school. In coaching, the therapist works only with the family. In mediation, the therapist works alternately with the family and the school. But in direct intervention, the therapist works conjointly with the family and school.

Harry Aponte's (1976a) "ecostructural" approach is an example of direct intervention in a conflict between a family and school. Aponte held the initial family session at the school and included in this session the student, parents, and relevant school personnel. The goal was to foster greater collaboration between the family and the school, facilitate conflict resolution, and encourage the development of specific plans to assist the student. Mary Eno (1985), while generally supporting a principle of minimal intervention in order to respect the boundaries between family and school, nevertheless endorsed direct intercession at the "interface" of the family and school in those cases when the "gentle leaning" of coaching was ineffective. Power and Bartholomew (1985) presented a case in which a series of direct interventions with the family and the school promoted a restructuring of a dysfunctional family–school relationship. Charles Fishman (1993) described a very intensive model of intervention called the "enhanced home–school partnership." According to this model, "parents become intimately involved in the child's education" (p. 183). This involvement could include daily communication with the school, or even accompanying the child to school to help the teachers elicit greater compliance from the child.

Advantages of Direct Intervention

Direct intervention has a number of advantages. First, since all the "key players" are together in one place, communication of information is more efficient, and it is easier to negotiate a shared definition of the problem that is acceptable to all. Second, rather than relying on reports of interactions between the family and school, the therapist can observe these interactions directly. Third, the therapist has more leverage to alter these interactional patterns. Finally, as long as both systems have agreed to utilize the therapist as a resource, the therapist can address dysfunctional interactions not only between the systems but also within each system.

Pitfalls of Direct Intervention

Therapists who choose this strategy must be skilled at tracking both content and process in large groups. It is not unusual for a family–school meeting to have a dozen participants, each having a different agenda. Therapists must be comfortable enough with their role in these meetings to allow all issues to be aired while preventing the meeting from degenerating into chaos. It can help if both the family and the school agree at the outset that the therapist will be in charge of the meeting.

   One disadvantage of direct intervention is that the parents might feel intimidated in a large meeting attended by many professionals. Parents express their intimidation in different ways. Some become overly submissive, others passively resistant, still others attack counter-phobically. The therapist should exercise caution in drawing conclusions about family dynamics from the way family members behave at these meetings, because this behavior might not be typical of the way they usually act, but rather a reaction to the unique context of the family–school meeting. Therapists can help parents feel less intimidated by encouraging the parents to speak first, actively soliciting their input, recounting ways in which they have tried to be helpful to the student in the past, and focusing on positive steps they could take to be helpful in the future.

   Another pitfall is that school personnel might feel intimidated and react defensively if they think that the therapist is aligned with the family against them. This reaction is understandable if the therapist has been working with the family for some time and only recently has initiated contact with the school. Therapists can avoid this pitfall by taking pains to join with the school at the outset of the meeting. To prevent family members from feeling betrayed or abandoned if the therapist seems to be more aligned with the school's point of view than they had anticipated, the therapist should explain his or her intentions to the family in advance.

In order for direct intervention to be effective, the following principles should be kept in mind:

- The therapist should make sure that both the family and school are open to the therapist's involvement.
- The purpose of the meeting should be framed as serving the needs of the student.
- The therapist should acknowledge the important contributions that the parents and school are each making to the student's welfare.
- The therapist should state explicitly that the goal of the meeting is to help the family and school work more effectively as a team for the student's sake.

Case Example: "You Know He Tries to Split Us Apart"

In the case of Dave Coletti, introduced at the beginning of this chapter, I concluded that lack of collaboration between family members and the school was blocking them from finding an effective solution to Dave's fighting. I suggested a meeting at school with the following goals: (1) to help the school counselor see Mrs. Coletti in a more positive light, (2) to help the parents and school personnel take a more consistent position toward Dave's fighting, and (3) to break the apparent coalition between Mr. Coletti and the school counselor by strengthening the parental team.

Prior to the school conference, I met with the parents to bring out the mother's voice in a way that was more likely to be heard by the father. I told the parents that I had telephoned the school and had learned that the school was exasperated with Dave and felt that there was no other option but to place him in the special program. However, I agreed with Mr. Coletti that it would not be good for Dave to go to this program. The parents and I would need to find a way of convincing the school that there were other viable alternatives.

I then invited Mrs. Coletti to express her ideas. She stated that she, too, agreed that Dave should remain in the regular classroom, but that she also understood that he was disruptive in class. I noted that the mother was more appreciative than the father of the school's dilemma, though she had been cast in the role of the "more difficult" parent by the school. I encouraged Mrs. Coletti to elaborate on her understanding of the school's dilemma and asked if I could invite her to express these ideas at the start of the school conference. I hoped that by articulating her appreciation of the school's position, Mrs. Coletti would elicit a more positive view from the school counselor.

Mrs. Coletti stated that she believed that Dave needed "more consistency." Often, there were no consequences at home for his disruptive behavior at school. Dave's father began to disagree; I reminded him that our goal was to keep Dave from placement. Maybe school personnel would be more willing to give Dave another chance if they felt that the parents would support them by enforcing consequences at home when Dave misbehaved at school. As is often the case, the frustrated parent softens toward the more lenient parent when she feels that the therapist understands her plight. Mrs. Coletti turned to her husband and said in a calm voice, "You know he tries to split us apart. He takes advantage of any disagreement between us." Mr. Coletti, now able to hear his wife, agreed and said that he would work with her and the school to enforce consequences at home.

At the school meeting, I began by stating that the goal of the meeting was to find a way to help Dave control himself better at school, so that he could remain in the regular classroom. As the parents and I had planned, I invited Mrs. Coletti to present her understanding of the school's dilemma, while Mr. Coletti took a backseat. Mrs. Coletti then asked school personnel if there was anything the school would like them to do to support their expectations of Dave. The principal replied that he appreciated the parents' involvement and would find it helpful if the parents could hold Dave accountable at home for his behavior at school. Before the parents could reply, the school counselor interjected, "Yes, but we mustn't lose sight of the fact that Dave is a very troubled boy who needs more than just discipline. He needs help."

The school counselor's statement implied that the triangle in the home was isomorphic to a triangle in the school. Mrs. Coletti and the principal were in the role of enforcers, while Mr. Coletti and the counselor were in the role of protectors. Each faction could try to enlist me against the other or triangle me in the conflict. The latter is what happened: Mr. Coletti turned to me and said, "Well, what do *you* think? Should we be harder on Dave, or do we need to be more permissive because he has problems that we don't fully understand?"

Fortunately, I had prepared for this move and was ready with a response: "I don't think the issue is whether to be tougher or more permissive with Dave. I think the issue is to make sure that all of the adults who care about him are working together as a team to help him do the best he can."

I picked up on Mrs. Coletti's nodding and asked the parents if they could find out from the principal what he had in mind when he asked them to reinforce at home the school's expectations of Dave. In response to their question, the principal said that it would be helpful if the parents could tell Dave that they understood that his fighting at school was a serious problem and that they supported the school's rules against it. The parents agreed and promised to contact the school every Friday to obtain reports about Dave's behavior, so that they could reinforce the school's expectations at home. I suggested that it be Mr. Coletti who would contact the principal to receive these reports: I hoped that this arrangement would engage father, a member of the "protective" faction, with the principal, a member of the "discipline" faction.

If I appeared to be siding with one position to the exclusion of the other, the excluded faction could redouble its efforts to be heard and thus perpetuate the polarization. I had to find a way to link the two factions together toward a common goal. In addition to supporting more consistency in handling Dave, I would also have to acknowledge the other faction's position: that Dave's fighting was not simply bad behavior. Rather, he resorted to fighting because he had no other way of expressing anger or resolving conflicts. Could the team work together to help Dave find other alternatives to fighting?

The principal suggested that the school counselor could meet with Dave to help him find different ways of handling conflict with teachers and other students. I supported this suggestion, and the school counselor agreed. I then pointed out that until Dave learned new ways of handling conflicts, he would probably continue to use old methods. One method he used to escape being held accountable for his own actions was to take advantage of any apparent disagreement between the authority figures and enlist one in a coalition against the other. This could happen, for example, if Dave complained to the counselor about a problem he was having at home with one of his parents.

All agreed that it would be helpful if the counselor discouraged Dave from complaining to her about his parents and instead focus on Dave's relationships with teachers and other students. She would direct Dave to bring family problems to me, and I would help him and his parents resolve their conflicts. To reinforce this message, the counselor would tell Dave that she would immediately notify Mrs. Coletti if he continued to bring up problems involving his parents.

The factions appeared to be dissolving. The parents and school personnel seemed to be working more effectively as a team. One more step was necessary. Remembering the principal's request, I suggested that Dave be invited into the meeting so that he could hear what had been decided. I asked if the principal could start by telling

Dave what the school expected of him. Then, Mr. Coletti would reinforce the principal's message by informing Dave that he would be in regular contact with the principal, and that there would be consequences at home for disruptive behavior at school. Next, Mrs. Coletti would verbalize agreement with his father's message, but then tell Dave that she understood that he needed to find other "outlets" for his anger, so that in controlling his fighting, he did not simply "hold in" his feelings. Finally, the counselor would offer to help Dave find other ways of dealing with conflicts at school, and tell him that she would not discuss problems Dave was having at home. The team also agreed to meet again in 1 month to review the plan and to make any necessary adjustments.

This case demonstrates how a carefully planned meeting involving the parents and school personnel dissolved coalitions, created more teamwork, and encouraged new patterns of interaction among the family, the school, and the adolescent. Sometimes, the parents and school are simply disengaged from one another, and the therapist need only facilitate greater engagement between them. At other times, the relationship between the parents and school is so fraught with anxiety that each system triangulates another party to help them deal with the other system. In this case, the therapist can help the parents and school deal directly with one another by working on less contentious issues before moving on to those issues in which their positions are more polarized.

PITFALLS AND COMPLICATIONS IN TREATING SCHOOL-RELATED PROBLEMS

Triangulation

Triangulation is a hazard whenever a therapist becomes involved in working with multiple systems. In work with families and schools, some common patterns of triangulation include the following:

1. One system (family or school) invites the therapist into a coalition against the other. For example, the parents may complain to the therapist about the school and vice versa. Either the parents or the school could put the therapist in the position of carrying messages to the other system. The school could disclose to the therapist information about the family that the school does not want the therapist to share with the parents.

2. The therapist unwittingly fosters a coalition with one system against the other. For example, the therapist, perhaps hoping to increase the alliance with the family, adopts the role of the family's protector against the school. Alternatively, the therapist could join with the school in blaming the parents for the student's school problems.

3. Both systems join forces against the therapist. For example, the family and school avoid their conflict with each other by scapegoating the therapist, or the parents and school repeatedly discount the therapist's input while complaining that therapy isn't helping. In some (rare) cases, the therapist might deliberately elect to precipitate this pattern as a strategic therapeutic maneuver. For example, if the therapist deems that greater involvement between the family and school is needed, she might deliberately insert herself in a triangle in order to induce the family and school to form a coalition with each other.

4. Conflicts in each system's relationship with the therapist are replicated isomorphically in the therapist's relationship with the other system. For example, the therapist's difficulty developing a relationship with an authoritarian father could be replicated in the therapist's difficulty developing a relationship with an authoritarian principal. A mother's tendency to confide in the therapist rather than in her husband could be replicated in a teacher confiding in the therapist rather than in the principal. In other cases, the relationship between the therapist and one system might be complementary to his or her relationship with the other system. For example, the therapist might adopt a submissive role with the school and a dominant role with the family. Or, the therapist might avoid conflicts with the family by scapegoating the school.

De-triangling

A therapist can avoid the pitfalls of triangulation by keeping the following principles in mind:

1. The therapist should clearly define his or her role, even when other parties might not be clear about their roles.
2. The therapist should strive to act at all times in ways consistent with the role he or she has defined for him- or herself.
3. The therapist should remain connected and concerned about the (possibly conflicting) agendas of the involved parties, without feeling that he or she needs to find an ideal solution that is acceptable to all. One of the most common ways that therapists become triangled is by being recruited into the role of savior. Therapists who accept this

role will often feel frustrated or inadequate if they are unable to resolve the impasse between the conflicting parties.

4. The therapist should avoid becoming invested in any particular outcome. To the extent that a therapist decides that a particular outcome of an impasse is necessary, the therapist runs the risk of becoming triangled into the impasse.

5. The therapist should strive to engage the family and the school in direct interaction with one another. When conflicts arise between the systems, as they inevitably do, the therapist should attempt to intervene by pushing the two conflicting systems together rather than allowing him- or herself to be pulled into a triangle.

When a School Requests a Consultation

While parents often take the initiative in seeking help for a child's school problem, sometimes it is the school that enlists the therapist's help with a problem. This arrangement poses its own potential pitfalls.

Therapists should make every effort to ascertain what is expected of them. If the therapist is hired by the school, then the therapist is working for the school, not the family (or, for that matter, the student). Nevertheless, it is important to make sure that the parents have been notified of the therapist's involvement. Meeting with minors without parental informed consent could violate ethical and legal guidelines.

Before accepting a position as consultant, the therapist should explore with the school its reasons for wanting a therapist as a consultant, its previous experiences with consultants, and what it hopes to gain from the consultation. Ideally, therapists should negotiate a role whereby they provide suggestions to the school regarding how to handle problematic situations involving students. The school is free to accept or reject these suggestions, but the school (not the consultant) retains the responsibility for the problem that precipitated the consultation.

Sometimes, a consultant is invited into a triangle because factions at the school have been unable to negotiate a resolution of a conflict between them. Signs that the consultant may have been invited into a triangle include the following:

1. The impasse seems to the consultant to be obviously resolved by a shift in position of one of the factions. Too obvious solutions should be suspect, more so if the participants seem sophisticated enough to arrive at these solutions on their own.

2. The consultant begins to feel indispensable to the school. The

school might attempt to prolong the consultant's involvement beyond the issues that had originally prompted the consultation. New issues continually arise that delay the consultant's exit from the system.

3. The consultant's role begins to expand beyond that specified at the outset of the consultation. This change can occur so gradually that the consultant might not recognize that it is happening. By the time a consultant realizes that his or her role has changed, it is often difficult to return to the original role.

4. The consultant is simultaneously revered and disqualified. The disqualification might take the form of the consultant's suggestions being ignored or halfheartedly followed. At the same time, the consultant's "input" might be accorded great value. Sometimes, one of the factions attempts to invite the consultant into a coalition by blaming the other faction for "not understanding" or "undermining" the consultant's input.

The best way to avoid these pitfalls is for consultants to negotiate at the outset a clear and mutually acceptable definition of their role. If efforts at de-triangling are not successful, consultants might be able to renegotiate their role, in effect, starting over. As a final resort, the therapist might need to resign from the position of consultant, preferably before another consultant is called (triangled) in to resolve the impasse between the original consultant and the school.

Involuntary School Referrals

Sometimes a therapist does not have a formal consulting arrangement with a school, but is used by the school as a resource to whom problematic cases are referred. While the family appears to accept the school's referral willingly, it is obvious upon meeting family members that they have come to treatment under duress.

Jorge Colapinto (1988) provides valuable guidance to therapists in these situations. He points out a "common pitfall in compulsory school referrals": focusing on internal family dynamics when the source of the problem is the relationship between the family and the school. Colapinto writes:

> People who have been compulsorily referred by the school may arrive at the agency grudgingly, and/or with less than a clear understanding of why they are being referred to therapy, let alone family therapy. They may feel defensive and prepared to meet somebody who is sitting on the same side as the teacher and principal. Frequently, families referred in this way already have a less than satisfactory relationship

with the school personnel, who sees them as uncooperative and neglectful of their parental functions. The parents guessed, if they did not hear, that the school thinks they *are* the problem. (p. 90, emphasis in original)

In working with families that are compulsorily referred to therapy by the school, Colapinto makes three recommendations:

1. The therapist should avoid the assumption that the school problem is serving a "function" for the family and that the family is covertly encouraging the problem. Rather, the therapist should assume that the family is maintaining the problem "not actively, but *passively*, by default—by not doing enough to deal with it. A certain pattern of interactions, with the potential to alleviate the problem, is missing" (Colapinto, 1988, p. 92). The therapist should not imply that the student's problems at school are caused by dysfunctional family dynamics, or that the family "needs" the student to fail in order to distract themselves from more threatening problems.

2. The therapist should acknowledge the parents' predicament and be sensitive to the shame they might feel for being blamed by the school for the child's problem. The therapist should carefully review with the parents the reasons for the referral and should not assume that they share or even understand the school's rationale for sending them to therapy.

3. Rather than attempting to uncover dysfunctional dynamics within the family, the therapist should focus on fostering better teamwork between the family and school. Colapinto advises a task-oriented emphasis on building collaboration between the family and school for the student's sake.

Colapinto's recommendations reinforce a theme that has been repeated in many variations throughout this chapter: A narrow focus on family dynamics can distract the therapist from seeing the complex interrelationships among the child, family, and school that could be contributing to the problem.

SUMMARY

In this chapter, I have argued that school-related problems are usually the result of many interacting factors. Often, the relationship between the parents and school is contributing to the problem. In these cases, I have recommended three different levels of involvement for the therapist—coaching, mediation, and direct intervention—each of which has advantages and pitfalls. In selecting among these methods, choose the one that that will have the maximum impact while being least intrusive on the family. A gentle nudge should be preferred over a forceful push, even if the latter, on first glance, appears necessary.

NOTE

1. However, authoritarian parenting might not have as much of a negative impact in some cultural groups. See Chapter 3 (p. 80).

CHAPTER 9

PROBLEMS OF "LEAVING HOME"

The high school senior who misses the deadline for filing college applications. The college freshman who "flunks out" after his first semester. The recent high school graduate who has no plans to attend college and no job. The college student who withdraws midway through her second semester because she "can't take the pressure."

————◆◆————

Cases like these are often viewed as problems of "leaving home." According to the theory of the family life cycle (Carter & McGoldrick, 1980), families face a significant transition at the end of adolescence when the children move out of the parental home. It is commonly believed that this step occurs following high school graduation, when the youngster either leaves for college or begins working full time. There are, however, reasons to question this assumption.

First of all, the process of "leaving home" is not as abrupt as the preceding account implies. Adolescents are going through a process of gradual individuation and increasing independence throughout the teenage years, and college students continue to maintain ties to the parental home by returning during weekends or vacations. In fact, as I address later, some problems of leaving home can be traced to a process that has been too abrupt rather than too prolonged.

Second, the culturally prescribed timetable that dictates high school graduation as the dividing line between dependence and independence on parents is simply not applicable to some adolescents and families.

Many adolescents are mature enough to handle independence and are ready to "leave home" before the prescribed time. Sometimes, problems that arise in families of 17 or even some 16 year-olds could result from a clash between the adolescent's genuine readiness for more independence and the restrictions of home and school. On the other hand, many adolescents are not ready to leave home at age 18. These adolescents, particularly boys, fall prey to our societal equation of maturity and independence, as Silverstein and Rashbaum (1994) point out:

> With all the focus on facilitating a departure, too little consideration is given to the possibility that getting sick, or getting into serious trouble, may be a young man's only means of being able to come home again, and perhaps a sign that he needs to *be* home. Unfortunately, the mental health field has managed to convince us that there is something wrong with any boy who is not ready to "leave the nest" on schedule. But human development is vastly more complex and variable than that of the birds who inspired this metaphor. (p. 160, emphasis in original)

The family's ethnic background and local community norms must also be taken into account. In certain cultures (e.g., Southern European), families value physical proximity and prefer children to remain at home until marriage (McGoldrick et al., 1982). In these families, transition from adolescence to young adulthood is generally less abrupt and is usually not accompanied by a physical separation from the parents. These families may find it difficult to accept a child's departure from home, and conflicts may arise when the adolescent tries to leave and the family discourages it.

Third, many young adults return to live in the parental home even after they have spent time living on their own. Sometimes, the motivation for returning home is financial: increased competition in the workplace has made it more difficult for young people to succeed financially. Young people are also marrying later than in previous decades. Can we really consider it a problem in "leaving home" if a young person who had demonstrated the capacity to live on his or her own later returns to "the nest"? I think not, and thus conclude that it is incorrect to think of the young person "leaving home" at all. Rather, what happens is that young persons gradually expand the sphere in which they can competently operate, at first to a college dorm, then perhaps to an apartment with roommates, then to living on their own, but at any time, they retain the option of returning to the parental home as needs or preferences dictate.

There are two other reasons why it's a mistake to assume that all problems that arise during late adolescence mean that the family is having difficulty making the transition from adolescence to the "launching" phase of the family life cycle. First of all, the family might come to therapy because of a problem that appears to have arisen *de novo* during the later years of adolescence, but upon further discussion with the family, it becomes apparent that the roots of the problem extend back many years. Perhaps there has been a history of academic difficulties, failure to meet responsibilities, or parental overprotectiveness that had been just mild enough for everyone to ignore until the time came for the adolescent to make a decision about what to do after high school graduation. Second, other contemporaneous factors might be creating stress for the family aside from the developmental stress of dealing with the departing adolescent. For example, the parents could be experiencing failing health. An older sibling might be going through marital problems and depending more on the parents who, distracted, withdraw too much from the adolescent at a time when he or she still needs their support. Or, the parents might be preoccupied with their own aging parents, whose increasing dependency on them coincides with the adolescent's graduation from high school.

Keeping these points in mind, I believe that there are certain signs that suggest that problems of late adolescence are tied to the family's difficulty making the developmental transition to the "launching" phase of the life cycle:

1. The parents are treating the young adult the way they would treat a much younger adolescent. Sometimes, parents work too hard to protect their child from failure and thus deprive the young person of the opportunity to learn how to handle problems independently. For example, if the adolescent's grades are dropping during senior year, the parents go into overdrive to monitor the youngster's homework, use concrete rewards or punishments for grades, or convene meetings with teachers that don't include the student.

2. Neither the parents nor the adolescent seem in a particular hurry for the youth to leave, and the adolescent seems stuck in his or her own development. For example, an 18-year-old boy of average intelligence and adequate social skills graduated from high school without any plans for seeking employment. Three months later, he's still watching soap operas, and no one in the family seems concerned.

3. An eldest or youngest child in the family develops symptoms that appear to have come on suddenly during the last year of high school, shortly after graduation, or upon leaving for college. Keep in mind, however, that these symptoms might have arisen not because the parents are holding the young person back, but because they are pushing him or her out too fast.

4. The family's primary concern is the adolescent leaving home, and there is no evidence of other significant issues in the family.

5. The young person makes several "false starts" or failed attempts to leave home, for example, failing out of several colleges or repeatedly moving in and out of the parental home.

PERSPECTIVES ON LEAVING HOME

The family therapy literature offers a number of theories to explain the adolescent's and family's difficulty with leaving home.

Maintenance of Homeostasis

According to this theory, the adolescent is unable to leave home because the child's presence is necessary to regulate the level of tension between the parents. This position is perhaps best exemplified by Jay Haley (1980):

> One way the young person can stabilize the family is to develop some incapacitating problem that makes him or her a failure, so that he or she continues to need the parents. The function of the failure is to let the parents continue to communicate through and about the young person, with the organization remaining the same. Once the young person and parents fail to disengage, the triangular stability can continue for many years, independent of the offspring's age, though the onset of the problem began at the age of leaving home. The "child" can be forty years old, and the parents in their seventies, still taking their crazy son or daughter from hospital to hospital and doctor to doctor. (p. 31)

Haley recommends that therapists push parents to require the adolescent to function more independently and set a deadline for the child to leave home. The therapeutic work focuses on helping the parents remain united and firm in their expectations. The therapist relentlessly pursues this agenda, even when the family raises other seemingly important concerns (e.g., marital conflict), and views attempts to divert attention to these issues as yet another effort to delay the adolescent's departure.

Hierarchical Incongruity

Cloé Madanes (1981), while agreeing that preserving homeostasis could be one dynamic underlying problems leaving home, suggested that the problem could also be viewed as a structural one, as an example of what she termed "hierarchical incongruity."

> Two incongruous hierarchies are simultaneously defined in the family. In one, the youth is incompetent, defective, and dependent on the parents for protection, food, shelter, and money, and the parents are in a superior position and provide for and take care of him. Yet simultaneously another hierarchy is defined in which the parents are dominated by the youth because of his helplessness or threats or dangerous behavior. If the parents are to be competent parents, they must demand from the youth the behavior that is appropriate for his age, but doing so may trigger extreme and dangerous behavior from the youth. If the youth behaves normally, he loses the power that the threats of extreme behavior gave him over his parents. (p. 123)

Madanes pointed out that parents' efforts to help the young person often reinforce the youth's helplessness, which elicits more helpfulness from the parents in an endless cycle. Similar to Haley, Madanes advises the therapist to challenge the parents to state explicitly what they expect of the young person and then to hold him or her accountable: "Discussion of rules and consequences are the basic work of the therapy" (p. 129).

Precipitous Disconnection

Taking a different view, Carl Whitaker (1975) argued that the young person's failure to separate from the family is the result of a rupture in family relationships that prevented the parents from providing the adolescent with the appropriate context for successful individuation:

> The usual symptomatic adolescent is an individual who has broken with his family in a precipitous, painful and unsatisfactory manner. Both he and the family are bleeding from the wounds of this operation. Often dropping out at such an early emotional age results in a more profound dependence and unresolvable ambivalence in the escapee and in the family system as well. If you accept this conception, then the treatment of adolescents is really a reentry problem and a debriefing problem. The adolescent is really a family dropout who has not stayed through his senior year, the year in which he would gain pre-adult status and which is ended by a graduation ceremony. He needs to reenter the family system and separate to try life on his own. (p. 206)

Whitaker advised the therapist to reengage the young person with the family and then help all family members to work through the issues that precipitated the adolescent's premature departure.

Restrictive Narratives

Writing from a narrative perspective, Eron and Lund (1993) suggested that a network of reciprocally confirming beliefs, expectations, and actions can transform a mild developmental difficulty with initial separation into a "narrative of failure." They cited an example of a college freshman who calls home often and expresses his worries about failing academically and socially. They write:

> Hearing their usually confident son's worry, they respond with concern. As the parents express their concern, their son, who prefers to view himself as independent, competent, and capable of managing his own affairs, begins to see his parents viewing him as incompetent. This only serves to undermine his confidence further. The situation spirals such that the parents begin to see their son as failing at becoming independent and themselves as having failed at having launched him. The worrisome phone calls continue and the parents finally suggest that he try a school closer to home and live with them. The young man becomes more convinced that his parents see him as incompetent and unable to manage independence. His timid behavior mirrors this view. At the point when the family enters treatment, the young man has dropped out of two more colleges that are closer to his home town, is unemployed, and is literally petrified to leave his parents' house; his symptoms are a metaphor for the failed transition. (p. 300)

Eron and Lund suggested that the way to "dissolve" this problem cycle is to reframe the problem as a "confidence problem" and to guide the family in the search for stories that emphasize the young man's strengths and prior evidence of his competence.

Parentification

According to Ivan Boszormenyi-Nagy and Muriel Spark (1973), an adolescent may not be able to leave home because he or she has been saddled with disproportionate responsibility for the welfare of her parents. Sometimes, the child's self-sacrifice on behalf of the parents can result in extreme symptoms, such as delinquency, psychosis, or suicide, which become the ostensible reason why the adolescent can't leave. These authors recommended that the therapist help the parents acknowledge the child's efforts on their behalf and help the child find more appropriate and less self-defeating ways of demonstrating care for them.

Contradictory Parental Messages

According to Heim Stierlin (1973; Stierlin, Levi, & Savard, 1971), the young person may be tied to his or her parents through more covert, unconscious processes such as projective identification. For example, parents who have not integrated their own terrifying impulses (such as aggression) might project these impulses onto the child, and then induce the child to act in accordance with these projections. In order for this defense to function, the child must be present, so the parent thwarts (usually unconsciously) the child's efforts to leave home. Successful treatment requires the parents to recognize and reown their split-off impulses, thus freeing the child from the bonds of the projective identification.

Stierlin (1973) also distinguished between *centripetal* and *centrifugal* family dynamics. Families in which centripetal dynamics predominate delay the adolescent's separation and block his or her moves toward autonomy, either by fostering the young person's dependency on the family or by inducing extreme guilt at any hint of separation. When centrifugal dynamics predominate, the family pushes the adolescent into premature autonomy and separation, which often results in failure, because the youth has not been sufficiently prepared for independence. Steirlin also identified a dynamic that represents a combination of the binding (centripetal) and expelling (centrifugal) dynamics, which he termed the "delegating mode." When the delegating mode is predominant, the young person is held on a "long leash," allowed to leave the family, but bound to act out to gratify vicariously the parents' own needs or fantasies.

Successful treatment depends upon the particular dynamic predominating in the family. For adolescents too tightly bound via centripetal dynamics, Stierlin recommended that the therapist work to encourage gradual separation. For those who have been prematurely expelled from the family, Stierlin advised reconnecting the adolescent and the family. Finally, for families in the delegating mode, Stierlin recommended an in-depth exploration and resolution of the "tangled skein of conflicting messages and loyalties" (1973, p. 62).

HOW TO ASSESS AND INTERVENE

I believe that each of these theories has something to offer for understanding the problems of "leaving home" and that a combination of them will be most useful in deciding how best to intervene with these problems. I wish to emphasize, however, that difficulties with leaving home do not necessarily imply dysfunctional family dynamics. The therapist's first task is to assess the problem and arrive at a formulation that best fits the family.

What's the Obstacle?

Sometimes a young person is having trouble adjusting to independent living, not because of family problems but because other obstacles are in his way. For example, a college sophomore was in danger of failing out of college. Talking with him and his family, there were no apparent difficulties associated with the developmental transition. Both parents seemed to be handling the boy's leave-taking well, and there did not appear to be marital conflicts. It did turn out, however, that the boy had a previously undiagnosed attention deficit disorder that made it difficult for him to concentrate on lectures. In addition, because he had managed to "get by" with little studying in high school, he had no idea how to prepare for tests. The boy agreed to take Ritalin, attended a class on study skills, managed to pass the semester and did well the following semester.

Whose Problem Is It?

The answer, of course, is "everyone's," but I think it's useful to try to sort out who in the family is experiencing the most distress. For example, a family presented with three problems: a daughter who had become intensely "homesick" and was unable to complete her college work; a mother with a history of depression, who would periodically retire to her room for weeks at a time; and marital conflict that was managed primarily through mutual avoidance. The family came to therapy asking for help for the daughter's problem.

When I met with the girl alone, it was obvious that she was not so much homesick as worried about her mother. I encouraged her to share her concern about her mother with her parents at the next family session. After she had done so, I turned to the parents and asked, "Can you convince your daughter that you can get along without her?"

Toward the end of a tearful discussion, during which I repeated my question four times, the mother agreed to treatment for her chronic depression and both parents agreed to marital therapy. Both parents thanked the girl for her concern and assured her that they would take better care of themselves.

Is the Youth Ready to Leave?

As noted earlier, some adolescents are pushed out of the family home long before they are ready. In some cases, the youth is simply not on the same timetable as his or her peers, yet may be embarrassed to discuss reservations about leaving home for fear of not meeting real or imagined parental expectations. For this reason, I recommend that the therapist always raise the option of postponing the leave-taking, and then carefully monitor the family's reaction.

For example, a high school senior was procrastinating on filling out his college applications while still professing a desire to go away to college in another state. He and his parents were locked in conflict around his "lack of responsibility." When I raised the possibility that the boy might not be sure whether he wanted to go to college right away, he at first rebuffed this idea, but as I pursued it, he hesitantly admitted that he was "confused" about what he wanted to do and wished he could have more time to think it over. Eventually, the boy decided to attend a 2-year college close to home.

Has the Family Prepared the Youth for Independence?

In other cases, the family has not prepared the adolescent for the separation. This often occurs when parents have been overly protective of the child. For example, a girl with a history of severe learning disabilities began to experience panic attacks 1 month before she was scheduled to leave for college. It turned out that she had never written a paper on her own, and that her mother had written all of her papers for her during high school. She was now understandably anxious that she could not handle the writing demands of the college she was planning to attend.

In another family, a very high achieving but shy young man who had done well through high school became depressed soon after leaving for college, 4 hours from home. The young man attributed his depression to missing his family and feeling lonely. The parents, well meaning but a bit naive, had not pushed this shy boy to expand his social network during high school, interpreting his preference for being alone as evidence of his studiousness. In this case, the goal was to block the parents from rescuing the boy. Instead, I urged them to encourage him to persist, reiterate their confidence in his ability to adjust to living away from home, and arrange for him to receive counseling at college. By the second semester, the boy reported feeling better, had made a few friends, and was looking forward to returning for his second year.

Keep the Momentum Going

By now, the reader might be a bit confused. Some of the time, as in the example just cited, I appear to be suggesting that the therapist encourage the separation, while at other times I appear to be suggesting that the therapist slow the process down. No confusion is intended. The principle is to examine the entire context in which the leave-taking is occurring, including the adolescent's stated goals, resources, and weaknesses.

In the case of the boy who was procrastinating on his college applications, it was clear to me that this boy really had not thought through the decision to attend college, and instead was being carried along by encouragement from teachers and parents. Thus, I believed that it was important to slow down the process to allow the boy a "moratorium" on the college decision rather than pushing for premature "foreclosure" based on the wishes of his family. In the case of the shy boy who became depressed when separated from his family, it was clear that this boy really wanted to attend college, had done well academically through high school, and simply wished that he could feel better so that he could make the most of his college experience. In this case, recalling the advice of Eron and Lund (1993; discussed earlier), I believed that the parents needed to "mirror" back to the boy their confidence that he could succeed if he persisted.

In any case, it is important to keep the family on the track toward increasing independence for the young person. This is not to say that the adolescent must be pushed in any particular direction, or even that the youth must be forced into a physical separation from the family. Rather, *the therapist should encourage the parents to help the young person make the next developmental step for which he or she is ready.* Stated another way, keep the momentum toward maturity going, either by unblocking a stuck process or by discouraging the parents from prematurely rescuing the adolescent.

Sometimes, engaging the family in therapy is the only recourse. A girl I had treated 1 year earlier for a mild depression called me the day after she returned to college after her winter break and frantically told me that she wanted to drop out and return home because she believed she had made the wrong decision about what college to attend. She said that her parents insisted that she consult with me before making her decision. It sounded to me like she had already made it. I gave her a little speech about tolerating "growing pains" and reaffirmed my confidence in her ability to succeed, wherever she chose to attend school. She listened politely and then resumed what I realized was a plea for my approval of her decision to come back home. In the end,

I decided to tell her that I would support whatever decision she made, but that since she had called to ask my opinion, I felt obliged to give it. I told her that there were merits to both staying at college and returning home. However, the worst thing she could do would be to come home without returning to therapy to try to understand her motives for making what appeared to be an impulsive decision.

She apparently took my statement as the endorsement she wanted. She returned home, and we resumed our work together. The next fall, she left home, but not for college. She pursued a dream she had kept secret all through her high school years: to move to Alaska and work as a tour guide. Some of the work of therapy was helping her parents "let go" of her enough so that she could tell them that she wasn't planning to fulfill their dream of her graduating from college.

In other cases, the therapist might have to push the process along more vigorously. Take the case of a young man who dropped out of college after his first year, took and promptly quit a series of jobs, and was now sitting at home while his widowed mother supported them both. I suspected that his mother was willing to condone the boy's behavior because she was worried how she would manage if he left home. This case appeared to fit Haley's (1980) paradigm (discussed earlier). I told the mother and the boy that I believed that he seemed to be taking advantage of her largess, and that she should keep a record of how much she was spending on his support so that he could repay her when he eventually got a job. Meanwhile, I encouraged the mother to develop her own social network, to accept offers to go out on dates, and to spend some evenings away from home, using the rationale that she needed to "prepare" for the boy's inevitable departure from home as soon as he "got on his feet again." As the mother's connections outside the family expanded, she began to demand more from the boy and eventually gave him the choice either to find a job within 30 days or to move out of the house. Now that she had taken a stand to support the boy's growing up, I shifted my support to the boy, coached him on job-seeking skills, and encouraged him to take aptitude and interest tests in order to define clearer career goals.

One of the ways that families can unwittingly thwart the process of leave-taking is to focus too intensely on one aspect of the process. Take the case of Tyrone, discussed in Chapter 6 as an example of "mild" problem behavior. Tyrone's mother was primarily concerned with what she called his "lack of responsibility," because he repeatedly came home late from dates with his girlfriend. I reframed the problem as one reflecting the difficulty Tyrone was having "saying good-bye" to his girlfriend, and then talked with him and his mother about the series of "good-byes" he was about to face as he prepared to leave for college.

If I had accepted that Tyrone's "lack of responsibility" was the problem, I might have precipitated a power struggle between him and his mother, which would enact a dynamic more characteristic of a younger adolescent and distract Tyrone from the important process of mourning the losses associated with leaving home.

This point is an important one that is often overlooked by families as the adolescent excitedly prepares to go away to college. Every leave-taking involves mourning. In their haste to support the adolescent's maturity, parents can fail to acknowledge the losses they and the adolescent are facing.

For example, a young man and his father were locked in combat regarding the expensive phone bill the boy had incurred talking nightly to his girlfriend, who was attending a month-long precollege orientation program 6 hours away. The boy had also not found a summer job and was, in the father's view, "pining away" for his girlfriend. During one of their typically unproductive arguments, the father cried, "I thought we had a great relationship, but I don't think so any more. You obviously care more about her than you care about my feelings."

I interjected at this point to offer a different explanation: The boy in fact cared a great deal about his father, and the fact that his relationship with his girlfriend seemed to be coming between them was evidence that the emotions connected with saying good-bye to her were so overpowering that they led him to act in a way that hurt his father. It was not that he didn't care enough about his father, I proposed, but that his mourning over the loss of his girlfriend was so intense that it impeded his judgment.

The boy agreed that no matter how hard he tried, he could think of little else than how much he missed his girlfriend. I asked him and his father to talk about how his dad might help him through this difficult experience. This discussion led us to consider the other losses this boy was about to face, including the loss of daily contact with his father, to whom he was strongly attached.

After several tearful conversations, the boy decided that he needed to end his relationship with his girlfriend because it was draining too much energy from the task of getting ready for college. We spent the final weeks of the summer helping him and his father plan a "ritual of leave-taking" that would include an opportunity for them to reminisce about the past, affirm their relationship in the present, and talk about how their relationship would change as the boy grew older.

Meanwhile, I talked with the boy about his relationship with his girlfriend and learned that he felt very insecure about her affection for him. His mother had left him and his father when the boy was 11. Though he continued to see his mother regularly, they were not close.

He and his mother had never talked about the divorce. I suggested that the intensity of the boy's longing for his girlfriend might be related to unresolved feelings of abandonment by his mother. He agreed that he had never felt sure about his mother's feelings for him, and that he frequently wondered "how a mother could just up and leave her kid like that."

I proposed that the "unfinished business" between him and his mother could be an obstacle to his leaving home successfully, since he might be tempted to keep "hanging on" in hopes of finally getting the affection from her that he had never received as a child. I suggested that we arrange a few sessions for him to talk with his mother about his feelings, not with the goal of necessarily receiving any particular response from her, but to help him acknowledge the loss and move on.

SUMMARY: FOUR PRINCIPLES

As I have emphasized in this chapter, when an adolescent and family appear to be stuck in the developmental process known as "leaving home," the therapist must carefully assess the context before assuming that his or her job is to force the separation. Sometimes (but not always) the adolescent's leaving home threatens a family's rigid organization, and the task of the therapy is to facilitate the reorganization of the family to allow the youth to leave. Other times, less malignant dynamics are at work, and it is these cases that I have tried to highlight in this chapter.

In closing and by way of summary, I suggest the following four steps for treating problems of leaving home:

1. Assess the adolescent's developmental readiness to leave home, and then support whatever steps seem appropriate given the young person's level of maturity.

2. Try to get the parents to take a supportive and encouraging stance with the adolescent, by which they mirror back their confidence that he or she will ultimately succeed at the goal he or she has chosen.

3. If you encounter resistance from the parents, it is likely that they are having difficulty "letting go" of the adolescent. It is essential that these issues be acknowledged and addressed, but only if the previous step has failed. Don't imply that the parents are holding the youth back before giving the parents a fair chance to support the transition.

4. Then, work on two fronts simultaneously: (a) Encourage the

adolescent to make small developmental steps despite the lack of support from the parents, and (b) help the parents deal with the individual or marital issues that might be impeding the developmental process. Working on (a) and ignoring (b) could undermine the young person's efforts to leave, while working on (b) and ignoring (a) can prolong the process and enable the parents to avoid confronting the anxiety about the child's departure.

CHAPTER 10

MULTIPROBLEM FAMILIES

B efore the session had even begun, Rosa appeared exhausted from trying to control her six children in the waiting room. Now, sitting in my office, she could hardly complete a sentence without having to reprimand one of the children. I had already heard about Rosa and her family. A single mother, she was referred by the Department of Child Protection after the school reported suspicious bruises on the legs of Inez, Rosa's 11-year-old daughter. During the preliminary investigation, Rosa admitted that she often slapped her children, but she denied abusing them. The child protection worker, however, assessed Rosa as a "high-risk parent" and informed her that she would be under observation and have to attend therapy.

Rosa had never been in therapy before, but she reported that her oldest child, Ramon, now 13, had seen a counselor for a few sessions after it was discovered that he had been sexually abused by one of Rosa's former boyfriends. Ramon continued to have nightmares and flagrantly disobeyed his mother, but Rosa had to discontinue the counseling because she was unable to afford the carfare to the therapist's office.

Rosa's six children ranged in age from 2 to 13. Only Ramon and Inez had the same father, who was now incarcerated for dealing drugs. The other four children all had different fathers. Two of these men were incarcerated, one for murder. Rosa was unsure of the whereabouts of the third, and the fourth had been expelled from her home when she discovered that he had abused Ramon. Rosa had admitted to the child protection worker that these men had beat her up, sometimes in the presence of the children. Her present boyfriend lived with his mother around the corner, but often spent nights at Rosa's tiny apartment, sleeping with her in the same room as three of the younger children. The three older children shared a sofa bed in the living room.

Rosa had lived on public assistance since she came to the mainland from Puerto Rico when she was 17. At that time, she already had one child and was pregnant with her second. She had two sisters who lived in the area; one was addicted to crack, and the other was married and worked part time. Rosa's father left her mother when Rosa was 9. She reported that her father was often drunk and would beat their mother and "touch" the girls, including Rosa. After her father left, Rosa's mother decided to come to the mainland, because she felt there was more opportunity for employment. Rosa's mother had a stroke 2 years ago and lived in a squalid nursing home too far from Rosa's house to permit regular visits.

Rosa had never worked outside the home. She still struggled with English, but proudly pointed out that she could read and often helped her children with their homework. She never finished high school, but hoped one day to earn her general equivalency diploma and then study cosmetology. She spent her day taking care of the two youngest children, who had not yet started school. Most days, her boyfriend, who was also unemployed, kept her company. She evaded my question about whether her boyfriend was hitting her, and she became defensive when I asked if he was using or selling drugs. She indignantly denied that she would allow drugs in her home, where her children could be exposed to them.

Ramon was doing poorly at school and received special help for what Rosa identified as a "learning problem." Inez was a good student but very quiet and withdrawn. The third child, Carlos, had been suspended three times since school started 2 months earlier, and was being considered for transfer to a special class for "kids with problems." Next in line was Enrique, who was in the first grade and had already been identified by the school as possibly having "attention disorder." He had been placed on a waiting list for evaluation by the school psychologist. Still at home were Carmen, age 4, and Rosita, age 2. Rosa admitted that she often had difficulty controlling the youngest children, and related a recent incident when she found Carmen playing with matches. She wanted both girls evaluated, because she believed they might have "an attention problem like Carlos."

Toward the end of the session, I asked Rosa what she would like to work on in therapy. She looked blankly at me and replied, "I don't know. I came here because I was told to come."

I suggested that perhaps I could help Rosa learn other ways of disciplining the children other than hitting them. Rosa agreed that this would be a good thing to work on. She then asked me if I knew how she could arrange to get a grant to pay for carfare so that she could visit her mother in the nursing home. I said I would look into it. We made an appointment for the same time the following week, and Rosa herded the children together for the ride home on the subway.

The next day, the child protection worker called me and asked for my "impressions" of the family. The worker told me that she felt that "something was going on" in this family, and she hoped I could find out what it was. She would need a written report from me "with recommendations" within 60 days. Two days later, I received a call from Ramon's school. Rosa had told them that I was "working with" Ramon. They were calling to ask my advice because they had run out of strategies for dealing with Ramon. They asked if I could come to a meeting at the school to discuss what they should do with him.

The following week, Rosa called an hour before the scheduled appointment to say that she could not come because Rosita was sick. We rescheduled for the following week at the same time. Rosa arrived 40 minutes late for the rescheduled appointment. We had barely started when I was buzzed by the receptionist and informed that my next family had arrived for their appointment. Rosa said that she understood and made another appointment for the following week.

Rosa did not appear for the appointment and did not call in advance. Since she had no phone, I was unable to reach her. The day after the appointment, the child protection worker called me to ask how the family was progressing and to remind me that my written report would be due in a few weeks. When I told the worker that it had been difficult to schedule a meeting time with the family, the worker said that she would visit the family at home and remind them that if they did not come to therapy, then there was a good chance that Inez would be "taken away" and "placed."

———◆———

Increasingly therapists are called upon to work with families, like Rosa's, who have multiple problems. Often these families are chaotic and fragmented, and may have long histories of dysfunction. Many of these families live in poverty and are supported by public assistance. Often they have come into contact with a variety of helping professionals such as counselors, social workers, child advocates, and foster parents.

It's hard to know where to begin to help these families. Their problems are so intertwined that it seems impossible to focus on one without tackling them all. Trying to coordinate the inputs of many different agencies, all of which have different agendas, can seem overwhelming. It's no wonder that many therapists feel as hopeless as these families feel.

Almost three decades ago, Salvador Minuchin and his colleagues broke new ground in working with multiproblem, low-income families with the publication of *Families of the Slums* (Minuchin, Montalvo, Guerney, Rosman, & Schumer, 1967). In this work, based upon their experiences at the Wiltwyck School for Boys, a correctional facility in New York, the authors described their attempts to develop a model of therapy that was more suited to urban low-income families than the ordinary techniques based on reflection and insight. The result of their efforts was the action-oriented model of treatment that became known as structural family therapy.

Harry Aponte (1976b) later expanded on this work by articulating the particular issues posed by therapy with low-income families:

> There is another problem that comes with poverty, and certainly not the exclusive possession of the poor, which is related to social organization. Social organization is an aspect of social ecology. It can be weakened at every socioeconomic level, but is particularly vulnerable to dysfunction under the social conditions linked to poverty and other forms of powerlessness. Some call the cluster of organizational problems that poor families often have *disorganization*; I prefer to call it *underorganization*, to suggest not so much an improper kind of organization, such as a deficiency in the degree of constancy, differentiation, and flexibility of the structural organization of the family system. This kind of internal underorganization is accompanied by a lack of organizational continuity of the family with the structure of its societal context, that is, its ecology. (Aponte, 1976b, p. 433, emphasis in original)

Aponte described the problems in these families in terms of *alignment*, *force*, and *boundary*:

> *Alignment* refers to the joining or opposition of one member of a system to another in carrying out an operation. *Force* defines the relative influence of each member on the outcome of an activity. *Boundary* tells who is included and excluded from the activity in question. (Aponte, 1976b, p. 434, emphasis in original)

In low-income families, alignments are either too weak or too rigid, power is loosely or rigidly distributed, and boundaries are impermeable or too diffuse. According to Aponte, the therapist must facilitate the development of a more effective organization in these families by creating appropriate alignments, efficient distribution of force, and stable but flexible boundaries.

In the two decades since Aponte's article was published, families who live in poverty have become even more disenfranchised. Low-income families are subject to disorganizing forces from both inside and outside. The rising rates of drug addiction, sexual abuse, adolescent pregnancy, and child neglect have taxed the already underorganized resources in these families. Furthermore, the environment in which these families live is hardly conducive to effective family functioning. Surrounded by violence, despair, homelessness, drug addiction, and want, these families understandably experience the world as a threatening place. In addition, these families are subject to another force that challenges their integrity as a social unit, one intended to be benevolent: the increasing role of social agencies in the lives of low-income families.

THE ROLE OF SOCIAL AGENCIES IN THE LIVES OF MULTIPROBLEM FAMILIES

In their well-intentioned efforts to help, social agencies often exacerbate the structural problems in low-income families (Colapinto, 1995). Most social service agencies have missions that target individuals (e.g., abused children, battered wives) and see their job as working to help these individuals rather than supporting the entire family. Low-income families who experience problems with their children are often subject to scrutiny by child protection agencies mandated by law to remove children from the home if there is evidence of abuse or neglect. Welfare laws encourage the peripheral status of fathers and husbands by cutting benefits if an able-bodied adult male resides in the household. The ascendance of "home-based" services (e.g., Markowitz, 1992; Seelig et al., 1992; Tavantzis et al., 1985), intended to make therapy more available to isolated families, can contribute to the deterioration of the boundary between the family and the social service team.

Therapists who work with low-income families must be prepared to confront the issues posed by the participation of the family in multiple extrafamilial systems. Therapists must broaden their lens beyond the family to the larger system that includes the family plus all of the systems that have become attached to the family over time. Often a problem that seems to be localized within the family can be linked to a problem between the family and the larger system (Imber-Black, 1991).

For example, a mother requested help with a defiant and oppositional adolescent girl. The mother, a single parent, had been reported to the county's Department of Child Protection for having slapped the girl during an argument some months ago. The mother complained that the child defied her rules, lied to her, and threatened to report her to the social worker from Child Protection whenever the mother tried to discipline her.

While the possibility of physical abuse must be investigated, it would be an error to ignore the potential impact of the larger system in contributing to the weak hierarchy in the family that led the mother to feel powerless. In exploring the role of the social worker from Child Protection, I realized that the social worker had unwittingly invited the adolescent into a coalition with her against the mother. The social worker, eager to establish a trusting relationship with the girl, had gone so far as to take her out to lunch and listen attentively as she recounted the "injustices" perpetrated on her by her mother. Concerned that the adolescent might be in danger of abuse, the social worker gave the girl her card and invited her to call at any time. Feeling empowered by her alignment with the social worker, the girl was actually more apt to be defiant toward her mother, which only increased the risk that her mother could lose control and physically abuse her. Meanwhile, the social worker, a single, childless woman 20 years the mother's junior, reported to me in supervision that she was frustrated because the mother seemed "resistant" to her suggestions about how to treat the girl. The social worker, dedicated and well intentioned, seemed oblivious to her contribution to the symptomatic cycle in this family.

It is a logical extension of the systems metaphor that the "supersystem" constituted by the family and social service agencies can be dysfunctional without the dysfunction being localized either within the family or within the agency (Imber-Black, 1991). A common example of a dysfunctional relationship between families and social service agencies is when one agency becomes triangled in a conflict between the family and another agency (Carl & Jurkovic, 1983). Sometimes it is the therapist who is triangled into a conflict between the family and social service agencies, such as Child Protection. In these cases, the simple fact that the therapist is involved can enable the family and the agency to avoid confronting their conflict directly.

Charles Fishman (1993) pointed out that *accommodation* is another dynamic that often characterizes the relationship between families and social service agencies. In an effort to help, the social service agency continually adjusts its expectations and strategies, while the family makes little change. Often, this accommodation progresses to the point that the agency is disempowered and has no leverage to effect change. This occurs, Fishman claims, because the social service agency is relatively more flexible than the family. When two systems come into contact, there is a tendency for the more flexible system to adapt to the less flexible one. In so doing, the more flexible system will begin to develop "symptoms" of its own, such as infighting among members of the team or a lack of clarity about its goals.

Conflicting Loyalties

Often, families have not directly requested services, but rather have been referred by another professional who believes that they could benefit from treatment. The family members dutifully comply, but might not understand why they have been sent to therapy. Sometimes families have their own expectations of therapy, and their agenda might conflict with the agenda of the referring agency. The therapist embarks on work with the family, only to discover later that he is caught in a triangle between the family and the referring agency. To assert the family's needs runs the risk of alienating the referral source, while to assert the agenda of the referral source can jeopardize therapy by undermining the therapeutic relationship with the family.

One venue in which this conflict can occur is in the foster care system. Many foster care agencies employ therapists to work with the children in their custody. Since the children in the agency's care have often experienced significant loss or trauma in their past, it is not unusual that they manifest symptoms suggesting that they should be referred for therapy. The therapist who thinks systemically, however, may be in a bind.

If the child has resided with the same foster parents for some time, and the child is manifesting symptoms, then it is possible that the foster parents and the child are participating in a symptomatic cycle. In this case, effective treatment will require the involvement of the foster parents. However, in many cases the foster parents do not see themselves as part of the problem. To the contrary, they see themselves as "heroes," who have rescued the child from unhappy circumstances and are giving the child a better home environment than he or she could ever hope to have had with the biological parents or in residential placement. To them, the problem certainly "belongs" to the child, and if they are involved at all, they see themselves as long-suffering victims or benevolent resources, not as participants in a symptomatic cycle.

If the therapist implies to the foster parents that they are contributing to the problem, they might redouble their efforts to prove that they are innocent and that the child, in fact, is the problem. This could lead to further scapegoating of the child and even, at times, covert messages to the child that he or she needs to be symptomatic in order to vindicate the foster parents. As the family and the therapist continue their conflict, the child's condition worsens. Eventually, the frustrated foster parents request that the foster care agency place the child with another family. Hearing of the conditions that prevailed in the original foster home, the new foster family is primed to repeat the same cycle.

Anticipating that the foster family could become frustrated and quit, the foster care agency might put overt or covert pressure on the therapist to stop implying that the foster family is part of the problem. They insist that the therapist see the child alone, to provide a "corrective emotional experience" that is intended to counterbalance the previous traumas the child had experienced. If the therapist resists, then she could lose her job with the agency.

One solution to this dilemma is, of course, educating foster care agencies about systemic concepts and helping them develop policies that are more conducive to working with families. In this vein, Minuchin (1984) has worked with state agencies to develop policies that are consistent with family systems concepts. But what is the therapist to do if the agency is not "enlightened" by systems thinking?

One possibility is to structure the therapy as a consultation to the referring person, who meets together with the foster family and the therapist to discuss the problem, the reason for referral, and the expectations of therapy. The foster parents might be engaged at this point as members of a team that will work with the therapist and the referring person to help the child with the problem. While this procedure runs the risk of forming a coalition with the foster parents against the child, it is certainly better than a power struggle with the foster parents over who is responsible for the problem. Eventually, as their trust in the therapist increases, the foster parents might be more willing to hear how they could be contributing to the problem.

Strengthening the Family's Boundaries

Helping families achieve more independence from the external agents that have become involved with their lives goes hand in hand with enhancing their abilities to function more effectively. Both goals must be addressed simultaneously. As families develop a greater repertoire of problem-solving capacities, they can function more and more independently of monitoring by external agencies. Similarly, to stimulate families to use their resources more creatively, it is important to discourage them from relying too much on external agencies for the solutions to their problems.

The therapist must help families create more appropriate relationships with the representatives of social service agencies. The therapist must help families to redefine themselves, to differentiate themselves from the often stressful environments in which they live, and from the agencies that sometimes intrude on their lives. External agents are most likely to intervene when the level of anxiety mounts and families are unable to contain it. Working to reinforce families' boundaries means that the therapist must strive to keep the level of anxiety within manageable limits by facilitating nonreactive listening among the family members, and between the family and the representatives of the social agencies.

Encouraging Autonomy and Inspiring Initiative

Therapy must help to empower families that have been disempowered by the system. These families do not see themselves as having much influence over what happens to them. They view the source of their problems as residing in others and the resolution of these problems as beyond their control. The concept that they can and should take responsibility for their own change seems to ring true to them in principle, but is difficult to implement in practice, because they feel so powerless to do anything that has much effect on their lives.

Family members in these circumstances often feel at the mercy of larger systems over which they have little influence. If the therapist tries to control or change the family, then the therapist is reinforcing this pattern. The therapist must instead help family members experience a sense that they can influence something that matters to them, that they can effect something significant in their lives.

Related to family members' experience of powerlessness is the belief that others are to blame for their problems. This belief is true to the extent that these families are often at the mercy of larger systemic forces over which they have little control. However, by abdicating responsibility for what happens to them, families simply become even more dependent on outside agencies. Thus, therapists must encourage family members to take responsibility for the decisions they make.

The therapist can be caught in a bind when family members do not seem able to protect a vulnerable child from physical harm. Here, the therapist might be torn between two options: taking decisive action to protect the child or empowering the family to take responsibility. If the therapist intervenes to protect the child (e.g., arranging to remove the child from the home), then the pattern of undermining the family's boundaries is reinforced. If the therapist delays action, hoping that the family members will eventually act, the child may be exposed to serious physical danger. Caught in this dilemma, the therapist can experience the same hopelessness and helplessness experienced by the family.

The *manner* in which the therapist takes action is crucial: It is essential for the therapist to involve families in the process of making decisions all along the way. Whenever decisions are to be made, the therapist should consult the family members and allow them to direct the therapist in the process. The therapist avoids acting unilaterally, but rather works under the direction of family members on their behalf. In this way, the therapist joins with the family by taking a temporary leadership position, but makes it clear that he or she is doing so under the family's direction.

RESPONDING TO CRISES AND REMAINING DIFFERENTIATED

Many family members believe that the purpose of therapy is to resolve crises and do not understand that therapy can help them address longer term issues. When there are no crises, family members miss sessions, since they have no immediate problem to discuss. Therapists can contribute to this pattern if they see their job as reducing stress on family members by solving problems for them.

When the family is in crisis, the therapist is mobilized to help the family find a solution. When a solution is found, the family returns to its precrisis state of relative stability. The postcrisis sessions (if the family even comes to them) are likely to seem directionless and ineffective, since the family's energies have been expended in dealing with the crisis. After the crisis has passed, the therapist does not push the family, perhaps fearing that any push will simply precipitate another crisis. The therapist has essentially colluded with family members by implicitly agreeing that the purpose of therapy is to help them restabilize after a crisis.

Crises generate anxiety for both families and therapists. The therapist, fearful that someone in the family could be harmed, might intervene in a way that reinforces family members' perception that it is the therapist's job (not theirs) to resolve the crisis. In some families, this tendency may be so pronounced that they actually exert *less* self-control while in therapy, since they assume (probably correctly) that the therapist will intervene if things get out of hand.

One way to disrupt this pattern is to utilize the family's crises as catalysts for change, an approach advocated by Brendler et al. (1991). Expanding upon Minuchin and Barcai's (1969) concept of therapeutic crisis induction, Brendler et al. argue that it is when the family is in crisis that a dysfunctional family structure is most open to change. Therapists can generate the necessary intensity for change by inducing crises that challenge the family to try new ways of solving problems.

Some therapists might balk at the idea of generating crises in families who already are underorganized, and whose main feature is that they apparently *lack* any coherent structure. However, even in these situations, it is important to remember that the "problem" is not the crisis per se, but rather the family's inability to handle it. By taking too active a role in problem solving, therapists can shortchange families by failing to challenge the basic structural weaknesses that impede their ability to arrive at effective solutions on their own.

Even if therapists are reluctant to induce crises, they can still capitalize on the momentum of naturally occurring crises. Simply by restraining themselves from taking too active a role in solving problems, therapists can utilize the anxiety generated by crises to motivate families to experiment with new ways of using their untapped resources.

Therapists who aim to shield families from feeling anxiety can actually impede their growth. Anxiety must be experienced before it can be creatively utilized as a vehicle for change. Kerr and Bowen (1988) argue that it is essential for therapists to have a higher level of differentiation of self than their patients. This means that the therapist must be better able than the family members to remain calm in the face of forces pulling for impulsivity and reactivity. Therapists will be in the best position for doing so if they do not fuse with families at times of crisis.

Unfortunately, it is not only families who pull therapists into crises. Other agencies, in their well-intentioned efforts to help, become activated when families are in crisis and, intending to "collaborate" with the therapist, might make demands on the therapist to provide "recommendations" for the family. Therapists must do their best to remain de-triangled at these times. The crisis belongs to the family, and the anxiety generated by the crisis is most appropriately experienced by them, not by the professionals involved. Some of the suggestions for avoiding triangulation in work with schools, discussed in Chapter 8, can be adapted to work with other social agencies.

SETTING AND PRIORITIZING GOALS

Difficulty Prioritizing Goals

Therapists who work with multiproblem families are often overwhelmed by the apparent chaos in these families. It is nearly impossible to focus on a finite set of goals, because there seems to be so much to do. The prospect of working on any single problem is stalemated by the presence of many others that are constantly demanding attention and competing for the family's limited resources.

These families might not see the relevance of setting goals. Unable to predict when the next crisis will hit, the needs of today take precedence over longer-term goals. There is little incentive to save, since any resources conserved for a future goal are likely to be diverted into the next crisis. There seems to be little point in trying to prevent crises, since frequent crises appear inevitable and unavoidable.

Eager to help, the therapist might try to persuade the family to concentrate on a specific goal that will be tackled in therapy. Family members, often at a loss themselves to specify an alternative goal, agree to work on the goal the therapist has suggested. However, since this goal is not particularly relevant to the family, they are unlikely to pursue it with the kind of enthusiasm the therapist expects. In this way, therapists become frustrated with families and conclude that they are unable to benefit from therapy.

One way to avoid this pitfall is for therapists to avoid taking too active a role in goal setting. Rather, therapists should help families define their own goals. Concrete images such as "scaling" (de Shazer, 1985) can help families articulate achievable goals. For example, if parents complain about the disobedience of a child, the therapist can ask the parents to rate the problem on a 10-point scale of increasing severity. If the parents rate the current severity of the problem as 6, the therapist then helps them define in concrete terms what would constitute a rating of 5, one step in the direction of improvement. Thus, rather than tackling what appears to be an unsurmountable problem all at once, the therapist works toward improvement one small step at a time.

Similarly, the therapist should pay careful attention to family members' beliefs about the process of change. How do family members believe change occurs? Do they believe that change is possible? Do they believe therapy can help them make these changes? Exploring previous changes and how they were made can guide this discussion. The therapist should attempt to utilize family members' own theories of change to facilitate the changes they wish to make.

The Problem with a Problem Focus

Therapists who insist that therapy be problem focused may find themselves frustrated when family members seem unable to concentrate on a single problem while putting other issues aside. If therapists insist on a problem focus with clear behavioral objectives, families might halfheartedly agree but then fail to follow through. A power struggle ensues, which stalemates the therapy and jeopardizes the fragile therapeutic relationship.

One solution to this dilemma is to abandon the idea that the purpose of therapy is to solve specific problems. Rather, the purpose of therapy is to enhance families' capacities to solve their own problems. This task is admittedly more difficult and takes more time. But it will have more lasting benefits for the family. The more active therapists are in solving problems for families, the less opportunity families have for learning to make better use of the resources at their disposal, however limited these resources seem to be.

Rather than asking, *What can I do to solve this problem?*, therapists should ask, *What is preventing this family from solving the problem? How can I help family members confront these obstacles and utilize their resources more creatively?* These questions orient therapists to helping families take the next attainable step in the process of achieving more independence.

The "Zone of Proximal Development"

In describing how children learn, Vygotsky (1978) defined the "zone of proximal development" as the next developmental step that a learner is ready to take. A skill is in the zone of proximal development if the child can perform the skill under the guidance of a teacher, but not yet independently. The goal is to move the learner into the zone of proximal development by gradually removing the amount of guidance provided by the teacher.

This concept can be applied to therapy with multiproblem families. These families perform some functions independently, while others can be accomplished only under the guidance of a therapist, and some functions are beyond what the therapeutic system can currently achieve. A therapy based on a growth orientation will assess the family's zone of proximal development and then develop a plan for helping the family move into this zone, thus expanding the family's capacity for independent problem solving.

There is always a zone of proximal development. The issue is not whether a family has one, but rather where it is. Therapists who are unable to identify a family's zone might be trying to take too large a step, or might be focusing too narrowly on a particular step that the family is not motivated to take. If therapists can be creative in utilizing families' resources, they will be able to help families perform increasingly more complicated tasks.

Accentuating Strengths and Divergence from Societal Narratives

Throughout this book, I have emphasized the idea that therapists should amplify existing family strengths as a way of solving problems. This principle is particularly important with members of multiproblem, low-income families, who are often unaware of their strengths. One of the main goals of therapy is to improve the capacity of families to appreciate their strengths and to utilize their resources creatively to solve their own problems. It is important, however, that therapists keep in mind that family members' cultural background will influence what qualities they consider strengths.

Many times, these families have been recruited into societal narratives about them. These narratives describe low-income families as unsophisticated, uneducated, powerless, irresponsible, and in need of supervision from others. Therapists, too, can be unwitting participants in these narratives, and might bring to therapy certain assumptions about work with low-income families. As a result, a therapist and family can participate in a problem-saturated narrative (White & Epston, 1990) that depicts low-income families as helplessly entangled in a web of problems from which there is little hope of escape. Therapists must be alert to opportunities to direct families' attention to "unique outcomes" or aspects of their experience that do not fit this dominant narrative. In doing so, therapists can assist families in constructing new narratives about themselves, in which they have more resources and more control over their own lives than the dominant societal narratives assert.

SETTING A STRUCTURE FOR THERAPY

Therapists might be unsure how much they can reasonably expect from families with few financial resources, who may be coming to therapy reluctantly. Believing that these families are tenuously committed to treatment, therapists might reduce their expectations and allow families considerable latitude on how therapy will proceed. Therapists might avoid confronting a family's routine lateness or inconsistent attendance, fearful that raising these issues could lead to a conflict that could drive the family from therapy. The family may interpret the therapist's inaction as confirmation that punctuality or consistency is not important.

On the one hand, it is necessary for the therapist to be patient. On the other hand, therapy can be rendered ineffective if certain minimum attendance criteria are not met. A family that attends one out of every four sessions on an irregular schedule will have great difficulty generating the momentum necessary for working on therapeutic goals. If a family arrives 30 or 40 minutes late, and the therapist extends the session, then the next family may feel slighted.

Gus Napier and Carl Whitaker (1978) pointed out that the therapist must win the "battle for structure" in the early stages of therapy. By this, they mean that therapists must specify the minimum conditions under which they feel they can effectively work with a particular family. Early in treatment, the therapist should negotiate a contract with the family, specifying who will attend therapy and how often sessions will occur. The therapist encourages the family members to think carefully about this contract before agreeing to it, because once they agree, the therapist intends to hold them to it.

Therapists should also make a distinction between the conditions under which they will "meet with the family," and the conditions under which "therapy" will take place. "Therapy" might require one set of conditions, such as the presence of all family members. However, the therapist can still "meet with the family" even when these conditions are not met, but then explain to the family that therapy cannot proceed since the minimum conditions for "therapy" have not been met. For example, in order to conduct "therapy" on the problem of an adolescent's rebelliousness, the therapist might contract with the family for three sessions of 2 hours each per month, to be attended by the adolescent, the single mother, and at least one other family member. If for one of these sessions the mother comes alone, the therapist can still meet with her, but explains that since the minimum conditions for therapy have not been met, he would not expect much therapeutic benefit from the session.

Failure to set a structure for therapy can have disastrous consequences. I have heard stories from supervisees about parents who have struck children during family sessions while the therapist watched helplessly. In one case, a mother routinely drank beer during the in-home family session. When the therapist requested that the mother desist, she refused to do so, asserting that the therapist had no right to tell her what she couldn't do in her own home. The therapist felt resentful and helpless, until he realized that he could not conduct therapy under these conditions and so informed the family, who used this opportunity to exit from treatment.

Ground Rules Are Important

Failure to set ground rules can replicate in the session the same chaos present in the family home. If children are unruly and parents shout at them or if family members repeatedly interrupt one another, everyone is apt to feel discouraged. Uncontrolled behavior in the therapy session only increases anxiety and promotes greater reactivity in an endless cycle. Failing to set a structure for therapy can contribute to the disempowerment of the family members, who may assume that the therapist should make and enforce the rules in his or her own office.

Rules regulating behavior in therapy sessions help families make the most of the resources at their disposal. Early in therapy, the therapist should negotiate with the family ground rules that are designed to reduce the chaos in the sessions. These rules may include, for example, that no one may speak while another person is speaking, that children must remain seated during the session, and that no shouting is allowed. All members of the family are asked to assent to these rules, and the parents are enlisted as allies in enforcing them.

VALUES, CONTROL, AND POWER

Values Clashes

Therapy can be stalled because of a clash of values between the therapist and the family. For example, some therapists might believe that therapy is best focused on distal issues or broad, "underlying" problems rather than on day-to-day crises. A family, on the other hand, might prefer to address more immediate concerns and might consider longer-term goals irrelevant. Therapists might believe that family members should work together for the welfare of all. Certain family members may not agree with this premise, holding that self-interest prevails over the common good. Therapists might believe that certain methods of disciplining children are more appropriate than others. Families might defend their methods of discipline as normative for their own culture. Therapists might believe that families should utilize their limited resources in particular ways rather than apparently "squandering" their funds. Families, on the other hand, might have different priorities for allocating their limited financial resources.

The line between therapeutic influence and inculcation of values is not so clearly drawn. As postmodern writers have pointed out, we can scarcely escape our own biases, and we are far more commonly engaged in a process of persuasion than we recognize (Gergen, 1991). Some authors have argued that therapists should denounce the role of "expert" and strive to dismantle the power differential between therapists and clients (e.g., Anderson & Goolishian, 1988; White, 1995).

Others have argued that it is not possible to conduct a values-free therapy. For example, Harry Aponte (1994) writes:

> The question is not one of *whether* the therapist's values will come face to face with the family's values in the crucible of therapy, but *how*. How can therapists work with their professional and personal values to benefit the families they treat? Negotiating the values that form the basis of problem definition, assessment, therapeutic interventions, and goal-setting becomes central to the therapeutic process. (p. 175, emphasis in original)

Aponte claims that values are always relevant to therapy. He exhorts us to acknowledge that we sometimes find it necessary to influence our clients' values and cautions us "to exercise no more influence over clients' values than is required to address clients' problems" (p. 184).

Sometimes it is appropriate to discuss values openly with families. At other times, it can be helpful to point out to families that their actions imply that they they want two incompatible things, and that pursuit of both simultaneously will assure that neither will be achieved. Families might be open to the idea that "one can't have one's cake and eat it too" and reorient their pursuits accordingly. Sometimes, therapists and families can "agree to disagree." But none of these discussions can take place unless the therapist creates a context in which families feel free to disagree openly with the therapist. If families fear reprisal for disagreeing with the therapist, they may pretend to agree but act otherwise.

The Limits of a Systemic Model

Many of the cherished concepts of systems theory need to be modified in order to be applicable to families who live in poverty. Feminist family therapists (e.g., Goldner, 1985, 1988; Luepnitz, 1988) have pointed out that the concepts of circularity and complementarity, integral to systems theory, assume that all members of the system have equal power. It is only by modifying a systems view with one informed by an awareness of hidden power differentials that therapists can avoid reinforcing the inequality among members of the system.

When working with low-income families, therapists must keep in mind the pervasive powerlessness experienced by these families by virtue of racial and economic discrimination in our society (see Minuchin, 1991). Failing to acknowledge these issues in the lives of these families puts the therapist at risk of perpetuating the social order by implying that these issues are not relevant. Therapists must recognize that the family is almost always "one down" relative to the social agencies that are involved with it. Similarly, within the family there may be power differentials based not only on gender but also on who controls the family's finances.

Interactions that appear dysfunctional to a therapist can appear adaptive when these issues are taken into account. For example, a therapist might notice that a mother fails to take a stand against the intrusive remarks and actions of her own mother. The therapist identifies this interaction as evidence of a dysfunctional hierarchy in the family and decides to enter into a therapeutic coalition with the mother in order to increase her authority in the system. It is only when the mother's mother refuses to return to therapy sessions that the therapist realizes his or her error. The mother lives rent-free in the grandmother's home, and the grandmother also contributes financial support to the mother and the grandchildren. Were the mother to leave the grandmother's home, she would sacrifice her own and her children's standard of living and jeopardize their safety by having to move to a dangerous neighborhood.

While the mother might be open to the possibility of renegotiating her relationship with her mother, it is the grandmother who determines how much this relationship will actually change. Had the therapist been aware of the mother's economic dependence on the grandmother, he or she might have taken a different approach. For example, rather than joining with the mother in a coalition against the grandmother, the therapist might have joined with the grandmother to help her see that her intrusive efforts to help her daughter contribute to her daughter's dependence on her. By recognizing the power differential in the family, it is no longer rendered invisible, and its implications can be fully explored. If the therapist had acknowledged the grandmother's tangible contributions to her daughter's and grandchildren's welfare, he or she might have had more leverage to induce the grandmother to wield her power more benevolently.

Powerlessness, subjugation, and violence are not simply "environmental stressors" in the lives of many low-income families. They are essential and often inescapable elements of the context in which these families live. A therapist who aspires to be "systemic" recognizes that each family's context is unique, constituted not only by the immediate interactions in the room but also by the family's own history, as well as the history and politics of the society in which the family lives (Boszormenyi-Nagy, Grunebaum, & Ulrich, 1991). Families are shaped not only by interactions among the family members, but also by value systems and political forces that keep them marginalized. As a relatively more powerful member of society simply by virtue of being well educated, if not male and/or Caucasian, the therapist is in a unique position either to support or subvert these societal discourses that strip power from individual family members, and from the family collectively.

CASE EXAMPLE: TWO TOKENS

After some research, I learned that Rosa could obtain a transportation grant that could help pay carfare to the nursing home where her mother was staying. I wrote Rosa a short note telling her that I had found out that some money could be available to her for transportation, and that I would tell her more about it when next we met. I also wrote that the child protection worker had been pressing me for information, and I wanted to discuss with Rosa what information (if any) I would release.

When a week had passed and I had not heard from Rosa, I phoned the child protection worker and asked if she could bring the family to the next therapy session. The worker protested that she was too busy to transport the family, and that it was up to the family to find transportation to the sessions. I then asked if I could accompany the worker to her next home visit. The worker gave me the time of the next scheduled visit and told me that if I wanted to be present, I could meet her at the family's home. I wrote another note to Rosa, stating that I would like to visit her at home. If she objected, she should call to tell me not to come. I then contacted the child protection worker to ask her for a specific list of the information she needed from me, as well as detailed criteria that her agency would use to decide if Rosa was complying with the department's mandates.

I did not hear from Rosa, so I arranged to be free for 2 hours on the date of the scheduled home visit. I planned to arrive at Rosa's apartment 30 minutes before the child protection worker was scheduled to arrive. I had received from the worker the list of information being requested and the criteria by which Rosa's fitness as a parent would be judged. I intended to discuss these items with Rosa during the 30 minutes prior to the worker's arrival.

Rosa greeted me like an old friend. Neither she nor I brought up the topic of the missed therapy appointments. She did, however, apologize for not responding to my "nice letter" and explained that she was very busy with the children and her mother. She ushered me into the small but clean living room and offered me a cup of tea.

Sipping tea together, I told Rosa how she could apply for the transportation grant. She was grateful and told me that she would try to come to therapy again. I asked her if she knew the purpose of the meeting with the child protection worker. Not surprisingly, she didn't really understand why we were meeting. I explained that I was being asked to provide evidence that Rosa was complying with treatment and making changes in the way she disciplined her children. I asked Rosa if she would help me decide what I should tell the worker. At first, Rosa protested, claiming, "I can't do that—I don't know anything."

I persisted, insisting that Rosa knew far more than I about what was best for her and for her family. Rosa then timidly suggested that perhaps I could help her convince the worker that she was really a good mother, and that she did not abuse her children. I saw this as an opportunity to share with Rosa the criteria I had received from the worker. At first defensive, Rosa eventually accepted the criteria, which included cooperating with the investigation, working to develop new parenting skills, and keeping the children safe.

I said that I thought I could help if Rosa would be willing to negotiate a contract to work with me toward meeting these criteria. I would tell the worker that I believed Rosa was actually making progress toward these goals even though she had been unable to attend therapy sessions regularly. With Rosa's help, I listed Rosa's strengths as a parent and cited several specific examples demonstrating that she loved and took care of her children.

I asked Rosa if she could attend therapy once per week. She hesitated and asked if it would be acceptable for her to come every other week. I said that Rosa should be the judge of how often she needed to come, keeping in mind that the child protection worker would be evaluating her based on the criteria we had just reviewed. Rosa became a bit defensive, arguing that she could not afford to come to therapy once per week.

I proposed that Rosa could attend therapy sessions at my office twice per month. Once per month, I would make a home visit and hold therapy at Rosa's apartment. In addition, once per week, Rosa would telephone me at a specific time, and I would also telephone Rosa at a specific time at her sister's house. The latter would require Rosa to ask her sister for help, something she was initially reluctant to do, until I convinced her that a stronger relationship with her sister could help her case with the child protection worker.

When the worker arrived a few minutes later, I noted with interest how coolly Rosa greeted her. She was nevertheless polite and offered the worker a cup of tea, which she declined. The worker immediately got down to business. She told Rosa that she knew that Rosa was not attending therapy, and that there was a strong possibility that her children would be taken from her. I asked the worker if Rosa could share with her what she and I had just been discussing. The worker looked surprised, but she agreed. Rosa then gave the worker a sketch of the plan we had devised, as I prompted her with reminders. The worker seemed satisfied, if skeptical. All agreed that another home visit would be scheduled in 3 months to evaluate Rosa's progress.

After the worker left, I congratulated Rosa on remaining calm even though I could see that she was not fond of the worker. I then brought up the phone calls I had received from Ramon's school. I told her that they were asking me for advice on how best to help Ramon in the classroom. Would Rosa like me to be involved in this way? She agreed that Ramon needed help and expressed her frustration with him. I asked what she thought could help Ramon do better in school. She came up with a few ideas, which I conspicuously wrote down. I then asked if Ramon could come to the next session, so that I could ask him if he had any additional ideas. Rosa agreed, and we parted cordially.

The next therapy session was scheduled for the following week. Immediately after returning to my office, I dashed off a short note reminding Rosa of the appointment and included two subway tokens for transportation. Rosa would need to handle the rest of the transportation cost herself. I mailed the note on the way home.

Rosa showed up on time for the family session, accompanied by Ramon and a modestly dressed, stately woman who appeared slightly older than she. Rosa introduced the visitor as her sister, Julia, and explained that Julia had offered to drive them to my office. Rosa offered to return the tokens, but I said she should keep them in her purse in case Julia was not available to drive them to our next appointment. Rosa asked if Julia could join the session, and I enthusiastically agreed. We discussed how we could help Ramon at school and came up with a few more ideas that I added to the list. At the end of the session, I asked Rosa if she would allow me to ask Julia for her telephone number, so that I had someone to call if I needed to reach Rosa between the sessions. Rosa agreed.

Over the next several weeks, my relationship with Rosa continued to improve. Though she occasionally missed therapy sessions, she remained about 80% faithful to the contract we had negotiated. One day, Rosa came to a session with a black eye, and it immediately occurred to me that Rosa might have missed previous therapy sessions because she was afraid that I would suspect that she was being beat up by her boyfriend.

When I first asked about her black eye, Rosa was evasive. I then asked her directly whether her boyfriend was hitting her. Rosa burst into tears and admitted that her boyfriend was violent and she was afraid of him. She couldn't move in with Julia, because he knew where she lived, and Rosa didn't think she or the children would be safe there. I suggested that we contact the child protection worker, tell her about Rosa's dilemma, and see if the worker could arrange for Rosa to go to a shelter for battered women.

A few weeks later, Rosa's mother's condition worsened. I suggested that one of their scheduled therapy sessions be held at the nursing home, an idea Rosa wholeheartedly supported. Julia was willing to drive us all to the nursing home. At the bedside of the frail, dying woman, I helped Rosa to grieve and say good-bye to her mother.

Though the family continued to have crises, though the children continued to have trouble at school, though Rosa continued to miss about one out of every four therapy sessions, she nevertheless provided the Department of Child Protection with satisfactory evidence of her fitness, and they closed her case. By then, however, Rosa had come to see me as a resource and agreed to continue in therapy even though it was no longer mandated.

SUMMARY

In this chapter, I have discussed the challenges of working with low-income, multiproblem families. The following are important principles to keep in mind to avoid therapist burnout and to empower the family to make the most of therapy:

- Stay calm and keep an appropriate emotional distance from the family, especially during crises.
- Help families appreciate their strengths and use them more effectively to solve their own problems. Avoid becoming a problem solver for the family. The "problem" is not the crisis per se, but rather the family members' inability to handle it on their own. Help families confront the obstacles that are impeding their ability to function more effectively.
- Rather than jumping in to defuse crises, use the momentum of the crisis to challenge the family to experiment with new ways of handling problems.
- If decisive action is necessary (e.g., removing a child from the home to avoid further abuse), try to do so in a way that does not disempower the family. Always involve family members in making decisions. As far as possible, act under the direction of the family and on its behalf.

- Set a structure for therapy and stick to it. Make and enforce ground rules in therapy sessions.
- When multiple social agencies are involved (as they almost always are), appreciate that these agencies have agendas of their own, that conflict among these agendas is common, and that representatives of these agencies have power over families. Watch out for triangulation. Help families to develop more effective relationships with the agencies as they work toward greater independence from them. Some of the suggestions for working with schools, discussed in Chapter 8, can be adapted to work with social agencies.
- Recognize that there is a thin line between therapeutic intervention and value inculcation. Communicate to the family members that you respect their points of view even if you don't agree with them. Invite them to express their disagreement openly rather than covertly through passive noncompliance.
- Keep in mind that racial, gender, and economic discrimination are not simply environmental stressors but powerful and inescapable elements of the complex social context in which these families live. Failure to acknowledge these forces in the lives of families can perpetuate injustice by implying that these issues are irrelevant. Interactions that at first appear dysfunctional may appear adaptive when power differentials within the family are taken into account.

EPILOGUE: THE ARCH

"I don't want to be here. I'm here only because my parents made me come. They said that I wasn't part of the family any more and if I wanted to get back in, I had to come here."

I asked the scruffy 16-year-old what he meant by not being "part of the family any more."

He just shrugged and said, "I don't know. It's just what they said. They'll feed me and give me a place to live but that's all."

I was surprised to hear this bland recital of what sounded like a major rejection by the family. I wondered how the situation at home had deteriorated to this point. The boy's mother sounded nice enough on the telephone a few days earlier when she called to ask me to see Steve.

"I know you work with families," she said, "but Steve said he wouldn't go with us. If he has to see someone, he wants to go alone. Will you do it?"

Sometimes you have to size up a clinical situation quickly, on the basis of very little information. The mother sounded sincere, and I thought perhaps I could convince Steve to allow the rest of the family to come in after I had a chance to connect with him. Before deciding, however, I needed more information. I asked Mrs. O'Brien to tell me more about the problem.

She related a not-unfamiliar story. Steve was a junior in a Catholic high school and was doing marginal work. He had just failed two subjects at midyear and didn't seem to care. What concerned her most, however, was that Steve had been in trouble with the police three times since the beginning of the school year: once for writing graffiti on a wall, once for stealing a cigarette lighter from a store, and once for pelting cars with eggs on Halloween. He was doing community service for the first charge and was awaiting hearings on the other two.

Mrs. O'Brien also suspected that Steve was smoking marijuana, though she didn't think that he was using any other drugs. She said that Steve's father had "read him the riot act" the night before, told him that if he didn't improve his grades, he'd be sent to public school, and grounded him for a month. They had tried family therapy before, but after a few visits Steve refused to attend. He was "open" to the idea of seeing "a counselor" now, but insisted that his parents not be part of the meetings.

I knew there were risks involved in agreeing to see Steve alone, but I decided to go ahead anyway. I realized that I could be inducted into a coalition with Steve against his parents, or that Steve could triangle me in his relationship with his parents by disclosing information to me that he didn't want them to know but that I thought they needed to know. I might fall into the trap of trying to replace his parents and he'd let me by having a better relationship with me than with them. Maybe we'd develop a bond that his parents could precipitously sever if his behavior did not improve, thus exposing him to the trauma of losing a relationship that had grown to be important to him.

On the other hand, though he was against therapy, Steve had expressed a clear preference to be seen alone. His parents were willing to agree that our sessions would be confidential, and that they would defer to my judgment regarding when they should be apprised of anything Steve had disclosed to me. They also recognized that it would take time for me to build a relationship with Steve, so they shouldn't necessarily expect to see any major changes right away. If they wanted therapy to end, for any reason, they would allow me at least one additional session to meet with Steve alone so that we could terminate comfortably.

Steve arrived promptly for his session late one January afternoon, a sturdy boy with wild hair that just grazed his shoulders, dressed in a torn T-shirt and shorts beneath his winter coat, and lime green high-top sneakers. He reluctantly shook the hand I offered him, sat down, and, without waiting to be asked, made his announcement about not wanting to be in therapy and needing to come in order to "get back in the family."

I told Steve that I appreciated knowing where I stood, and that I sympathized with the bind he was in. I asked him if there was anything he wanted to talk about, not really surprised when he smirked and replied in the negative, glaring at me as if daring me to offend him. I got the same response when I asked him if he wanted to ask me any questions about myself.

Feeling a little anxious now, I related to Steve what his mother had told me on the phone and asked him if he had any comment. Another smirk and grunt. I asked him why he didn't want his parents to come to therapy.

"We tried it once," he said with a frisson of contempt in his voice, "but it didn't do any good. My parents won't change."

I got another grunt when I asked him how he wanted his parents to change. I then asked him if he had ever talked with a therapist or counselor alone.

"Once," he said, "they made me go see this other guy. I sat down and he asked me why I was there, and I said I didn't know. He asked me if I wanted to work on anything, and I said no, so he told me I could leave. I was there about 10 minutes. I don't think he liked me very much."

I had no way of knowing if Steve realized that he had given me some good advice on how not to do therapy with him. I couldn't repeat my colleague's mistake, even if Steve was baiting me to dismiss him from my office in frustration. It was up to me to find a way to have a relationship with him.

I asked him about school. "What's it like there?" I asked, with genuine curiosity. I hadn't worked with any kids who had attended his school, and I had some fond and not-so-fond memories of my own high school, an all-male Catholic prep school, similar to the one Steve was attending.

Perhaps sensing my real curiosity, Steve seemed to let his guard down a bit. He said he liked the school, but he hated taking Latin, and he thought some of the teachers were "jerks." I asked him if there were any classes he liked. He told me that he liked art and added that he had been taking art classes on weekends since he was in elementary school. His smirk in response to my question about participation in school sports told me not to go there, but he added on his own that he was on the Chess Team and often went out of town to play tournaments with the team. Jumping at what seemed to be an opening, I suggested that maybe we could play a game of chess at our next session.

"No thanks," Steve sneered.

I asked him how he liked going to an all-boys school, and he said that he didn't mind because he had no trouble meeting girls outside of school. He didn't have a girlfriend right now, though, and he didn't care to.

"There's plenty of time for that," he said. "Right now I just like hanging out with my friends."

I asked him what he liked doing with his friends.

"Just hanging out," he said, "playing a little ball, listening to music, you know."

Risking our fragile conversation, I asked if he ever smoked any "weed" with his friends. I was surprised when he answered, without a beat. "Yeah, sometimes," he said, "but not as much as my parents think."

The conversation continued in this way for the next 30 minutes, and by the end of our session, I had learned quite a bit about Steve. In addition to what I have already related, I also learned that he got straight A's in math, that he liked math and found it challenging, that he had been working 20 hours per week at a gas station since he was in the ninth grade, and had even begun saving money in an IRA. He grunted when, at the end of our session, I said I'd see him next week at the same time, but I really didn't doubt that he'd be back.

Not only did Steve come back the following week, but he came on time every week for the next 3 months. His grades had improved, and though he wasn't exactly delightful to live with, he occasionally had dinner with the family, did his chores more or less regularly, and followed the house rules most of the time. It was his parents who suggested that maybe Steve didn't need to come any more. He was doing so much better, and he was involved in a lot of activities during the last month of school. Steve, of course, "didn't mind" stopping, since (he reminded me) he didn't want to come in the first place. But we had had some interesting conversations over those 3 months.

Reflecting on our time together, I remembered that the first breakthrough came when I decided that I'd open up a bit more than I usually do about my own life and my own experiences as a teenager attending a Catholic high school not unlike his own. Steve actually started asking me questions, an event that I chose to interpret as his beginning to have an interest in me. I told Steve that I enjoyed talking with him.

He parried back, "Yeah, sure, you're getting paid for it."

"You're right. I am getting paid," I admitted. "But I'm not paid to like you. And I do. And I don't like everyone I work with."

Steve didn't answer, but for the first time he was speechless, not silent.

At our sixth session, I asked Steve how he was feeling about our meetings.

"Just like I thought," he replied. "A waste of time and money. I'm not going to change, and you can't make me change."

A bit surprised, I asked Steve if he thought that I was trying to change him. He answered, "That's what you're supposed to be doing, ain't it?"

I even surprised myself at the spontaneity of my reply: "Maybe. But I'm not doing it with you. I'm just trying to get to know you. So far, I like what I see and even if I could (and I can't), I wouldn't want to change you."

A few sessions later, Steve sardonically remarked that "you adults" were interested only in "showing us kids that we gotta do whatever you say."

I asked him to elaborate, and he told me that the weekend before, he and his friends were "hanging out" in a parking lot, just tossing a football around, and they were chased away by the police.

"We weren't using drugs or anything, I swear," Steve said with indignation. "The cop thought we were going to cause trouble just because we were a bunch of teenagers."

Steve went on to tell me other such experiences, and I began to remember some long-forgotten feelings from my own youth, when I felt that I didn't have any rights, that I was a "second-class citizen" in an adult world.

It occurred to me that Steve was a member of a minority group, and, like many minorities, he was subject to prejudice based on stereotypes. I thought about this idea a lot after the session, and when we met the following week, I thanked Steve for teaching me this valuable lesson. I apologized to him "on behalf of all adults" for the times we were disrespectful and unreasonable in our dealings with teenagers. Steve glared at me suspiciously.

"I really mean it," I added. "And I just needed to say that to you whether you believe me or not."

He fidgeted in his chair, and I thought I might have seen a glisten of moisture in his eyes.

Our sessions had a spontaneous quality. I never knew what would be the topic of the day. One week, we debated politics; I took the role of asking questions that forced Steve to articulate his position. Another week, Steve gleefully told me about his mock campaign for the class presidency. Toward the end, he finally showed me some of his artwork. I asked questions (again, genuinely curious) and told him what I liked about his work.

So what did we accomplish? I was glad that Steve wasn't a managed care case, because I don't know how I would have provided adequate justification for the "medical necessity" of his treatment or the treatment goals I was pursuing. All I knew was that we were developing a relationship, I genuinely liked this boy (though I was never sure why), and he seemed to be calming down. He was beginning to differentiate himself from his peers and take less affront at his parents' expectations of him.

He never mentioned it, but I assume he "got back in" the family. When his dad (whom Steve always spoke of with a mixture of contempt and fear) asked me if Steve could stop coming to therapy, I sensed a very different tone in Mr. O'Brien's voice, one that told me that he was less frantic, more confident that Steve would be OK.

I'll remember Steve as one of my best teachers. He taught me to be more spontaneous in my sessions, to draw on parts of myself that I don't usually draw on in therapy. At various times, I was peer (when I told him stories of my own adolescence), adult (when I apologized for the way adults treated kids, when I told him what it feels like to be an adult, what our fears and insecurities are), student (when I thanked him for helping me to see the prejudice kids experience just for being kids), advocate (when I offered to speak with his parents on his behalf), and, yes, even therapist (when I helped him articulate his feelings of humiliation at having to show his homework to his father every night, which led to his confronting his father verbally rather than in passive-aggressive refusal to comply with his father's directive).

Because I was forced to abandon my typical therapeutic stance in order to offer this boy a lifeline that he was willing to grasp, because I had to admit that I couldn't force Steve to change, I was left only to be myself, to respond to him not out of any theoretical or technical principles, but out of my genuine liking and care for him. What he had for those 15 sessions was my undivided attention, my honesty, my willingness to be vulnerable, my unconditional acceptance of him—all ultimately based on my conviction that I had something to offer him if he would just stick it out long enough.

Steve taught me that, after all is said and done, after all the pages are read and written, theory and principles can take us only so far. The rest comes from the heart of therapy, the relationship, one firmly supported by the ARCH—Acceptance, Respect, Curiosity, and Honesty.

REFERENCES

Adams, G., Gullotta, T., & Montemayor, R. (Eds.). (1992). *Adolescent identity formation*. Newbury Park, CA: Sage.

Alexander, J. F. (1973). Defensive and supportive communications in normal and deviant families. *Journal of Consulting and Clinical Psychology, 40,* 223–231.

Alexander, K. L., & Eckland, B. K. (1975). School experience and status attainment. In S. E. Dragastin & G. H. Elder (Eds.), *Adolescence in the life cycle: Psychological change and social context.* Washington, DC: Hemisphere.

Allgood-Merten, B., Lewinsohn, P. M., & Hops, H. (1990). Sex differences and adolescent depression. *Journal of Abnormal Psychology, 99,* 55–63.

American Psychiatric Association. (1994). *Diagnostic and statistical manual of mental disorders* (4th ed.). Washington, DC: Author.

Ames, C., & Archer, J. (1988). Achievement goals in the classroom: Students' learning strategies and motivational processes. *Journal of Educational Psychology, 80,* 260–270.

Anderson, C. M. (1983). A psychoeducational program for families of patients with schizophrenia. In W. R. McFarlane (Ed.), *Family therapy in schizophrenia.* New York: Guilford Press.

Anderson, H., & Goolishian, H. A. (1988). Human systems as linguistic systems: Preliminary and evolving ideas about the implications for clinical theory. *Family Process, 27,* 371–393.

Aponte, H. (1976a). The family–school interview: An eco-structural approach. *Family Process, 15,* 303–311.

Aponte, H. (1976b). Underorganization in the poor family. In P. Guerin (Ed.), *Family therapy: Theory and practice.* New York: Gardner.

Aponte, H. (1994). *Bread and spirit: Therapy with the new poor.* New York: Norton.

Apter, T. (1990). *Altered loves: Mothers and daughters during adolescence.* New York: Ballantine.

Archer, S. L. (1989). Gender differences in identity development: Issues of process, domain, and timing. *Journal of Adolescence, 12,* 117–138.

Asseltine, R. H., Jr., Gore, S., & Colton, M. E. (1994). Depression and the social developmental context of adolescence. *Journal of Personality and Social Psychology, 67,* 252–263.

Atkinson, B., & Heath, A. (1990). Further thoughts on second-order family therapy: This time it's personal. *Family Process, 29,* 145–155.

Attie, I., & Brooks-Gunn, J. (1989). The development of eating problems in adolescent girls: A longitudinal study. *Developmental Psychology, 25,* 70–79.

Barkley, R. A., Guevremont, D. C., Anastopoulos, A. D., & Fletcher, K. E. (1992). A comparison of three family therapy programs for treating family conflicts in adolescents with attention-deficit/hyperactivity disorder. *Journal of Consulting and Clinical Psychology, 60,* 450–462.

Bartholomew, K. L. (1984). "I would eat for her if I could": Guiding the paradox in an anorectic system. *Journal of Strategic and Systemic Therapies, 3,* 57–65.

Bateson, G. (1972). *Steps to an ecology of mind.* New York: Ballantine.

Bateson, G., Jackson, D. D., Haley, J., & Weakland, J. H. (1956). Toward a theory of schizophrenia. *Behavioral Science, 1,* 251–264.

Bem, S. (1975). Sex-role adaptability: One consequence of psychological androgyny. *Journal of Personality and Social Psychology, 31,* 634–643.

Bergman, S. J. (1995). Men's psychological development: A relational perspective. In R. F. Levant & W. S. Pollack (Eds.), *A new psychology of men.* New York: Basic Books.

Berman, A. L., & Jobes, D. A. (1991). *Adolescent suicide: Assessment and intervention.* Washington, DC: American Psychological Association Press.

Berndt, T. (1979). Developmental changes in conformity to peers and parents. *Developmental Psychology, 15,* 608–616.

Bingham, C. R., & Crockett, L. J. (1996). Longitudinal adjustment patterns of boys and girls experiencing early, middle, and late sexual intercourse. *Developmental Psychology, 32,* 647–658.

Blair, C., Freeman, C., & Cull, A. (1995). The families of anorexia nervosa and cystic fibrosis patients. *Psychological Medicine, 25,* 985–993.

Blos, P. (1962). *On adolescence: A psychoanalytic interpretation.* New York: Free Press.

Blos, P. (1967). The second individuation process of adolescence. *Psychoanalytic Study of the Child, 22,* 162–186.

Bogdan, J. L. (1984). Family organization as an ecology of ideas: An alternative to the reification of family systems. *Family Process, 23,* 375–388.

Boszormenyi-Nagy, I., Grunebaum, J., & Ulrich, D. (1991). Contextual therapy. In A. S. Gurman & D. P. Kniskern (Eds.), *Handbook of family therapy* (Vol. 2). New York: Brunner/Mazel.

Boszormenyi-Nagy, I., & Spark, M. (1973). *Invisible loyalties.* New York: Harper & Row.

Bowen, M. (1978). *Family therapy in clinical practice.* Northvale, NJ: Aronson.

Bowlby, J. (1988). *A secure base: Clinical applications of attachment theory.* London: Routledge.

Brendler, J., Silver, M., Haber, M., & Sargent, J. (1991). *Madness, chaos, and violence: Therapy with families at the brink.* New York: Basic Books.

Brent, D. A., Kolko, D. J., Allan, M. J., & Brown, R. V. (1990). Suicidality in affectively disordered adolescent inpatients. *Journal of the American Academy of Child and Adolescent Psychiatry, 29,* 586–593.

Brier, N. (1989). The relationship between learning disability and delinquency: A review and reappraisal. *Journal of Learning Disabilities, 22,* 546–553.

Brody, E. B. (1975). Adolescents as a United States minority group in an era of social change. In A. J. Esman (Ed.), *The psychology of adolescence: Essential readings.* New York: International Universities Press.

Bronfenbrenner, U. (1977). Toward an experimental ecology of human development. *American Psychologist, 32,* 513–531.

Brooks, G. R., & Silverstein, L. B. (1995). Understanding the dark side of masculinity: An interactive systems model. In R. F. Levant & W. S. Pollack (Eds.), *A new psychology of men.* New York: Basic Books.

Brooks-Gunn, J., & Reiter, E. (1990). The role of pubertal processes. In S. Feldman & G. Elliott (Eds.), *At the threshold: The developing adolescent.* Cambridge, MA: Harvard University Press.

Brown, B. B. (1990). Peer groups and peer cultures. In S. Feldman & G. Elliott (Eds.), *At the threshold: The developing adolescent.* Cambridge, MA: Harvard University Press.

Brown, B. B., Mounts, N., Lamborn, S. D., & Steinberg, L. (1993). Parenting practices and peer group affiliation in adolescence. *Child Development, 64,* 467–482.

Brown, L. M., & Gilligan, C. (1992). *Meeting at the crossroads.* New York: Ballantine.

Bruch, H. (1982). Anorexia nervosa: Therapy and theory. *American Journal of Psychiatry, 139,* 1531–1538.

Bruch, H. (1988). *Conversations with anorexics.* New York: Basic Books.

Bruner, J. (1987). Life as narrative. *Social Research, 54,* 11–32.

Buchanan, C., Eccles, J., & Becker, J. (1992). Are adolescents the victims of raging hormones?: Evidence for activational effects of hormones at adolescence. *Psychological Bulletin, 111,* 62–107.

Buhrmester, D., & Furman, W. (1987). The development of companionship and intimacy. *Child Development, 58,* 1101–1113.

Cairns, R., Cairns, B., & Neckerman, H. (1989). Early school dropout: Configurations and determinants. *Child Development, 60,* 1437–1452.

Carl, D., & Jurkovic, G. J. (1983). Agency triangles: Problems in agency-family relationships. *Family Process, 22,* 441–451.

Carlat, D. J., Camargo, C. A., Jr., & Herzog, D. B. (1997). Eating disorders in males: A report on 135 patients. *American Journal of Psychiatry, 154,* 1127–1132.

Carr, M., Borkowski, J. G., & Maxwell, S. E. (1991). Motivational components of underachievement. *Developmental Psychology, 27,* 108–118.

Carter, B. (1988). Fathers and daughters. In M. Walters, B. Carter, P. Papp, & O. Silverstein (Eds.), *The invisible web: Gender patterns in family relationships.* New York: Guilford Press.

Carter, E. A., & McGoldrick, M. (Eds.). (1980). *The family life cycle: A framework for family therapy.* New York: Gardner.

Caspi, A., & Moffitt, T. E. (1991). Individual differences are accentuated during periods of social change: The sample case of girls at puberty. *Journal of Personality and Social Psychology, 61,* 157–168.

Cass, V. (1979). Homosexual identity formation: A theoretical model. *Journal of Homosexuality, 4,* 219–235.

Chalfant, J. C. (1989). Learning disabilities: Policy issues and promising approaches. *American Psychologist, 44,* 392–398.

Chamberlain, P., & Rosicky, J. G. (1995). The effectiveness of family therapy in the treatment of adolescents with conduct disorders and delinquency. *Journal of Marital and Family Therapy, 21,* 441–459.

Chao, R. (1994). Beyond parental control and authoritarian parenting style: Understanding Chinese parenting through the cultural notion of training. *Child Development, 65,* 1111–1119.

Cohen, J. (1985). Learning disabilities in adolescence: Developmental considerations. *Adolescent Psychiatry, 12,* 177–196.

Colapinto, J. (1988). Avoiding a common pitfall in compulsory school referrals. *Journal of Marital and Family Therapy, 14,* 89–96.

Colapinto, J. (1995). Dilution of family process in social services: Implications for treatment of neglectful families. *Family Process, 34,* 59–74.

Colby, A., Kohlberg, L., Gibbs, J., & Lieberman, M. (1983). A longitudinal study of moral judgment. *Monographs of the Society for Research in Child Development, 48* (Serial No. 200).

Cole, D. A., & McPherson, A. E. (1993). Relation of family subsystems to adolescent depression: Implementing a new family assessment strategy. *Journal of Family Psychology, 7,* 119–133.

Cole-Detke, H., & Kobak, R. (1996). Attachment processes in eating disorder and depression. *Journal of Consulting and Clinical Psychology, 64,* 282–290.

Coleman, E. (1990). Toward a synthetic understanding of sexual orientation. In D. P. McWhirter, S. A. Sanders, & J. M. Reinisch (Eds.), *Homosexuality/heterosexuality: Concepts of sexual orientation.* New York: Oxford University Press.

Compas, B. E., Ey, S., & Grant, K. E. (1993). Taxonomy, assessment, and diagnosis of depression during adolescence. *Psychological Bulletin, 114,* 323–344.

Cook, L. D. (1979). The adolescent with a learning disability: A developmental perspective. *Adolescence, 14,* 697–707.

Cramer, P. (1979). Defense mechanisms in adolescence. *Developmental Psychology, 15,* 476–477.

Crisp, A. H. (1983). Some aspects of the psychopathology of anorexia nervosa. In P. L. Darby, P. E. Garfinkel, D. M. Garner, & D. V. Coscina (Eds.), *Anorexia nervosa: Recent developments in research.* New York: Liss.

Csikszentmihalyi, M., & Larson, R. (1984). *Being adolescent.* New York: Basic Books.

Culbertson, F. M. (1997). Depression and gender: An international review. *American Psychologist, 52,* 25–31.

Darling, N., & Steinberg, L. (1993). Parenting style as context: An integrative model. *Psychological Bulletin, 113,* 487–496.

DeBaryshe, B.D., Patterson, G. R., & Capaldi, D. M. (1993). A performance model for academic achievement in early adolescent boys. *Developmental Psychology, 29,* 795–804.

Denborough, D. (1996). Step by step: Developing respectful and effective ways of working with young men to reduce violence. In C. McLean, M. Carey, & C. White (Eds.), *Men's ways of being.* Boulder, CO: Westview.

de Shazer, S. (1985). *Keys to solution in brief therapy.* New York: Norton.

Dickerson, V. C., & Zimmerman, J. (1992). Families with adolescents: Escaping problem lifestyles. *Family Process, 31,* 341–354.

Dishion, T., Patterson, G., Stoolmiller, M., & Skinner, M. (1991). Family, school, and behavioral antecedents to early adolescent involvement with antisocial peers. *Developmental Psychology, 27,* 172–180.

Dornbusch, S., Carlsmith, J., Bushwall, S., Ritter, P., Leiderman, P., Hastoff, A., & Gross, R. (1985). Single parents, extended households, and the control of adolescents. *Child Development, 56,* 326–341.

Dornbusch, S. M., Ritter, P. L., Leiderman, P. H., Roberts, D. F., & Fraleigh, M. J. (1987). The relation of parenting style to adolescent school performance. *Child Development, 58,* 1244–1257.

Dubow, F. F., Kausch, D. F., Blum, M. D., Reed, J., & Bush, E. (1989). Correlates of suicidal ideation and attempts in a community sample of junior high and high school students. *Journal of Clinical Child Psychology, 18,* 158–166.

Dunphy, D. (1963). The social structure of urban adolescent peer groups. *Sociometry, 26,* 230–246.

Dweck, C., & Licht, B. (1980). Learned helplessness and intellectual achievement. In J. Garber & M. Seligman (Eds.), *Human helplessness.* New York: Academic Press.

Eccles, J. S., Midgley, C., Wigfield, A., Buchanan, C. M., Reuman, D., Flanagan, C., & McIver, D. (1993). Development during adolescence: The impact of stage-environment fit on young adolescents' experiences in schools and families. *American Psychologist, 48,* 90–101.

Efran, J. S., Lukens, M. D., & Lukens, R. J. (1990). *Language, structure, and change: Frameworks of meaning in psychotherapy.* New York: Norton.

Elkaim, M. (1997). *If you love me, don't love me.* Northvalc, NJ: Aronson.

Elkind, D. (1967). Egocentricism in adolescence. *Child Development, 38,* 1025–1034.

Elliott, D. S., & Ageton, S. S. (1980). Reconciling race and class differences in self-reported and official estimates of delinquency. *American Sociological Review, 45,* 95–110.

Elmen, J. (1991). Achievement orientation in early adolescence: Developmental patterns and social correlates. *Journal of Early Adolescence, 11,* 125–151.

Eno, M. M. (1985). Children with school problems: A family therapy perspective. In R. L. Ziffer (Ed.), *Adjunctive techniques in family therapy.* New York: Grune & Stratton.

Entwisle, D. (1990). Schools and the adolescent. In S. Feldman & G. Elliott (Eds.), *At the threshold: The developing adolescent.* Cambridge, MA: Harvard University Press.

Epstein, J. (1983). The influence of friends on achievement and affective outcomes. In J. Epstein & N. Karweit (Eds.), *Friends in school.* New York: Academic Press.

Erikson, E. (1950). *Childhood and society.* New York: Norton.

Erikson, E. (1959). Identity and the life cycle. *Psychological Issues, 1,* 1–171.

Erikson, E. (1968). *Identity: Youth and crisis*. New York: Norton.

Eron, J. B., & Lund, T. W. (1993). How problems evolve and dissolve: Integrating narrative and strategic concepts. *Family Process, 32,* 291–309.

Evans, C., & Street, E. (1995). Possible differences in family patterns in anorexia nervosa and bulimia nervosa. *Journal of Family Therapy, 17,* 115–131.

Eveleth, P., & Tanner, J. (1976). *Worldwide variation in human growth*. New York: Cambridge University Press.

Faigel, H. D., Sznajderman, S., Tishby, O., & Turel, M. (1995) Attention deficit disorder during adolescence: A review. *Journal of Adolescent Health, 16,* 174–184.

Feldman, S., & Elliott, G. (Eds.). (1990). *At the threshold: The developing adolescent*. Cambridge, MA: Harvard University Press.

Fisch, R., Weakland, J. H., & Segal, L. (1982). *The tactics of change: Doing therapy briefly*. San Francisco: Jossey-Bass.

Fisher, L. (1986). Systems-based consultation with schools. In L. C. Wynne, S. H. McDaniel, & T. T. Weber (Eds.), *Systems consultation: A new perspective for family therapy*. New York: Guilford Press.

Fishman, H. C. (1988). *Treating troubled adolescents: A family therapy approach*. New York: Basic Books.

Fishman, H. C. (1993). *Intensive structural therapy: Treating families in their social context*. New York: Basic Books.

Fontaine, J. H., & Hammond, N. L. (1996). Counseling issues with gay and lesbian adolescents. *Adolescence, 31,* 817–830.

Fordham, S., & Ogbu, J. U. (1986). Black students' school success: Coping with the "burden of acting white." *Urban Review, 18,* 176–206.

Forehand, R., Wierson, M., Thomas, A. M., Armistead, L., Kempton, T., & Neighbors, B. (1991). The role of family stressors and parent relationships on adolescent functioning. *Journal of the American Academy of Child and Adolescent Psychiatry, 30,* 316–322.

Frasciello, L. M., & Willard, S. G. (1995). Anorexia nervosa in males: A case report and review of the literature. *Clinical Social Work Journal, 23,* 47–58.

Frauenglass, S., Routh, D. K., Pantin, H., & Mason, C. (1997). Family support decreases influence of deviant peers on Hispanic adolescents' substance use. *Journal of Clinical Child Psychology, 26,* 15–23.

Freedman, J., & Combs, G. (1996). *Narrative Therapy: The social construction of preferred realities*. New York: Norton.

Freud, A. (1958). Adolescence. *Psychoanalytic Study of the Child, 13,* 255–278.

Friedman, E. (1987). How to succeed in therapy without really trying. *Family Therapy Networker, 11,* 26–31.

Fromm-Reichmann, F. (1948). Notes on the development of treatment of schizophrenics by psychoanalytic psychotherapy. *Psychotherapy, 11,* 263–274.

Fulgini, A., & Eccles, J. (1993). Perceived parent–child relationships and early adolescents' orientation toward peers. *Developmental Psychology, 29,* 622–632.

Gallatin, J. (1975). *Adolescence and individuality*. New York: Harper & Row.

Garland, A. F., & Zigler, E. (1993). Adolescent suicide prevention: Current research and social policy implications. *American Psychologist, 48,* 169–182.

Gastfried, D. R., Biederman, J., & Jellinek, M. S. (1984). Desipramine in the treatment of adolescents with attention deficit disorder. *American Journal of Psychiatry, 141,* 906–908.

Gergen, K. (1991). *The saturated self: Dilemmas of identity in contemporary life.* New York: Basic Books.

Gilbert, S., & Thompson, J. K. (1996). Feminist explanations of the development of eating disorders: Common themes, research findings, and methodological issues. *Clinical Psychology: Science and Practice, 3,* 183–202.

Gilligan, C. (1982). *In a different voice.* Cambridge, MA: Harvard University Press.

Gilligan, C., Lyons, N. P., & Hanmer, T. J. (Eds.). (1990). *Making connections: The relational worlds of adolescent girls at Emma Willard School.* Cambridge, MA: Harvard University Press.

Ginsburg, G. S., & Bronstein, P. (1993). Family factors related to children's intrinsic/extrinsic motivational orientations and academic performance. *Child Development, 64,* 1461–1474.

Gittelman, R., Mannuzza, S., Shenker, R., & Bonagura, N. (1985). Hyperactive boys almost grown up: I. Psychiatric status. *Archives of General Psychiatry, 42,* 937–947.

Goldner, V. (1985). Feminism and family therapy. *Family Process, 24,* 31–47.

Goldner, V. (1988). Generation and gender: Normative and covert hierarchies. *Family Process, 27,* 17–33.

Gordon, S., & Gilgun, J. (1987). Adolescent sexuality. In V. Van Hasselt & M. Hersen (Eds.), *Handbook of adolescent psychology.* New York: Pergamon.

Gottesman, I. I. (1991). *Schizophrenia genesis: The origins of madness.* New York: Freeman.

Gottfredson, M. R., & Hirschi, T. (1994). A general theory of adolescent problem behavior: Problems and prospects. In R. Ketterlinus & M. E. Lamb (Eds.), *Adolescent problem behaviors.* Hillsdale, NJ: Erlbaum.

Green, R. J. (1989). "Learning to learn" and the family system: New perspectives on underachievement and learning disorders. *Journal of Marital and Family Therapy, 15,* 187–203.

Gutstein, S. E., Rudd, M. D., Graham, J. C., & Rayha, L. L. (1988). Systemic crisis intervention as a response to adolescent crises: An outcome study. *Family Process, 27,* 201–211.

Haley, J. (1976). *Problem-solving therapy.* San Francisco: Jossey-Bass.

Haley, J. (1980). *Leaving home: The therapy of disturbed young people.* New York: McGraw-Hill.

Hall, G. S. (1904). *Adolescence.* New York: Appleton.

Halmi, K. A. (1995). Changing rates of eating disorders: What does it mean? *American Journal of Psychiatry, 152,* 1256–1257.

Hamlett, K. W., & Curry, J. F. (1990). Anorexia nervosa in adolescent males: A review and case study. *Child Psychiatry and Human Development, 21,* 79–94.

Hare-Mustin, R. T. (1987). The problem of gender in family therapy theory. *Family Process, 26,* 15–27.

Hare-Mustin, R. T. (1994). Discourses in the mirrored room: A postmodern analysis of therapy. *Family Process, 33,* 19–35.

Harrop, C. E., Trower, P., & Mitchell, I. M. (1996). Does the biology go around the symptoms?: A Copernican shift in schizophrenia paradigms. *Clinical Psychology Review, 16,* 641–654.

Hart, B. I., & Thompson, J. M. (1996). Gender role characteristics and depressive symptomatology among adolescents. *Journal of Early Adolescence, 16,* 407–426.

Harter, S. (1990). Self and identity development. In S. Feldman & G. Elliott (Eds.), *At the threshold: The developing adolescent.* Cambridge, MA: Harvard University Press.

Hauser, S. T., Powers, S. I., Noam, C. G., Jacobson, A. M., Weiss, B., & Follansbee, D. J. (1984). Familial contexts of adolescent ego development. *Child Development, 55,* 195–213.

Hill, J., & Lynch, M. (1983). The intensification of gender-related role expectations during early adolescence. In J. Brooks-Gunn & A. Petersen (Eds.), *Girls at puberty.* New York: Plenum.

Hirschi, T. (1969). *Causes of delinquency.* Berkeley: University of California Press.

Hoffman, L. (1981). *Foundations of family therapy: A conceptual framework for systems change.* New York: Basic Books.

Holinger, P. C., Offer, D., Barter, J. T., & Bell, C. C. (1994). *Suicide and homicide among adolescents.* New York: Guilford Press.

Hunter, F., & Youniss, J. (1982). Changes in functions of three relations during adolescence. *Developmental Psychology, 18,* 806–811.

Imber-Black, E. (1991). A family-larger system perspective. In A. S. Gurman, & D. P. Kniskern (Eds.), *Handbook of family therapy* (Vol. 2). New York: Brunner/Mazel.

Inaszu, J. K., & Fox, G. L. (1980). Maternal influences on the sexual behavior of teenage daughters. *Journal of Family Issues, 1,* 81–102.

Inhelder, B., & Piaget, J. (1958). *The growth of logical thinking from childhood to adolescence.* New York: Basic Books.

Jack, D. C. (1991). *Silencing the self: Women and depression.* New York: HarperCollins.

Jessor, R., & Jessor, S. L. (1977). *Problem behavior and psychological development: A longitudinal study of youth.* San Diego: Academic Press.

Joanning. H., Quinn, W., Thomas, F., & Mullen, R. (1992). Treating adolescent drug abuse: A comparison of family systems therapy, group therapy, and family drug education. *Journal of Marital and Family Therapy, 18,* 345–356.

Johnston, L., Bachman, J., & O'Malley, P. (1994). *Monitoring the future: Questionnaire responses from the nation's high school seniors, 1993.* Ann Arbor, MI: Institute for Social Research.

Jordan, J. V. (1991). Empathy and self boundaries. In J. V. Jordan, A. G. Kaplan, J. B. Miller, I. P. Stiver, & J. L. Surrey, *Women's growth in connection: Writings from the Stone Center.* New York: Guilford Press.

Jordan, J. V., Kaplan, A. G., Miller, J. B., Stiver, I. P., & Surrey, J. L. (1991). *Women's growth in connection: Writings from the Stone Center.* New York: Guilford Press.

Josselson, R. (1987). *Finding herself: Pathways to identity development in women.* San Francisco: Jossey-Bass.

Kandel, D. (1978). Homophily, selection, and socialization in adolescent friendships. *American Journal of Sociology, 84,* 427–436.

Kandel, D. B., & Davies, M. (1982). Epidemiology of depressive mood in adolescents. *Archives of General Psychiatry, 39,* 1205–1212.

Kaplan, A. G. (1991). The "self-in-relation": Implications for depression in women. In J. V. Jordan, A. G. Kaplan, J. B. Miller, I. P. Stiver, & J. L. Surrey, *Women's growth in connection: Writings from the Stone Center.* New York: Guilford Press.

Kaplan, A. G., Klein, R., & Gleason, N. (1991). Women's self development in late adolescence. In J. V. Jordan, A. G. Kaplan, J. B. Miller, I. P. Stiver, & J. L. Surrey, *Women's growth in connection: Writings from the Stone Center.* New York: Guilford Press.

Katchadourian, H. (1990). Sexuality. In S. Feldman & G. Elliott (Eds.), *At the threshold: The developing adolescent.* Cambridge, MA: Harvard University Press.

Kegan, R. (1982). *The evolving self.* Cambridge, MA: Harvard University Press.

Kendall, P. D. (Ed.). (1991). *Child and adolescent therapy: Cognitive-behavioral procedures.* New York: Guilford Press.

Kerr, M., & Bowen, M. (1988). *Family evaluation.* New York: Norton.

Kinsey, A., Pomeroy, W., & Martin, C. (1948). *Sexual behavior in the human male.* Philadelphia: Saunders.

Kite, M. (1984). Sex differences in attitudes towards homosexuals: A meta-analytic review. *Journal of Homosexuality, 10,* 69–81.

Kline, C. L. (1972). The adolescents with learning problems: How long must they wait? *Journal of Learning Disabilities, 5,* 262–284.

Kohlberg, L. (1963). The development of children's orientations toward a moral order. *Vita Humana, 6,* 11–33.

Kopeikin, H. S., Marshall, V., & Goldstein, M. J. (1983). Stages and impact of crisis-oriented family therapy in the aftercare of acute schizophrenia. In W. R. McFarlane (Ed.), *Family therapy in schizophrenia.* New York: Guilford Press.

Krieder, D., & Motto, J. (1974). Parent–child role reversal and suicidal states in adolescence. *Adolescence, 9,* 365–370.

Larson, R., & Richards, M. (1994). *Divergent realities: The emotional lives of mothers, fathers, and adolescents.* New York: Basic Books.

Lau, S. (1989). Sex role orientation and domains of self-esteem. *Sex Roles, 21,* 415–422.

Lau, S., & Cheung, P. C. (1987). Relations between Chinese adolescents' perception of parental control and organization and their perception of parental warmth. *Developmental Psychology, 23,* 726–729.

Leff, J., & Vaughn, C. (1981). The role of maintenance therapy and relatives' expressed emotion in relapse of schizophrenia: A two-year follow up. *British Journal of Psychiatry, 139,* 102–104.

Leon, G. R., Fulkerson, J. A., Perry, C. L., & Early-Zald, M. B. (1995). Prospective analysis of personality and behavioral vulnerabilities and gender influences in the later development of disordered eating. *Journal of Abnormal Psychology, 104,* 140–149.

Lerner, R. M. (1978). Nature, nurture, and dynamic interactionism. *Human Development, 21,* 1–20.

Levant, R. F. (1995). Toward the reconstruction of masculinity. In R. F. Levant & W. S. Pollack (Eds.), *A new psychology of men*. New York: Basic Books.

Levin, L., & Schonberg, K. (1987). Familial violence among adolescents who attempt suicide. *Journal of Adolescent Health Care, 8,* 302.

Lewinsohn, P. M., Rohde, P., & Seeley, J. R. (1996). Adolescent suicidal ideation and attempts: Prevalence, risk factors, and clinical implications. *Clinical Psychology: Science and Practice, 3,* 25–46.

Liddle, H. A. (1993). Engaging adolescents in family therapy: Some early phase skills. In T. S. Nelson & T. S. Trepper (Eds.), *101 interventions in family therapy*. New York: Haworth.

Liddle, H. A., & Dakoff, G. A. (1995). Efficacy of family therapy for drug abuse: Promising but not definitive. *Journal of Marital and Family Therapy, 21,* 511–543.

Lidz, T., Cornelison, A., Fleck, S., & Terry, D. (1957). Intrafamilial environment of schizophrenic patients: II. Marital schism and marital skew. *American Journal of Psychiatry, 114,* 241–248.

Lowenstein, L. G. (1994). Anorexia nervosa in boys: A review of the recent literature and a case treated in a therapeutic community. *Family Therapy, 21,* 233–240.

Luepnitz, D. A. (1988). *The family interpreted: Feminist theory in clinical practice*. New York: Basic Books.

Lusterman, D. (1985). An ecosystemic approach to family-school problems. *American Journal of Family Therapy, 13,* 22–30.

Maccoby, E. (1990). Gender and relationships: A developmental account. *American Psychologist, 45,* 513–520.

Mackey, S. K. (1996). Nurturance: A neglected dimension in family therapy with adolescents. *Journal of Marital and Family Therapy, 22,* 489–508.

Madanes, C. (1981). *Strategic family therapy*. San Francisco: Jossey-Bass.

Madanes, C. (1984). *Behind the one-way mirror: Advances in the practice of strategic therapy*. San Francisco: Jossey-Bass.

Magnusson, D., Strattin, H., & Allen, V. L. (1985). Biological maturation and social development: A longitudinal study of some adjustment processes from midadolescence to adulthood. *Journal of Youth and Adolescence, 14,* 267–283.

Mannuzza, S., & Gittelman, R. (1984). The adolescent outcome of hyperactive girls. *Psychiatry Research, 13,* 19–29.

Mannuzza, S., Klein, R. G., Bonagura, N., & Malloy, P. (1991). Hyperactive boys almost grown up: V. Replication of psychiatric status. *Archives of General Psychiatry, 48,* 77–83.

Marcia, J. (1966). Development and validation of ego identity status. *Journal of Personality and Social Psychology, 3,* 551–558.

Marcia, J. (1976). Identity six years after: A follow-up study. *Journal of Youth and Adolescence, 5,* 145–150.

Markowitz, L. M. (1992). Making house calls. *Family Therapy Networker, 16,* 26–37.

Markstrom-Adams, C. (1989). Androgyny and its relation to adolescent psychological well-being: A review of the literature. *Sex Roles, 21,* 469–473.

Markus, H., & Nurius, P. (1986). Possible selves. *American Psychologist, 41,* 954–969.

Marshall, W. (1978). Puberty. In F. Falkner & J. Tanner (Eds.), *Human growth* (Vol. 2). New York: Plenum

Massad, C. (1981). Sex role identity and adjustment during adolescence. *Child Development, 52,* 1290–1298.

McCord, J. (1990). Problem behaviors. In S. Feldman & G. Elliott (Eds.), *At the threshold: The developing adolescent.* Cambridge, MA: Harvard University Press.

McGoldrick, M., Pearce, J. K., & Giordano, J. (Eds.). (1982). *Ethnicity and family therapy.* New York: Guilford Press.

McLean, C. (1996). Boys and education in Australia. In C. McLean, M. Carey, & C. White (Eds.), *Men's ways of being.* Boulder, CO: Westview.

McLean, C., Carey, M., & White, C. (Eds.). (1996). *Men's ways of being.* Boulder, CO: Westview.

Meilman, P. W. (1979). Cross-sectional age changes in ego identity status during adolescence. *Developmental Psychology, 15,* 230–231.

Micucci, J. A. (1995). Adolescents who assault their parents: A family systems approach to treatment. *Psychotherapy, 32,* 154–161.

Miller, J. B. (1991). The construction of anger in women and men. In J. V. Jordan, A. G. Kaplan, J. B. Miller, I. P. Stiver, & J. L. Surrey, (Eds.), *Women's growth in connection: Writings from the Stone Center.* New York: Guilford Press.

Minuchin, S. (1974). *Families and family therapy.* Cambridge, MA: Harvard University Press.

Minuchin, S. (1984). *Family kaleidoscope.* Cambridge, MA: Harvard University Press.

Minuchin, S. (1991). The seductions of constructivism. *Family Therapy Networker, 15,* 47–50.

Minuchin, S., & Barcai, A., (1969). Therapeutically induced crisis. In J. H. Masserman (Ed.), *Science and psychoanalysis* (Vol. 14). New York: Grune & Stratton.

Minuchin, S., & Fishman, H. C. (1981). *Family therapy techniques.* Cambridge, MA: Harvard University Press.

Minuchin, S., Lee, W., & Simon, G. W. (1996). *Mastering family therapy: Journeys of growth and transformation.* New York: Wiley.

Minuchin, S., Montalvo, B., Guerney, B. G., Rosman, B. L., & Schumer, F. (1967). *Families of the slums.* New York: Basic Books.

Minuchin, S., & Nichols, M. P. (1993). *Family healing: Strategies for hope and understanding.* New York: Free Press.

Minuchin, S., Rosman, B. L., & Baker, L. (1978). *Psychosomatic families: Anorexia nervosa in context.* Cambridge, MA: Harvard University Press.

Moore, K., Peterson, J., & Furstenberg, F., Jr. (1986). Parental attitudes and the occurrence of early sexual activity. *Journal of Marriage and the Family, 48,* 777–782.

Mueller, C., Field, T., Yando, R., & Harding, J. (1995). Under-eating and over-eating concerns among adolescents. *Journal of Child Psychology and Psychiatry and Allied Disciplines, 36,* 1019–1025.

Mullis, I., Dossey, J., Campbell, J., Gentile, C., O'Sullivan, C., & Latham, A. (1994). *NAEP 1992 trends in academic progress.* Washington, DC: U.S. Department of Education.

Muus, R. E. (1996). *Theories of adolescence* (6th ed.). New York: McGraw-Hill.

Napier, A. Y., & Whitaker, C. A. (1978). *The family crucible.* New York: Harper & Row.

Newcomer, S., & Udry, J. (1984). Mothers' influence on the sexual behavior of their teenage children. *Journal of Marriage and the Family, 46,* 477–485.

Nichols, M. P. (1987). *The self in the system: Expanding the limits of family therapy.* New York: Brunner/Mazel.

Nolen-Hoeksema, S. (1987). Sex differences in unipolar depression. *Psychological Bulletin, 101,* 259–282.

Oetting, E. R., & Beauvais, F. (1987). Peer cluster theory, socialization characteristics, and adolescent drug use: A path analysis. *Journal of Counseling Psychology, 34,* 205–213.

Offer, D., & Offer, J. B. (1975). *From teenager to young manhood.* New York: Basic Books.

Offer, D., Ostrov, E., & Howard, K. I. (1981). The mental health professional's concept of the normal adolescent. *Archives of General Psychiatry, 38,* 149–152.

Offer, D., & Schonert-Reichl, K. A. (1992). Debunking the myths of adolescence: Findings from recent research. *Journal of the American Academy of Child and Adolescent Psychiatry, 31,* 1003–1014.

O'Hanlon, B., & Wilk, J. (1987). *Shifting contexts: The generation of effective psychotherapy.* New York: Guilford Press.

Omer, H. (1994). *Critical interventions in psychotherapy.* New York: Norton.

Osherson, S., & Krugman, S. (1990). Men, shame and psychotherapy. *Psychotherapy, 27,* 327–339.

Papp, P. (1983). *The process of change.* New York: Guilford Press.

Paré, D. A. (1995). Of families and other cultures: The shifting paradigm of family therapy. *Family Process, 34,* 1–19.

Parry, A. (1991). A universe of stories. *Family Process, 30,* 37–54.

Parry, A., & Doan, R. E. (1994). *Story re-visions: Narrative therapy in the postmodern world.* New York: Guilford Press.

Pennington, B. F. (1991). *Diagnosing learning disorders: A neuropsychological framework.* New York: Guilford Press.

Petersen, A. C., Compas, B. E., Brooks-Gunn, J., Stemmler, M., Ey, S., & Grant, K. E. (1993). Depression in adolescence. *American Psychologist, 48,* 155–168.

Petersen, A. C., Sarigiani, P. A., & Kennedy, R. F. (1991). Adolescent depression: Why more girls? *Journal of Youth and Adolescence, 20,* 247–271.

Pfeffer, C. R. (1981). The family system of suicidal children. *American Journal of Psychotherapy, 35,* 330–341.

Pipher, M. (1994). *Reviving Ophelia: Saving the selves of adolescent girls.* New York: Putnam.

Pittman, F. (1993). *Man enough: Fathers, sons and the search for masculinity.* New York: Berkley.

Plass, P. S., & Hotaling, G. T. (1995). The intergenerational transmission of running away: Childhood experiences of the parents of runaways. *Journal of Youth and Adolescence, 24,* 335–348.

Pleck, J. H. (1981). *The myth of masculinity.* Cambridge, MA: MIT Press.

Pleck, J. H. (1995). The gender role strain paradigm: An update. In R. F. Levant & W. S. Pollack (Eds.), *A new psychology of men.* New York: Basic Books.

Pleck, J. H., Sonnenstein, F. L., & Ku, L. C. (1994). Problem behaviors and masculinity ideology in adolescent males. In R. Ketterlinus & M. E. Lamb (Eds.), *Adolescent problem behaviors.* Hillsdale, NJ: Erlbaum.

Pollack, W. S. (1995). No man is an island: Toward a new psychoanalytic psychology of men. In R. F. Levant & W. S. Pollack (Eds.), *A new psychology of men.* New York: Basic Books.

Power, T. J., & Bartholomew, K. L. (1985). Getting uncaught in the middle: A case study in family-school system consultation. *School Psychology Review, 14,* 222–229.

Price, J. A. (1996). *Power and compassion: Working with difficult adolescents and abused parents.* New York: Guilford Press.

Quadrel, M. J., Fischhoff, B., & Davis, W. (1993). Adolescent (in)vulnerability. *American Psychologist, 48,* 102–116.

Remafedi, G. (Ed.). (1994). *Death by denial: Studies of suicide in gay and lesbian teenagers.* Boston: Alyson.

Richman, J. (1979). The family therapy of attempted suicide. *Family Process, 18,* 131–142.

Robin, A. L., Siegel, P. T., Koepke, T., Moye, A. W., & Tice, S. (1994). Family therapy versus individual therapy for adolescent females with anorexia nervosa. *Journal of Developmental and Behavioral Pediatrics, 15,* 111–116.

Rohner, R. P., & Pettengill, S. M. (1985). Perceived parental acceptance-rejection and parental control among Korean adolescents. *Child Development, 56,* 524–528.

Romeo, F. F. (1994). Adolescent boys and anorexia nervosa. *Adolescence, 29,* 643–647.

Rosen, H., & Kuehlwein, K. T. (Eds.). (1996). *Constructing realities: Meaning-making perspectives for psychotherapists.* San Francisco: Jossey-Bass.

Rosenthal, R., & Jacobson, L. (1968). *Pygmalion in the classroom: Teacher expectations and pupils' intellectual development.* New York: Holt, Rinehart & Winston.

Rourke, B. P., Young, G. C., & Leenaars, A. A. (1989). A childhood learning disability that predisposes those afflicted to adolescent and adult depression and suicide risk. *Journal of Learning Disabilities, 22,* 169–175.

Russell, G. F. M., Szmulker, G. I., Dare, C., & Eisler, I. (1987). An evaluation of family therapy in anorexia nervosa and bulimia nervosa. *Archives of General Psychiatry, 44,* 1047–1056.

Sargent, J. (1987a). Integrating family and individual therapy for anorexia nervosa. In J. E. Harkaway (Ed.), *Eating disorders.* Rockville, MD: Aspen.

Sargent, J. (1987b). *Talking to you* [Videotape]. (Available from Videotape Rentals, Philadelphia Child Guidance Center, 34th Street and Civic Center Boulevard, Philadelphia, PA 19104)

Sargent, J., Liebman, R., & Silver, M. (1985). Family therapy for anorexia nervosa. In D. M. Garner & P. E. Garfinkel (Eds.), *Handbook of psychotherapy for anorexia nervosa and bulimia.* New York: Guilford Press.

Savin-Williams, R. (1994). Verbal and physical abuse as stressors in the lives of lesbian, gay male, and bisexual youths: Associations with school problems, running away, substance abuse, prostitution, and suicide. *Journal of Consulting and Clinical Psychology, 62,* 261–269.

Savin-Williams, R., & Berndt, T. (1990). Friendship and peer relations. In S. Feldman & G. Elliott (Eds.), *At the threshold: The developing adolescent.* Cambridge, MA: Harvard University Press.

Scales, P., & McEwin, C. (1994). *Growing pains: The making of America's middle school teachers.* Columbus, OH: National Middle School Association.

Schnarch, D. M. (1991). *Constructing the sexual crucible: An integration of sexual and marital therapy.* New York: Norton.

Schwartz, R. C. (1987). Our multiple selves. *Family Therapy Networker, 11,* 25–31.

Schwartz, R. C. (1995). *Internal family systems therapy.* New York: Guilford Press.

Seelig, W. R., Goldman-Hall, B. J., & Jerrell, J. M. (1992). In-home treatment of families of severely disturbed adolescents in crisis. *Family Process, 31,* 135–149.

Selekman, M. (1993). *Pathways to change: Brief therapy solutions with difficult adolescents.* New York: Guilford Press.

Selman, R. (1980). *The growth of interpersonal understanding: Developmental and clinical analyses.* New York: Academic Press.

Selvini Palazzoli, M. (1986). Towards a general model of psychotic games. *Journal of Marital and Family Therapy, 12,* 339–349.

Selvini-Palazzoli, M., Boscolo, L., Cecchin, G., & Prata, G. (1978). *Paradox and counterparadox.* New York: Aronson.

Selvini-Palazzoli, M., Boscolo, L., Cecchin, G., & Prata, G. (1980). Hypothesizing–circularity–neutrality: Three guidelines for the conductor of the session. *Family Process, 19,* 3–12.

Selvini-Palazzoli, M., & Viaro, M. (1988). The anorectic process in the family: A six stage model as a guide for individual therapy. *Family Process, 27,* 129–148.

Shaver, P., Furman, W., & Buhrmester, D. (1985). Transition to college: Network changes, social skills, and loneliness. In S. Duck & D. Perlman (Eds.), *Understanding personal relationships: An interdisciplinary approach.* London: Sage.

Shedler, J., & Block, J. (1990). Adolescent drug use and psychological health: A longitudinal inquiry. *American Psychologist, 45,* 612–630.

Sherman, R., & Fredman, N. (1986). *Handbook of structured techniques in marriage and family therapy.* New York: Brunner/Mazel.

Silbereisen, R., Petersen, A., Albrecht, H., & Kracke, B. (1989). Maturational timing and the development of problem behavior: Longitudinal studies in adolescence. *Journal of Early Adolescence, 9,* 247–268

Silverstein, O., & Rashbaum, B. (1994). *The courage to raise good men.* New York: Penguin.

Simmons, R., Burgeson, R., Carlton-Ford, S., & Blyth, D. A. (1987). The impact of cumulative change in early adolescence. *Child Development, 58,* 1220–1234.

Simmons, R., & Rosenberg, F. (1975). Sex, sex roles, and self image. *Journal of Youth and Adolescence, 4,* 229–258.

Singer, M. T., Wynne, L. C., & Toohey, M. L. (1978). Communication disorders and the families of schizophrenics. In L. C. Wynne, R. L. Cromwell, & S. Matthysse (Eds.), *The nature of schizophrenia*. New York: Wiley.

Smetana, J. (1989). Adolescents' and parents' reasoning about actual family conflict. *Child Development, 59,* 1052–1067.

Smolak, L., Levine, M., & Gralen, S. (1993). The impact of puberty and dating on eating problems among middle school girls. *Journal of Youth and Adolescence, 22,* 355–368.

Staples, R. (1992). African American families. In J. M. Henslin (Ed.), *Marriage and family in a changing society*. New York: Free Press.

Staver, N. (1953). The child's learning difficulty as related to the emotional problems of the mother. *American Journal of Orthopsychiatry, 23,* 131–140.

Steiger, H. (1989). Anorexia nervosa and bulimia in males: Lessons for a low-risk population. *Canadian Journal of Psychiatry, 34,* 419–424.

Stein, J. H., & Reiser, L. W. (1994). A study of white middle-class adolescent boys' responses to "semenarche" (the first ejaculation). *Journal of Youth and Adolescence, 23,* 373–384.

Steinberg, L. (1987a). Single parents, stepparents and the susceptibility of adolescents to antisocial peer pressure. *Child Development, 58,* 269–275.

Steinberg, L. (1987b). The impact of puberty on family relations: Effects of pubertal status and pubertal timing. *Developmental Psychology, 23,* 451–460.

Steinberg, L. (1990). Autonomy, conflict, and harmony in the family relationship. In S. Feldman & G. Elliott (Eds.), *At the threshold: The developing adolescent*. Cambridge, MA: Harvard University Press.

Steinberg, L. (1996). *Adolescence* (4th ed.). New York: McGraw-Hill.

Steinberg, L., Fletcher, A., & Darling, N. (1994). Parental monitoring and peer influences on adolescent substance use. *Pediatrics, 93,* 1060–1064.

Steinberg, L., Lamborn, S., Darling, N., Mounts, N., & Dornbusch, S. (1994). Over-time changes in adjustment and competence among adolescents from authoritative, authoritarian, indulgent, and neglectful families. *Child Development, 65,* 754–770.

Steinberg, L., Lamborn, S., Dornbusch, S. M., & Darling, N. (1992). Impact of parenting practices on adolescent achievement: Authoritative parenting, school achievement and encouragement to succeed. *Child Development, 63,* 1266–1281.

Steinberg, L., & Silverberg, S. (1986). The vicissitudes of autonomy in early adolescence. *Child Development, 57,* 841–851.

Steinberg, L., & Steinberg, W. (1994). *Crossing paths: How your child's adolescence triggers your own crisis*. New York: Simon & Schuster.

Steiner-Adair, C. (1990). The body politic: Normal female adolescent development and the development of eating disorders. In C. Gilligan, N. P. Lyons, & T. J. Hanmer (Eds.), *Making connections: The relational worlds of adolescent girls at Emma Willard School*. Cambridge, MA: Harvard University Press.

Stern, S., Whitaker, C. A., Hagemann, N. J., Anderson, R. B., & Bargman, G. J. (1981). Anorexia nervosa: The hospital's role in family treatment. *Family Process, 20,* 395–408.

Stierlin, H. (1973). A family perspective on adolescent runaways. *Archives of General Psychiatry, 29,* 56–62.

Stierlin, H., Levi, L. D., & Savard, R. L. (1971). Parental perceptions of separating children. *Family Process, 10,* 411–427.

Surrey, J. L. (1991). Eating patterns as a reflection of women's development. In J. V. Jordan, A. G. Kaplan, J. B. Miller, I. P. Stiver, & J. L. Surrey, *Women's growth in connection: Writings from the Stone Center.* New York: Guilford Press.

Surrey, J. L. (1997). What do you mean by mutuality in therapy? In J. V. Jordan (Ed.), *Women's growth in diversity: More writings from the Stone Center.* New York: Guilford Press.

Swarr, A. E., & Richards, M. H. (1996). Longitudinal effects of adolescent girls' pubertal development, perceptions of pubertal timing and parental relations on eating problems. *Developmental Psychology, 32,* 636–646.

Szapocznik, J., Kurtines, W. M., Foote, F. H., Perez-Vidal, A., & Heris, O. (1983). Conjoint versus one-person family therapy: Some evidence for the effectiveness of conducting family therapy through one person. *Journal of Consulting and Clinical Psychology, 51,* 889–899.

Tannenbaum, L., & Forehand, R. (1994). Maternal depressive mood: The role of the father in preventing adolescent problem behaviors. *Behaviour Research and Therapy, 32,* 321–325.

Tanner, J. (1972). Sequence, tempo, and individual variation in growth and development of boys and girls aged twelve to sixteen. In J. Kagan & R. Coles (Eds.), *Twelve to sixteen: Early adolescence.* New York: Norton.

Tavantzis, T. N., Tavantzis, M., Brown, L. G., & Rohrbaugh, M. (1985). Home-based structural family therapy for delinquents at risk of placement. In M. P. Mirkin, & S. L. Koman (Eds.), *Handbook of adolescents and family therapy.* New York: Gardner.

Tolan, P. H., Cromwell, R. E., & Brasswell, M. (1986). Family therapy with delinquents: A critical review of the literature. *Family Process, 25,* 619–649.

Treboux, D., & Busch-Rossnagel, N. (1990). Social network influences on adolescent sexual attitudes and behaviors. *Journal of Adolescent Research, 5,* 175–189.

Vygotsky, L. S. (1978). *Mind in society: The development of higher psychological processes.* Cambridge, MA: Harvard University Press.

Waller, J. V., Kaufman, M. R., & Deutsch, F. (1940). Anorexia nervosa: A psychosomatic entity. *Psychosomatic Medicine, 2,* 3–16.

Walters, M., Carter, B., Papp, P., & Silverstein, O. (Eds.). (1988). *The invisible web: Gender patterns in family relationships.* New York: Guilford Press.

Weeks, G. R., & L'Abate, L. (1982). *Paradoxical psychotherapy: Theory and practice with individuals, couples, and families.* New York: Brunner/Mazel.

Weiner, I. B. (1971). Psychodynamic aspects of learning disability: The passive-aggressive underachiever. *Journal of School Psychology, 9,* 246–251.

Wender, E. H. (1995). Attention-deficit hyperactivity disorders in adolescence. *Journal of Developmental and Behavioral Pediatrics, 16,* 192–195.

Whitaker, C. A. (1975). The symptomatic adolescent: An AWOL family member. In M. Sugar (Ed.), *The adolescent in group and family therapy.* New York: Brunner/Mazel.

White, M. (1983). Anorexia nervosa: A transgenerational system perspective. *Family Process, 22,* 255–273.

White, M. (1986). Negative explanation, restraint, and double description: A template for family therapy. *Family Process, 25,* 169–184.

White, M. (1987). Anorexia nervosa: A cybernetic perspective. In J. E. Harkaway (Ed.), *Eating disorders.* Rockville, MD: Aspen.

White, M. (1993). Deconstruction and therapy. In S. Gilligan & R. Price (Eds.), *Therapeutic conversations.* New York: Norton.

White, M. (1995). *Re-authoring lives: Interviews and essays.* Adelaide, South Australia: Dulwich Centre.

White, M., & Epston, D. (1990). *Narrative means to therapeutic ends.* New York: Norton.

Winnicott, D. W. (1965). *The maturational process and the facilitating environment.* London: Hogarth Press.

Wynne, L., Ryckoff, I., Day, J., & Hirsch, S. (1958). Pseudomutuality in the family relations of schizophrenics. *Psychiatry, 21,* 205–220.

Yoshikawa, H. (1994). Prevention as cumulative protection: Effects of early family support and education on chronic delinquency and its risks. *Psychological Bulletin, 115,* 28–54.

Young, H., & Ferguson, L. (1979). Developmental changes through adolescence in the spontaneous nomination of reference groups as a function of decision context. *Journal of Youth and Adolescence, 8,* 239–252.

Ziffer, R. L. (1985). The utilization of psychological testing in the context of family therapy. In R. L. Ziffer (Ed.), *Adjunctive techniques in family therapy.* New York: Grune & Stratton.

INDEX

("f" indicates a figure, "n" indicates a note, "t" indicates a table)

Stress, adolescent coping
   mechanisms, 137
Structural family therapy, 2–3,
   280–281
   anorexia, 97–98
Suicidal ideation, presenting
   problem, 14, 135–140
Suicide. *See also* Treatment,
   depression and suicidality
   adolescents and, 136, 138–139,
      141, 151–152
   contributing factors, 141
   fantasy technique, 149
"Suicide watch," 144
Supersystem dysfunction, 282
Supervision, parental, 172
Surrey, Janet, on anorectics, 96
Symptomatic cycle, 3, 13, 17–20, 18f
   adolescent problem behavior,
      173f, 173–174
   anorexia, 101–104, 103f
   contracting, 28–31
   disruption of, 21, 22f, 23, 32–48, 50
   disruption techniques, 32–48
   identification of, 24–28
   psychosis, 215, 216f
Synthesis, gay identity stage, 69
Systemic family therapy, 3
Systems theory, low-income families
   and, 293

T

Teachers, impact on academic
   performance, 235
"Technical eclecticism," 3
Techniques, as tools, 2
"Tell me/Don't tell me bind,"
   33–34, 101, 151
"Test limits," mild problem
   behavior, 174
"Testing the waters," 152
Thematic Apperception Test (TAT),
   125
Theory, orientation toward, 2
Therapeutic contract, importance of,
   10

Therapeutic crisis induction, 286
Therapeutic relationship,
   determinant of success, 3
Therapist
   reaction to stalemates, 46–48
   role
      in conflict resolution, 48–49
      with low-income families, 281,
         284–290, 292–293
      as school consultant, 259–260
      self as tool, 300–305
      signs of inappropriate role, 199
Therapy. *See also* Family therapy;
   Individual therapy
   purpose of, 4
   stages and phases of, 16
   structural requirements for,
      290–292
   success of, 4
"Third-person perspective," 63, 171
Tolerance, gay identity stage, 69
"Transitional object," peer group, 64
Treatment
   depression and suicidality,
      144–148
   eating disorder, 104–106
   leaving home, 275–276
   low-income families, 284–290
   problem behavior, 176–194
   psychosis, 206–211, 211–228
Treatment contract
   anorexia, 105, 106–110, 133
   psychosis, 216
Triangulation, 12, 26
   anorexia and, 98
   coaching and, 248–249
   problem of multiple systems,
      257–258
   use of other professionals, 46–47

U

Unbalancing, technique of, 31, 36
Underachievement. *See also*
   School-related problems
   contributing factors of, 231–244,
      232t, 244–245